Cindi Bagan, PT

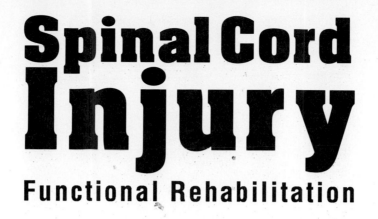

Spinal Cord Injury

Functional Rehabilitation

Spinal Cord Injury

Functional Rehabilitation

Martha Freeman Somers, MS, PT
Assistant Professor
Physical Therapy Educational Department
Medical University of South Carolina
Charleston, South Carolina

Illustrated by Susan Gilbert

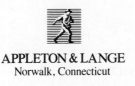

APPLETON & LANGE
Norwalk, Connecticut

0-8385-8649-X

Copyright © 1992 by Appleton & Lange
A Publishing Division of Prentice Hall

98 99 00 01 / 10 9 8 7

Prentice Hall International (UK) Limited, *London*
Prentice Hall of Australia Pty. Limited, *Sydney*
Prentice Hall Canada, Inc., *Toronto*
Prentice Hall Hispanoamericana, S.A., *Mexico*
Prentice Hall of India Private Limited, *New Delhi*
Prentice Hall of Japan, Inc., *Tokyo*
Simon & Schuster Asia Pte. Ltd., *Singapore*
Editora Prentice Hall do Brasil Ltda., *Rio de Janeiro*
Prentice Hall, *Englewood Cliffs, New Jersey*

Library of Congress Cataloging-in-Publication Data

Somers, Martha F.
    Spinal cord injury : functional rehabilitation / Martha F. Somers ;
illustrated by Susan Gilbert.
      p.   cm.
    ISBN 0-8385-8649-X
    1. Spinal cord—Wounds and injuries—Patients—Rehabilitation.
2. Spinal cord—Wounds and injuries—Physical therapy.   I Title.
    [DNLM: 1. Spinal Cord Injuries—rehabilitation.   WL 400 S694s]
    RD594.3.S63   1991
    617.4′82044—dc20
    DNLM/DLC
    for Library of Congress   91-22113
                                                           CIP

Acquisitions Editor: Scott Percy Horton
Production Editor: Sandra K. Huggard
Designer: S. M. Byrum

To Dave,
who would be mortified if I wrote something schmaltzy here,
so I'll leave it at that.

Contents

Preface

The goal of rehabilitation after spinal cord injury is to facilitate a person's return to a lifestyle that is as healthy, fulfilling, and independent as possible. Physical therapists play a central role in this process, working with recently injured people to maximize physical capabilities and mobility. Three major elements are required for a therapist to fulfill this role most effectively.

The first requirement is a basic understanding of spinal cord injuries and issues relevant to disability. Pertinent areas of knowledge include pathology, mechanisms of injury, medical/surgical management, physical sequelae, the prevention and management of complications, functional potentials, psychosocial impact, wheelchair-accessible architectural design, equipment options, and disability-related civil rights. This knowledge base is needed for optimal program planning and implementation.

The second requirement is a knowledge of the physical skills involved in functional activities and of the process involved in acquiring these skills. It is not enough merely to know the eventual outcome, which may take months to accomplish. The therapist must know how to break down a functional task into its component parts and to work on these components while developing the strength and flexibility required for the task. Many a therapist has been baffled when faced, on the one hand, with a text that explains the maneuvers that a cord-injured person performs to transfer and, on the other hand, with a newly injured person who can barely remain conscious while sitting upright, much less even begin to perform the skills shown in the book.

The third major element required for effective participation in rehabilitation is an approach to the cord-injured person that promotes self respect and encourages autonomy. Unfortunately, this element is often overlooked. Although we health professionals have as our stated goals the independent functioning of our patients, we often unwittingly encourage dependence. Many practices prevalent in health care serve to encourage "compliance" and to discourage autonomous behavior. If the rehabilitation effort is to be successful, the social environment of the rehabilitation unit must be structured in a way that fosters the development of self-reliant attitudes and behaviors.

There are several books on the market that address the topic of rehabilitation following spinal cord injury. However none of them encompasses all of the above-described elements. *Spinal Cord Injury: Functional Rehabilitation* was written to provide such a comprehensive treatment of the subject. The reader will gain a basic knowledge base relevant to spinal cord injuries and will develop an understanding of both the physical skills required for functional activities and the therapeutic strategies for achieving these skills. As or more importantly, the reader will gain an appreciation for the importance of psychosocial adaptation after spinal cord injury and will develop some insight into the impact that rehabilitation professionals can have in this area.

A Few Words About Words

"What's in a name? A rose by any other name would smell as sweet."

William Shakespeare

Maybe so, Bill, but I bet if you labeled that rose "radioactive," not too many people would get close enough to take a whiff.

Language has a profound impact on attitudes and values. Our perceptions of and judgments about others are both expressed and perpetuated by the words we use. The health care system in the United States is replete with the use of belittling and dehumanizing language. Health professionals label people by their diagnoses, calling people "head injuries," "CP kids," "cords," and so on. When we do this, we define people by their disabling conditions, reducing them to one-dimensional shadows of people. (How can a *person* be a *spinal cord*?) Another common practice among health professionals involves referring to people as "patients" when this term no longer applies. Most of us think of ourselves (and other able-bodied people) as *patients* only while we are utilizing the services of another clinician. As soon as we walk out of the health professional's office, we cease being *patients* and revert to our accustomed roles. When thinking/writing/speaking about disabled people, however, we often refer to them as *patients* whether or not they are utilizing the services of health professionals. The implication is that these people remain dependent upon health professionals indefinitely. Once a patient, always a patient.

In writing this text I have attempted to avoid using language that dehumanizes or belittles people with spinal cord injuries. Instead of labeling people by their diagnoses, I have chosen language that affirms their personhood. Thus rather than referring to a "C6 quadriplegic," for example, I have referred instead to a "person (or individual) with C6 quadriplegia."

In like manner, I gave much thought to eliminating the word "patient" from the text. "Patient" has implications of dependency and powerlessness. Another word may more appropriately convey the role of the person undergoing rehabilitation. But what word to use? "Client" evokes images of business suits and impersonal, formal interactions. I personally like "student," but I didn't think it would fly. Readers, especially health professional students, may find the term confusing. For the lack of a better term, I have retained the word "patient" but have attempted to avoid its overuse.

And then there's gender. The world is inhabited by both males and females. Both sexes sustain spinal cord injuries, and both sexes are involved in their rehabilitation. I gave some thought to avoiding using only the masculine pronoun in the text. But hundreds of pages of "he or she," "himself or herself," and "his or her" would have been tiresome at best. Again for the lack of a better alternative, I have used masculine pronouns throughout the text. The one exception is Chapter 16, the chapter on sexuality and sexual functioning. I chose to refer to both sexes throughout this chapter in an attempt to counteract the tendency of some rehabilitation professionals to ignore or to minimize the impact of spinal cord injury on the sexual functioning and sexuality of women.

As a result of my attempts to minimize the use of "patient" and to affirm the sexuality of women with spinal cord injuries, I may at times have resorted to some verbal gymnastics. I beg the reader's indulgence if I did so.

Acknowledgments

THANKS TO:

the various people who both fired my interest and taught me about working with people with spinal cord injuries: Don Neumann, Bob Meyers, Darrell Bennett, Joyce Krantz, Janet Ngai, Irene McClay, Mike Radakovich, Andrea Behrman, Dave Somers, Toula Latto, Jill Carter, and the patients/students/clients with whom I have worked.

Julia Freeman-Woolpert, who first introduced me to normalization principles.

the numerous family, friends, and colleagues who provided encouragement, suggestions, and editorial assistance in the writing of this book. In this group are included Andrea Behrman, Julia Freeman-Woolpert, Dave Somers, Dave and Connie Freeman, Patty Freeman, Jim Morrow, Karen Clayton, Mary Miedaner, Chris McAdam, Jim Robinson, Dave Morrisette, Jack Thomas, Sandy Brotherton, Lisa Saladin, Luis Leflore, and countless students.

Stephany Scott, my editor, who has provided limitless enthusiasm and support and who with a firm and steady hand has held up the light at the end of the tunnel.

Susan Gilbert, who somehow managed to translate my chicken scratches (or windshield smears) in to fantastic illustrations.

Finally, a special thanks to Dave and Jessie Somers for the support that they gave and the sacrifices that they have made while I wrote this book.

List of Charts

1

Introduction

Damage to the spinal cord has profound and global effects. Paralysis of voluntary musculature can lead to reduced mobility as well as impairment of vocational, avocational, and self-care abilities. Spinal cord injury can also affect the functioning of the sensory, respiratory, cardiovascular, gastrointestinal (GI), genitourinary (GU), and integumentary systems. A host of debilitating and potentially life-threatening physical complications can result.

The psychosocial sequelae of spinal cord injury are equally important. Bodily changes, altered sexual functioning, impaired mobility, incontinence, and functional dependence all constitute seemingly overwhelming losses with which cord-injured people must come to terms. Moreover, spinal cord injuries cause previously "normal" people to become "handicapped" and thus to become subject to society's prejudices regarding disabled people.

Although spinal cord injury is one of the most serious injuries that a person can survive, it is possible to return to a healthy, happy, and productive life after even the most severe of cord injuries. Achieving this outcome, however, is a monumental task that requires the coordinated efforts of the cord-injured person, his or her family, and a specialized multidisciplinary team of professionals. From the moment of injury onward, specialized care is essential for maximization of health as well as psychosocial and functional adaptation.

REHABILITATION FOLLOWING SPINAL CORD INJURY

Goals of Rehabilitation
The ultimate goal of rehabilitation after spinal cord injury is to enable a newly injured person to return to as healthy, fulfilling, and independent a lifestyle as possible. This requires growth in a variety of areas.

Psychosocial Adjustment. To return to a happy and fulfilling life following spinal cord injury, an individual must come to terms with his losses and formulate a new identity. The individual must also learn how to cope in a society in which he is now a member of a devalued minority. This psychological and social adjustment may be the most crucial area of growth after spinal cord injury.

Physical Skills. During rehabilitation, a cord-injured person learns how to perform a variety of physical activities. Through functional training, he gains skills required for self-care and mobility in the home and community.

Health Maintenance. Health maintenance is an active process after spinal cord injury. Virtually constant vigilance is required to avoid complications such as decubiti and urinary tract infections. If an individual is to stay healthy following spinal cord injury, he must learn how the body works, how to prevent and detect complications, and what to do when they occur.

Vocational and Avocational Adjustment. In many instances paralysis makes it impossible to return to a job held prior to the spinal cord injury. Recreational activities enjoyed prior to the injury may also be impossible. Return to an independent and fulfilling lifestyle requires adaptation in both of these areas.

Services Required
Spinal cord injury necessitates specialized and comprehensive rehabilitation services; a multidisciplinary team is required to enable people to achieve their optimal levels of functioning. Rehabilitation involves the coordinated efforts of counselors, nurses, occupational therapists, physical therapists, physicians, recreation therapists, and vocational counselors. Each of these professionals should have expertise in rehabilitation after spinal cord injury.

General hospitals are not able to provide the comprehensive care required following spinal cord injury. Ideally a patient will be transferred to a specialized center as soon as possible after injury.

Rehabilitation Approach

One of the major purposes of a rehabilitation program is for the individual to achieve independence. That means independence from family members, independence from friends, and *independence from the rehabilitation team.*

Requirements for Independent Functioning. There are three basic requirements that must be met for a person to function independently: knowledge, ability, and attitude.

Knowledge is critical to self-direction. Knowledge in the following areas will promote independence after spinal cord injury: the body's functioning following cord injury, prevention and management of complications, treatment alternatives, legal rights, equipment options, architectural accessibility, and services and resources available in the community. Armed with this knowledge, a cord-injured person can be self-reliant.

A variety of abilities are required for independent functioning. Physical abilities enable people to perform functional tasks without assistance. If a person lacks the physical capacity to perform a given activity, autonomous functioning requires the ability to gain and to direct assistance from another person. Other abilities involved in independent functioning include skills in problem solving, social interaction, and self-advocacy.

Finally, an independent attitude is essential for autonomous functioning. Unless a disabled person is motivated to function independently, he will never do so.

Fostering Independence. A rehabilitation program must address each of these areas—knowledge, skill, and attitude—if the cord-injured person is to function independently. The first two requirements, knowledge and skill, are most readily filled. Training and educational programs can be designed to provide information and to develop skills.

The development of an independent outlook is more problematic. It is an area more likely to be neglected and most easily undermined. We as health professionals often seem to do everything we can to develop a *dependent* attitude in our patients: we push their wheelchairs even when they are capable of doing it themselves; we feed them, bathe them, dress them, make decisions for them; and we "pro-

tect" them from full knowledge of their physical conditions. Every day in blatant and subtle ways, we tell them that they are dependent and that they *need* our help.

To foster an independent attitude, the entire rehabilitation team must emphasize the disabled person's autonomy and personal responsibility. From the day of injury onward, the cord-injured person should be included in decision making and in self-care as much as possible.

The patient *must be involved* in his rehabilitation. He should be provided with all relevant information and work as a partner with clinicians to set goals, to problem solve, and to make decisions. The patient should be responsible for the rehabilitation program, for taking initiative, for directing, and for participating fully in it.

Autonomous behaviors do not always appear spontaneously when a patient is given the opportunity to direct his care. A variety of factors can cause initial reluctance or inability to participate actively in rehabilitation. Many cord-injured people learn dependence in the weeks or months following their injuries when they are placed in the traditional role of dependent and passive patient. Many feel incapable of self-direction because of their preexisting beliefs about disabled people. Others may simply feel overwhelmed. Finally, a certain number may have been passive and dependent prior to their injuries. Whatever the cause of a patient's reluctance or inability to participate actively in his program, the rehabilitation team must work with the patient to encourage and to develop his capacity to take responsibility for himself.

SUMMARY

Spinal cord injury has a profound impact on a person's ability to care for himself, to move from place to place, and to participate in his accustomed social, vocational, and avocational activities. Injury to the spinal cord also makes a person vulnerable to social discrimination and a variety of physical complications.

Return to a healthy, fulfilling, and independent life following spinal cord injury requires the acquisition of a knowledge base and various physical and psychosocial abilities. It also requires the preservation or development of a sense of autonomy and personal responsibility. The purpose of rehabilitation after spinal cord injury is to foster growth in all of these areas.

SUGGESTED READING

The following books contain first-hand accounts of disability and rehabilitation.

Brightman, A. (1984). *Ordinary moments: The disabled experience*. Baltimore: University Park Press.

Callahan, J. (1989). *Don't worry, he won't get far on foot*. New York: Vintage Books.

Corbet, B. (1980). *Options: Spinal cord injury and the future*. Denver, CO: A.B. Hirschfeld Press.

Maddox, S. (1987). *Spinal network*. Boulder, CO: Spinal Network.

2

Spinal Cord Injuries

Every year an estimated 7,800 people in the United States sustain spinal cord injuries.[1] There are presently approximately 220,000 spinal cord-injured individuals alive in this country (DeVivo, Fine, Maetz, & Stover, 1980; Kennedy, Stover, & Fine, 1986; NSCIA, 1988).

Motor vehicle accidents are the most common cause (47.7%) of spinal cord injury (Kennedy et al., 1986). Motorcycle accidents cause a disproportionate number of these vehicular accident-related injuries, accounting for approximately 7% of all spinal cord injuries (Young, Burns, Bowen, & McCutchen, 1982). Motor vehicle accidents are followed by falls or falling objects (20.8%), sports (14.2%), and acts of violence (14.6%). The remaining 14.6% of spinal cord injuries comes from a variety of causes. The incidence of the different causes of cord injury varies with sex, race, and age, being influenced by the activities and hazards prevalent in each population (Kennedy et al., 1986).

The vast majority of spinal cord injuries, approximately 80%, are sustained by males. Most are between 16 and 30 years of age at the time of injury. Nineteen is the most common age of injury (Kennedy et al., 1986). The prevalence of spinal cord injuries among young males is not the result of any anatomical or physiological vulnerability peculiar to this population. It is simply due to the fact that these are the people who are most prone to participating in such high-risk activities as driving too fast (and too drunk), riding motorcycles, playing football, and diving into unfamiliar waters where stumps and boulders are hidden beneath the surface.

ANATOMY REVIEW

An understanding of spinal cord injuries and their management requires a basic knowledge of the anatomy of the vertebral column, spinal cord, the cord's vascular supply, and spinal nerves.

Vertebral Column

Most spinal cord injuries are the result of trauma to the vertebral column, which contains 7 cervical, 12 thoracic, 5 lumbar, 5 sacral, and 4 coccygeal vertebrae. The cervical, thoracic, and lumbar vertebrae are separated by intervertebral discs and are connected and stabilized by ligaments. The sacral and coccygeal vertebrae are fused.

A typical vertebra consists of a body, located anteriorly, and an arch. The spinal cord is encased within the vertebral foramen, formed by the vertebral bodies and arches. Figure 2–1 illustrates the components of a vertebra.

The vertebral column is stabilized by ligaments. The anterior longitudinal ligament is attached to the anterior aspect of the vertebral bodies and limits extension. The posterior longitudinal ligament is attached to the posterior aspect of the vertebral bodies and limits flexion (Yashon, 1986). The ligamenta flava, supraspinous ligament, interspinous ligaments, and articular capsules stabilize the posterior arch (deGroot & Chusid, 1988; Denis, 1983).

The three-column model of the spine (Fig. 2–2) helps to understand the degree of instability that results from different ligamentous or boney injuries. This model was first proposed for the thoracolumbar spine (Denis, 1983) but is also applicable to the cervical region (Allen, 1989; Harris, Edeiken-Monroe, & Kopaniky, 1986). In this model the spine is conceptualized as consisting of three columns. At a given spinal segment, the anterior column consists of the anterior part of the vertebral body, the anterior longitudinal ligament, and the anterior anulus fibrosus.[2] The middle column includes the posterior wall of the vertebral body, the posterior longitudinal

---

[1] This estimation is probably low due to underreporting of cases in which people either sustain minimal neurological damage or die soon after injury (Kennedy et al., 1986).

[2] The anulus fibrosus is the fibrous outer portion of the intervertebral disc.

5

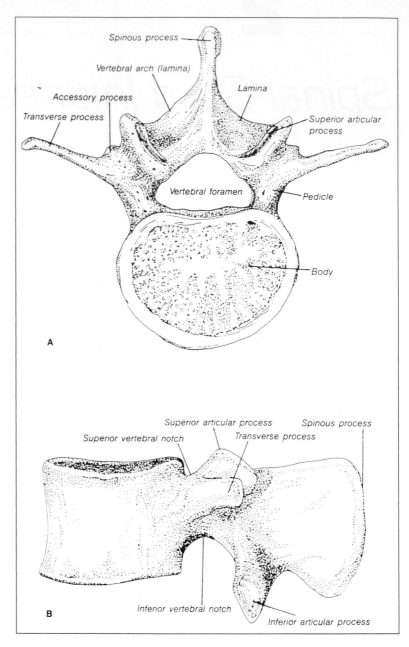

Figure 2-1. Components of a vertebra. **A.** Superior view of a typical midlumbar vertebra. **B.** Lateral view of a typical midlumbar vertebra. *(Reproduced with permission from Galli, R., Spaite, D., & Simon, R. [1989]. Emergency orthopedics: The spine [p. 160]. Norwalk, CT: Appleton & Lange.)*

ligament, and the posterior anulus fibrosus. The posterior column consists of the vertebral arch and the supraspinous ligament, interspinous ligament, capsule, and ligamentum flavum. Each column contributes to the overall stability of the spinal column. Instability of the spine occurs only when two or more columns sustain damage (Denis, 1983).

Spinal Cord

The spinal cord extends from the medulla oblongata just above the foramen magnum to the level of the L1 or L2 vertebra (deGroot & Chusid, 1988; Thelan, Davie, & Urden, 1990; Yashon, 1986). It is located within the vertebral foramen, also called the vertebral canal. The cord is protected anteriorly by the vertebral bodies and by the vertebral arches laterally and posteriorly.

Seen in transverse section, the spinal cord has an H-shaped area of gray matter centrally (Fig. 2–3). This gray matter is composed of cell bodies, small projection fibers, and glial support cells (Thelan et al., 1990). The dorsal (posterior) horn of the gray matter is predominately sensory. The ventral (anterior) horn contains the bodies of lower motor neurons innervating skeletal muscles. The lateral horn, present only in the thoracic and upper lumbar

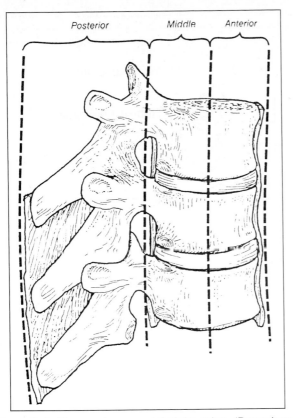

Figure 2–2. Three-column model of the spine. *(Reproduced with permission from Galli, R., Spaite, D., & Simon, R. [1989]. Emergency orthopedics: The spine [p. 162]. Norwalk, CT: Appleton & Lange.)*

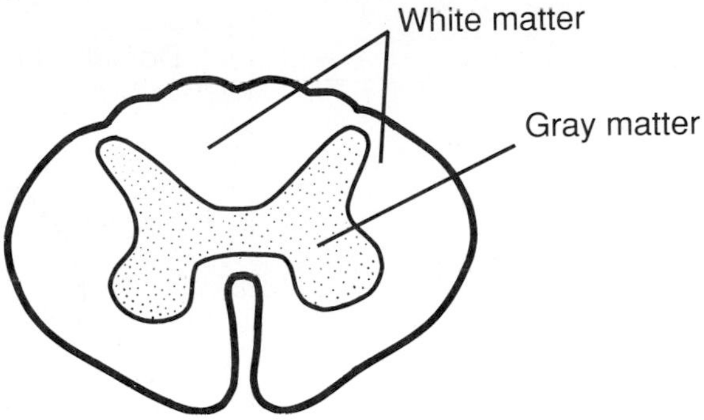

Figure 2–3. Schematic cross-section of the spinal cord. *(Reproduced with permission from deGroot, J., & Chusid, J. [1988]. Correlative neuroanatomy (20th ed.) [p. 32]. Norwalk, CT: Appleton & Lange.)*

regions, contains the cell bodies of preganglionic sympathetic fibers (deGroot & Chusid, 1988).

The gray matter of the spinal cord is surrounded by white matter consisting of ascending and descending fibers. Fibers carrying similar sensory information or motor functions travel together in tracts (Fig. 2–4 and Chart 2–1). Additionally, the fibers within at least some tracts are organized somatotopically: fibers are grouped with others traveling to or from the same cord segment (Fig. 2–5; deGroot & Chusid, 1988).

Chart 2–1. Major Spinal Pathways[a]

	Motor Tracts	
Name	**Travels in Cord Ipsilateral or Contralateral to Muscles it Innervates**	**Type of Control**
Lateral corticospinal	Ipsilateral	Voluntary motion (limbs)
Ventral corticospinal	Contralateral	Voluntary motion (axial)
Vestibulospinal	Both	Postural reflexes
Rubrospinal	Ipsilateral	Voluntary motion (limbs)
Pontine reticulospinal	Both	Modulation of spinal reflexes
Medullary reticulospinal	Both	Modulation of spinal reflexes
	Sensory Tracts	
Lateral spinothalamic	Contralateral	Sharp pain, temperature, light touch
Dorsal columns	Ipsilateral	Proprioception, 2-point discrimination, stereognosis, vibration, fine touch
Spinoreticular	Ipsilateral	Deep pain

[a] deGroot & Chusid (1988); Martin (1989); Meyer (1989a)

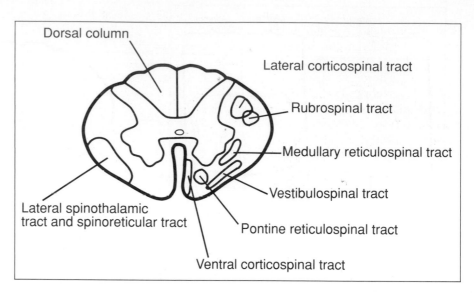

Figure 2–4. Major ascending and descending fiber tracts in the spinal cord. Ascending tracts are shown on the left; descending tracts are shown on the right.

Vascular Supply

The spinal cord receives its blood supply from a single anterior artery and from two posterior spinal arteries. The posterior arteries are joined by communicating vessels. Except in the area of the conus medullaris (the tapering caudal end of the cord), the anterior and posterior spinal arteries are not interconnected (Meyer, 1989). The anterior spinal artery supplies the anterior two thirds of the spinal cord, including the gray matter and the anterior and anterolateral white matter. The posterior arteries supply the posterolateral and posterior white matter of the spinal cord (McLeod & Lance, 1989; Meyer, 1989).

In the cervical region the anterior spinal artery is supplied primarily by the vertebral arteries and the intracranial vessels from which they arise. The posterior spinal arteries in this region are supplied by the vertebral arteries and the posterior inferior cerebellar arteries. In the thoracic and lumbar regions, the anterior and posterior spinal arteries are fed by segmental arteries that arise from the aorta. The largest of these arteries, the vessel of Adamkiewicz, supplies the anterior spinal artery at some point between T8 and L4. It is an important contributor to spinal circulation (deGroot & Chusid, 1988; McLeod & Lance, 1989; Meyer, 1989).

Spinal Nerves

There are 8 cervical, 12 thoracic, 5 lumbar, 5 sacral, and 1 coccygeal pairs of spinal nerves. Each spinal nerve has a dorsal (sensory) and a ventral (primarily

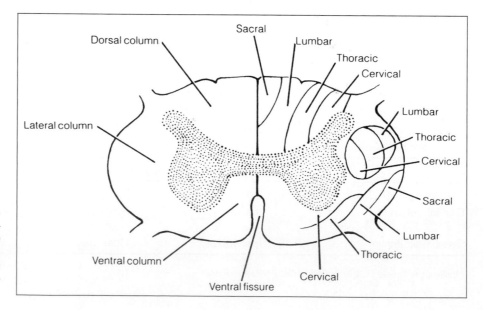

Figure 2–5. Somatotopic organization in the spinal cord. *(Reproduced with permission from deGroot, J., & Chusid, J. [1988]. Correlative neuroanatomy (20th ed.) [p. 43]. Norwalk, CT: Appleton & Lange.)*

motor) root that arise from a single cord segment. The C1 through C7 spinal nerves exit the vertebral foramen above the correspondingly numbered vertebrae. The C8 spinal nerve exists below the C7 vertebra. (There are 8 cervical nerves and only 7 cervical vertebrae.) The spinal nerves of T1 and below exit below the correspondingly numbered vertebrae (Fig. 2–6; deGroot & Chusid, 1988).

Because the spinal cord is shorter than the vertebral column, spinal nerves must travel caudally before exiting the vertebral canal. Distal to the

conus medullaris, the spinal nerves form the cauda equina (Fig. 2–6).

MECHANISMS OF VERTEBRAL INJURIES

Most spinal cord injuries occur as the result of direct or indirect trauma to the vertebral column. Approximately 10% of these spinal cord injuries occur with no detectable vertebral injury. In adults this is most likely to occur in individuals with preexisting narrow spinal canals or spondylosis (Cook, 1988; Rogers, 1989). Children can sustain spinal cord injury without any detectable damage to the vertebral column because their spinal columns are more mobile than those of adults (Pang & Pollack, 1989).

Most injuries of the vertebral column involve either a single level or a limited number of contiguous vertebrae. In 3% to 5% of cases of vertebral injury, however, the spinal column sustains damage at two or more levels that are separated by undamaged vertebrae. The secondary level of injury is often located at the rostral or caudal extremes of the spine. Multiple, noncontiguous, vertebral injuries are associated with severe trauma. They occur most commonly in association with injuries of the upper and middle thoracic spine (Cook, 1988; Rogers, 1989). Noncontiguous injuries rostral to a known injury are a matter of concern because if undetected and not treated properly, they may result in higher damage to the spinal cord with resulting paralysis and sensory loss at a higher level. Caudally located, noncontiguous injuries can impact on muscle tone and bowel, bladder, and genital functioning (Beric, Dimitrijevic, & Light, 1987).

Spinal column injuries are rarely caused by direct trauma to the vertebrae; most result from forces that create violent motions of the head or trunk (Rogers, 1989). The magnitude and direction of the traumatic force determines the type and extent of boney and ligamentous damage. The degree to which the vertebrae, soft tissues or both impinge upon the cord, the cord's vascular supply, or the spinal nerves determines the extent of neurological damage that results.

Laboratory studies have demonstrated that forces applied in different directions lead to distinct patterns of boney and ligamentous damage. Other factors that affect vertebral injury include the position of the person's head, neck, and trunk at the time of injury; the magnitude, rate of application, and duration of injuring force; and the point of application of the injuring force (Crowell, Edwards, & White, 1989). Outside of the laboratory, most injuries probably result from a combination of forces.

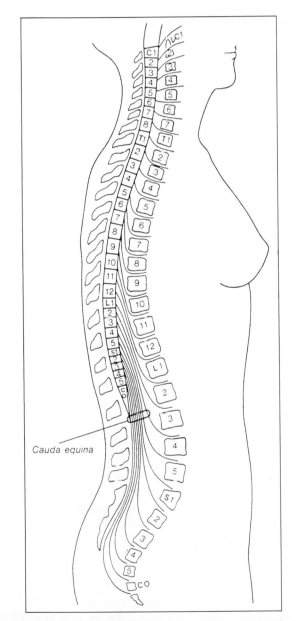

Figure 2–6. Schematic diagram of the spatial relationship of the vertebrae, spinal cord, nerve roots, and cauda equina. *(Reproduced with permission from Galli, R., Spaite, D., & Simon, R. [1989]. Emergency orthopedics: The spine [p. 163]. Norwalk, CT: Appleton & Lange.)*

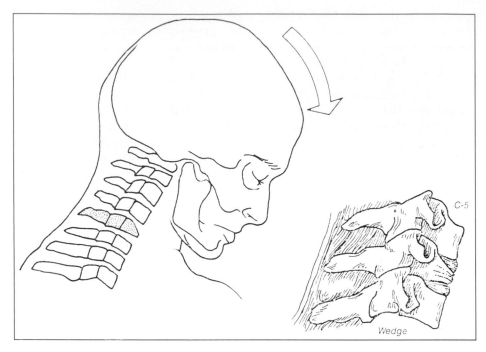

Figure 2–7. Wedge fracture resulting from flexion injury to the cervical spine. *(Reproduced with permission from Galli, R., Spaite, D., & Simon, R. [1989]. Emergency orthopedics: The spine [p. 108]. Norwalk, CT: Appleton & Lange.)*

Moreover, the forces involved in a given person's injury are usually unknown; they can only be inferred from a history of the accident and the pattern of vertebral and ligamentous injury found. Despite these limitations, information gleaned from laboratory studies is useful for understanding the causative mechanisms of vertebral column injury (Harris et al., 1986; Meyer, 1989; Rogers, 1989).

Cervical Injuries

Because of its relatively poor mechanical stability, the cervical spine is more vulnerable to trauma than other areas of the vertebral column (Meyer, 1989; Yashon, 1986). Moreover, injury to the spine in this region is likely to result (40% incidence) in damage to the cord (Cook, 1988). As a result of these factors, a disproportionate number (approximately 53%) of spinal cord injuries occur in the cervical region (Fine, Kuhlemeier, DeVivo, & Stover, 1979; Kennedy et al., 1986).

Most survivors of cervical spinal cord injuries have cord damage at the lower cervical levels; vertebral fractures at C1 and C2 are rarely associated with significant neurological deficits (Cook, 1988). This is largely due to a combination of two factors. The vertebral canal is large at the craniovertebral junction, with the spinal cord occupying only 50% of the available space. Thus it is possible for 50% of the canal's area to be intruded upon by displaced boney elements without damage to the spinal cord. In addition, when the spinal cord *is* injured at this level, the injury is not likely to be survived. Com-

plete cord injuries at C1 and C2 interrupt the diaphragm's innervation, making survival possible only if resuscitation is provided immediately (Fine et al., 1979; Meyer, 1989; Rogers, 1989).

The forces most frequently causing vertebral injury in the cervical spine are flexion, vertical loading, and extension. These forces may be accompanied and modified by rotation, lateral flexion or both.

Flexion. Flexion injuries of the cervical spine have the highest incidence of neurological injury (Meyer, 1989). This type of injury is most commonly the result of rapid deceleration, as occurs in head-on collisions (Thelan et al., 1990).

When the neck is flexed violently, the vertebral column is subjected to compression force anteriorly and distraction force posteriorly (Cook, 1988; Harris et al., 1986). Hyperflexion may result in damage to soft tissue, vertebrae, or a combination of the two (Harris et al., 1986). With the exception of clay-shoveler fractures,[3] the posterior ligamentous complex sustains damage in all flexion injuries (Cook, 1988; Harris et al., 1986).

Compression of the anterior aspect of the vertebral column can result in collapse of the anterior aspect of a vertebra, called a wedge fracture (Fig. 2–7; Cook, 1988; Crowell, Edwards, & White, 1989; Harris et al., 1986). This type of fracture is usually

---

[3] A clay-shoveler fracture is an avulsion fracture of the spinous process of C6, C7, or T1 (Harris et al., 1986).

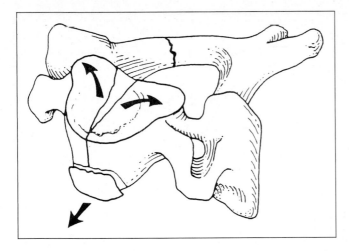

Figure 2–8. Flexion teardrop fracture accompanied by sagitally oriented fracture of the vertebral body with posterior displacement of the boney fragments into the neural canal. *(Reproduced with permission from Crowell, R., Edwards, W., & White, A. [1989]. Mechanisms of injury in the cervical spine: Experimental evidence and biomechanical modeling. In* The cervical spine *(2nd ed.) [p. 72]. Philadelphia: Lippincott.)*

stable (Cook, 1988) and typically does not result in neurological injury (Crowell et al., 1989).

A more serious injury that can result from compression of the anterior aspect of the vertebral column is a teardrop fracture. In this injury a triangular fragment is split from the vertebral body anteriorly. Flexion teardrop fractures are associated with severe ligamentous disruption (Harris et al., 1986) and are often accompanied by a sagitally oriented fracture of the vertebral body with posterior displacement of the boney fragments into the neural canal (Fig. 2–8; Crowell et al., 1989). Severe damage to the cord typically results from flexion teardrop fractures (Crowell et al., 1989; Harris et al., 1986; Rogers, 1989).

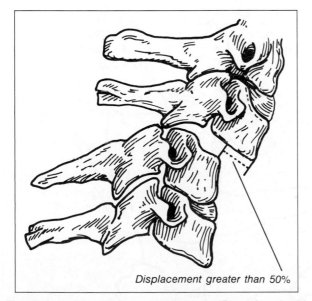

Displacement greater than 50%

Figure 2–9. Bilateral facet dislocation. *(Reproduced with permission from Galli, R., Spaite, D., & Simon, R. [1989]. Emergency orthopedics: The spine [p. 118]. Norwalk, CT: Appleton & Lange.)*

Damage to the ligaments stabilizing the cervical spine can also have grave results. When posterior distractive forces resulting from hyperflexion, possibly in combination with rotation (Crowell et al., 1989), cause total disruption of the intervertebral ligaments and intervertebral disc, the vertebrae are free to dislocate. Typically distraction and shearing forces drive the superior vertebra forward. The dislocated vertebra's inferior facets lodge in front of the superior facets of the subjacent vertebra, and the facets "lock" (Fig. 2–9). A dislocation with bilateral locked facets is extrememy unstable and usually results in severe neurological damage (Cook, 1988; Harris et al., 1986; Rogers, 1989).

Flexion With Rotation. Flexion and rotation forces, possibly in combination with lateral flexion and shearing (Cook, 1988), can result in the dislocation and locking of a single facet joint (Fig. 2–10). This displacement is made possible by disruption of the facet joint capsule and posterior ligaments (Rieser, Mudiyam, & Waters, 1985).

Unilateral facet dislocations are usually stable. This type of injury is associated with neurological damage, usually Brown-Séquard syndrome or nerve root damage, approximately 30% of the time (Cook, 1988; Harris et al., 1986).

Vertical Compression. Axial loading through the straightened (slightly flexed) cervical spine results in burst fractures (Crowell et al., 1989; Harris et al., 1986). Burst fracture in the cervical spine is most often the result of striking the head while diving into shallow water (Fig. 2–11). In this type of accident, a burst fracture occurs most frequently at C4 or C5, with complete quadriplegia resulting (Buchanan, 1987a).

A burst fracture is a comminuted fracture of the vertebral body; the vertebral body is crushed.

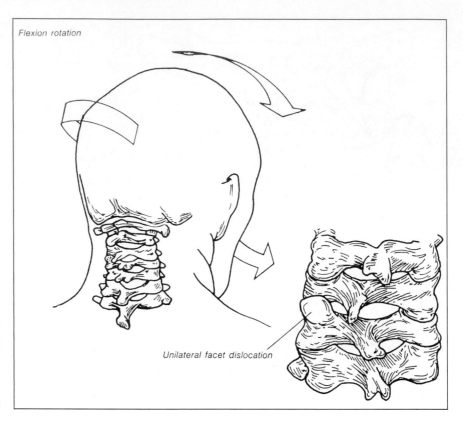

Flexion rotation

Unilateral facet dislocation

Figure 2–10. Unilateral facet dislocation resulting from combined flexion and rotation of the cervical spine. *(Reproduced with permission from Galli, R., Spaite, D., & Simon, R. [1989]. Emergency orthopedics: The spine [p. 109]. Norwalk, CT: Appleton & Lange.)*

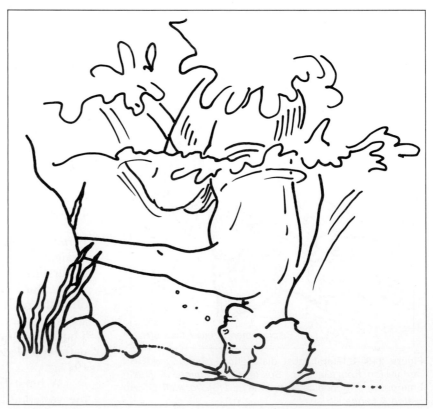

Figure 2–11. Common mechanism of injury of burst fracture in cervical spine: striking head while diving into shallow water.

Neurological damage occurs when boney fragments are driven posteriorly into the spinal canal (Fig. 2–12). Burst fractures are accompanied by fractures of the vertebral arch (Harris et al., 1986).

Extension Injuries. Extension injuries often occur when someone strikes his chin or forehead in a fall or is struck from behind when riding in a vehicle (Fig. 2–13). The most common location for an extension injury is C4-5 (Buchanan, 1987a).

When the neck is extended violently, the cervical spine is subjected to distraction force anteriorly and compression force posteriorly (Cook, 1988). These forces can result in boney or ligamentous damage or both.

The posterior compressive forces involved in an extension injury can result in fractures on one (unilateral) or both (bilateral) sides of the vertebral arch, often in two adjacent vertebrae. A unilateral fracture is most common (Allen, 1989; Cook, 1988). When a bilateral fracture occurs, the vertebral body can dislocate (Harris et al., 1986).

Severe anterior distractive forces can cause rupture of the anterior longitudinal ligament and discovertebral bond. A small fragment of the anterior vertebral body may be avulsed in the process (Fig. 2–14). When hyperextension results in severe ligamentous disruption anteriorly, the superior vertebra dislocates posteriorly. This injury is called a hyperextension dislocation, sprain, or strain. The spinal cord is compressed by the vertebral body and disc fragments anteriorly and the ligamentum flava and laminae posteriorly (Fig. 2–15; Cook, 1988; Galli, Spaite, & Simon, 1989; Harris et al., 1986).

When the cervical spine is hyperextended, neurological damage can occur without any boney or ligamentous damage. This occurs most frequently in the presence of osteophytic changes or a congenitally small canal (Peterson & Altman, 1989). Spinal cord damage secondary to hyperextension injury is often confined to the central aspect of the cord.

Hyperextension of the cervical spine is most likely to lead to cord damage if the person is elderly. Degenerative changes in the vertebrae of people in this age group make them more vulnerable to extension injuries. Osteophytes projecting posteriorly from the vertebral bodies can impinge upon the spinal cord when the neck is hyperextended by a relatively mild force. Because of the mild trauma involved, cervical cord injury in these cases is often overlooked by examining physicians. Symptoms may be attributed to hysteria, malingering, cerebrovascular accident, or other neurological or cardiovascular disorder (Crawford & Shepherd, 1989; Peterson & Altman, 1989).

Lateral Flexion. Violent lateral flexion leads to compression on one side of the vertebral column and distraction on the other. The compressive

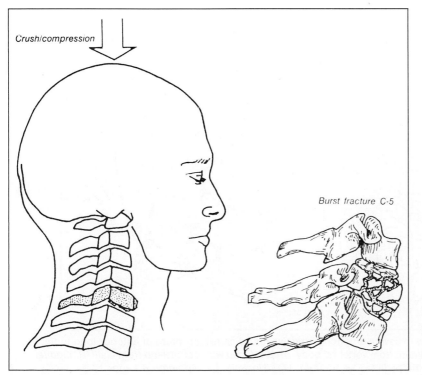

Crush/compression

Burst fracture C-5

Figure 2–12. Burst fracture resulting from compression (axial loading) of the cervical spine. *(Reproduced with permission from Galli, R., Spaite, D., & Simon, R. [1989]. Emergency orthopedics: The spine [p. 110]. Norwalk, CT: Appleton & Lange.)*

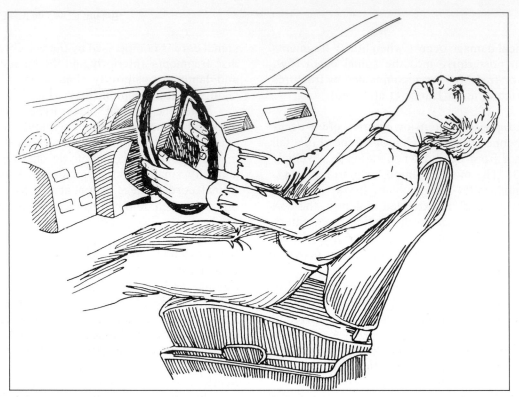

Figure 2–13. Common mechanism of extension injury in cervical spine: vehicle struck from behind. *(Reproduced with permission from Galli, R., Spaite, D., & Simon, R. [1989]. Emergency orthopedics: The spine [p. 137]. Norwalk, CT: Appleton & Lange.)*

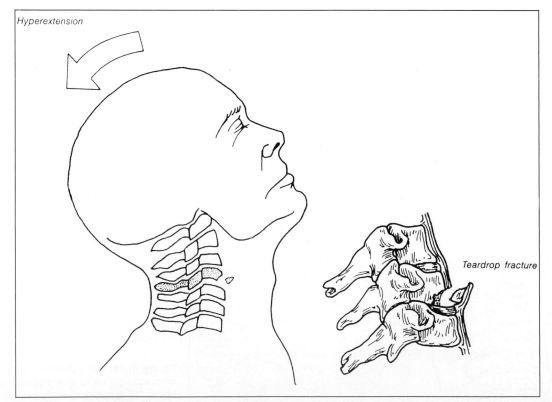

Hyperextension

Teardrop fracture

Figure 2–14. Hyperextension injury with severe anterior distractive forces causing rupture of anterior longitudinal ligament and avulsion of anterior fragment from vertebral body. *(Reproduced with permission from Galli, R., Spaite, D., & Simon, R. [1989]. Emergency orthopedics: The spine [p. 111]. Norwalk, CT: Appleton & Lange.)*

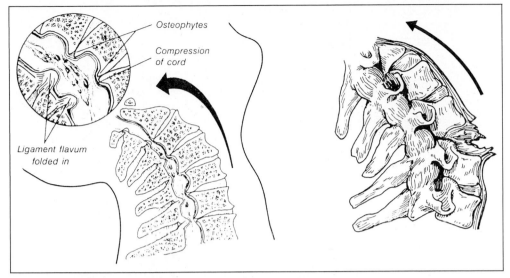

Figure 2–15. Hyperextension sprain. The spinal cord is compressed by the vertebral body, disc fragments, or osteophytes and/or anteriorly and the ligamentum flavum and laminae posteriorly. *(Reproduced with permission from Galli, R., [p. 123] Spaite, D., & Simon, R. [1989]. Emergency orthopedics: The spine [p. 123]. Norwalk, CT: Appleton & Lange.)*

forces, occurring on the side toward which the spine laterally flexes, can result in lateral wedging of the vertebral body and fracture of the vertebral arch. Distractive forces on the contralateral side can cause ligamentous disruption. Lateral flexion injuries can lead to severe spinal cord damage and are often associated with brachial plexus injuries (Allen, 1989).

Pure lateral flexion injuries are rare (Allen, 1989). More commonly, lateral flexion combines with and modifies the effects of other forces to produce spinal injury (Cook, 1988; Harris et al., 1986).

Thoracic Injuries
The rib cage provides the T1 through T10 spine with great stability. As a result, extreme violence is required to injure the spine in this region. Thoracic spinal cord injuries are less common than cervical injuries but are more likely to be complete (Fine et al., 1979; Kennedy et al., 1986). This is probably due to the magnitude of force required to injure the thoracic spine, the small size of the vertebral canal in this region, and the relatively poor vascular supply of the upper thoracic cord (Fine et al., 1979; Meyer, 1989). Trauma to the lower thoracic spine can injure the vessel of Adamkiewicz, a major source of the thoracolumbar cord's vascular supply. The resulting neurological damage can ascend as high as T4 (Meyer, 1989).

Thoracic injuries are often caused by gunshot wounds, vehicular accidents, and falls (Meyer, 1989). The most common site of injury to the thoracolumbar spine is the T12-L1 junction (Yashon, 1986). This is where the relatively rigid thoracic spine meets the relatively flexible lumbar spine (Cook, 1988; Galli et al., 1989).

The spatial arrangement of boney and neural tissue in the low thoracic and upper lumbar regions is such that vertebral injury can result in diverse patterns of neurological damage. All of the lumbar and sacral cord segments lie between the upper border of the T10 vertebral body and the level of L1 or L2. Additionally, spinal nerves from higher cord levels lie adjacent to the cord within the vertebral canal in this region as they travel caudally before exiting. As a result, the neural canal at a given vertebral level may enclose more than one cord level as well as spinal nerves from several higher levels (Fig. 2–16). Vertebral damage can result in trauma to any or all of this neural tissue or in no neurological damage.

The basic mechanics of vertebral and ligamentous injury of the spine described above in reference to cervical injuries are similar throughout the spinal column. For example, extreme motions in the sagittal or frontal planes cause compression of the vertebrae in the direction of the motion and distraction of the opposite boney and ligamentous elements. The patterns of injury typical of the thoracic spine are described below.

Flexion. Most fractures of the thoracic vertebrae are wedge compression fractures caused by compression of the anterior aspects of the vertebral bodies (Fig. 2–17). The thoracic region may be prone to this type of fracture because the normal

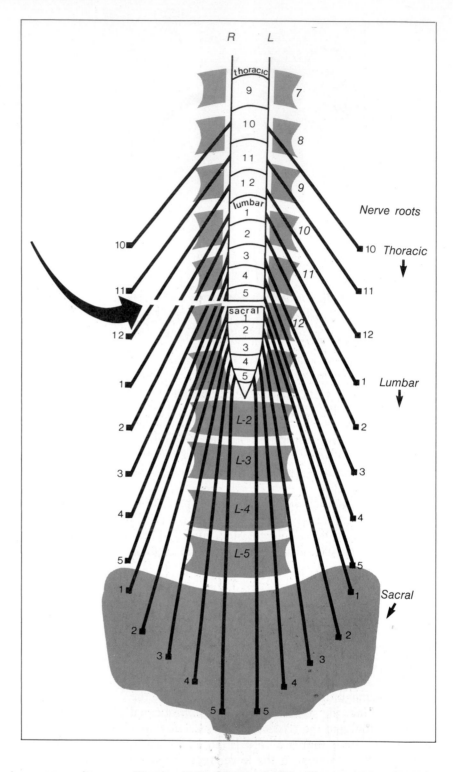

Figure 2–16. Schematic diagram of the anatomic basis of "mixed" injuries in lumbosacral region. Injury to the 12th thoracic vertebra has transected the cord between the lumbar and the sacral segments; the roots are lost on the right side, "spared" on the left side. Variations of these patterns occur in different patients even with identical boney injuries. *(Reproduced with permission from Galli, R., Spaite, D., & Simon, R. [1989]. Emergency orthopedics: The spine [p. 213]. Norwalk, CT: Appleton & Lange.)*

kyphotic curve converts vertical compression forces to flexion (Cook, 1988). The incidence of neurological damage occurring with this type of injury varies with the severity of the fracture (Meyer, 1989).

In severe cases of flexion injury, a wedge compression fracture is combined with damage to the posterior vertebral or boney elements or both

(Denis, 1983; Meyer, 1989). The posterior damage is caused by distraction forces created when the vertebra pivots on its intact middle column (Denis, 1983).

Flexion With Rotation. When rotation is combined with flexion (Fig. 2–18), rotational shearing is added to the anterior compressive and posterior distrac-

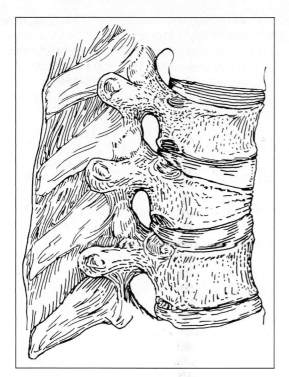

Figure 2–17. Wedge fracture resulting from flexion of the thoracic spine (*ribs removed for visualization*). *(Reproduced with permission from Galli, R., Spaite, D., & Simon, R. [1989]. Emergency orthopedics: The spine [p. 216]. Norwalk, CT: Appleton & Lange.)*

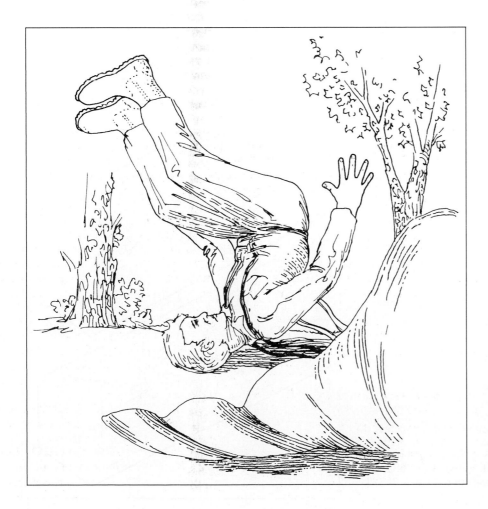

Figure 2–18. Fall onto upper back and one shoulder produces flexion-rotation forces on the spine. *(Reproduced with permission from Galli, R., Spaite, D., & Simon, R. [1989]. Emergency orthopedics: The spine [p. 217]. Norwalk, CT: Appleton & Lange.)*

tive forces created by flexion. This combination of forces can disrupt all three columns of the spine. Flexion-rotation injuries can lead to fracture dislocations with anterior compression of the vertebral body, damage to the anterior longitudinal ligament, disruption of the disc, a horizontal fracture (slice fracture) through the vertebral body, and fractures of the posterior arch. Fractures of transverse processes and ribs are frequently associated with these injuries. Neurological damage is common following flexion-rotation injuries, resulting from dislocation of the vertebrae, entry of boney fragments into the spinal canal, or both (Cook, 1988; Denis, 1983; Meyer, 1989).

Vertical Compression. The thoracic spine may be subjected to vertical compression when a person is struck by a falling object or falls and lands on his upper thoracic spine, buttocks, or feet. Falls most frequently result in burst fractures of T10, T11, or T12 (Buchanan, 1987a; Meyer, 1989).

Burst fractures of thoracic vertebrae are similar to cervical burst fractures. The vertebral body is crushed, and the laminae fracture. Retropulsion of boney fragments into the vertebral canal often leads to cord damage (Denis, 1983; Meyer, 1989).

Extension or Lateral Flexion. The thoracolumbar spine is rarely injured by isolated extension or lateral flexion forces (Cook, 1988; Meyer, 1989; Yashon, 1986). When injuries occur from these forces, they involve disruption of the anterior ligaments and lateral wedging of the vertebral body, respectively (Denis, 1983; Meyer, 1989).

Lumbar Injuries

The lumbar segment of the spinal column is of intermediate stability: it is more flexible than the tho-

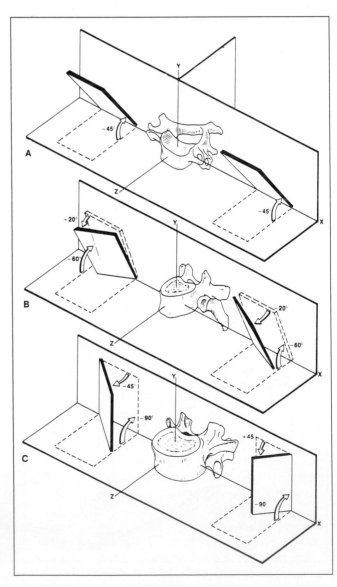

Figure 2–19. Orientation of facet joints (rough estimates). **(A)** Cervical. **(B)** Thoracic. **(C)** Lumbar: vertical orientation of facet joints makes pure dislocation in the lumbar region rare. *(Reproduced with permission from White, A., & Panjabi, M. [1978]. Clinical biomechanics of the spine [p. 30]. Philadelphia: Lippincott.)*

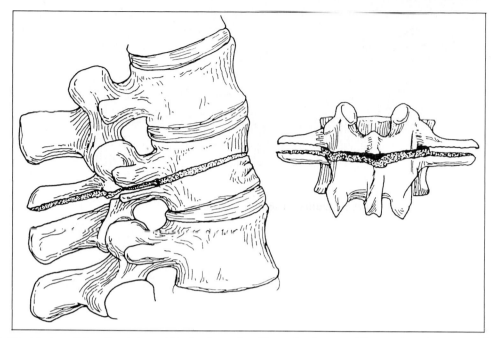

Figure 2–20. Flexion-distraction injury of the lumbar spine. Boney fractures and ligamentous tears associated with these injuries are horizontally oriented. *(Reproduced with permission from Galli, R., Spaite, D., & Simon, R. [1989]. Emergency orthopedics: The spine [p. 222]. Norwalk, CT: Appleton & Lange.)*

racic spine but less flexible than the cervical spine. Although it lacks the stability provided by the thoracic cage, the lumbar spine is supported by strong paraspinal and abdominal musculature (Cook, 1988).

Common causes of injury to this region include falls, vehicular accidents, gunshot wounds, and direct impact from heavy objects (Meyer, 1989; Rieser et al., 1985). Injury occurs most frequently at the thoracolumbar junction.

Neurological damage resulting from trauma to the lumbar spine is usually incomplete (Fine et al., 1979). This is in part due to the relatively good vascular supply and large vertebral canal in this region. In addition, caudal to L1 or L2, the cord is not present in the vertebral canal. The cauda equina, the sole neurological element within the neural canal in this region, is less sensitive than the spinal cord to trauma (Meyer, 1989; Yashon, 1986).

Flexion. The mechanism and patterns of injury from violent flexion of the lumbar spine are comparable to those of flexion injury in the thoracic spine. Wedge compression fractures due to flexion, often not associated with neurological damage, are frequent at L1 (Denis, 1983).

Flexion With Rotation. The orientation of the intervertebral facet joints in the lumbar spine (Fig. 2–19) provides a good deal of anteroposterior stability. The restricted mobility allowed by these joints, combined with strong joint capsules, makes pure dislocation rare in the lumbar region (Cook, 1988; Yashon, 1986). Violent flexion rotation is more likely to result in fracture dislocation, as occurs in the thoracic spine. These fracture dislocations usually result in neurological injury (Bedbrook, 1981; Cook, 1988).

Flexion With Distraction. Combined flexion and distraction forces are typical of, but not limited to, "seat-belt injuries" associated with old-fashioned lap belts worn without shoulder restraints. In this type of injury the lumbar spine is flexed violently about a fulcrum located at the anterior abdominal wall. Flexion about this anteriorly-located fulcrum results in extreme distractive forces on the middle and posterior columns of the spine (Cook, 1988; Denis, 1983).

Spinal column damage in this type of injury can occur at one or two levels (Denis, 1983). It may be limited to the ligaments and discs or may include vertebral fractures (Cook, 1988). The boney fractures and ligamentous tears associated with flexion-distraction injuries are horizontally oriented (Fig. 2–20). The posterior aspect of the vertebral body, annulus fibrosus, vertebral arch, and posterior longitudinal ligament may be torn by the distractive forces, and the anterior aspect of the vertebral body may compress. Disruption of the middle and posterior columns allows dislocation or subluxation to occur (Denis, 1983). About 15% of these injuries

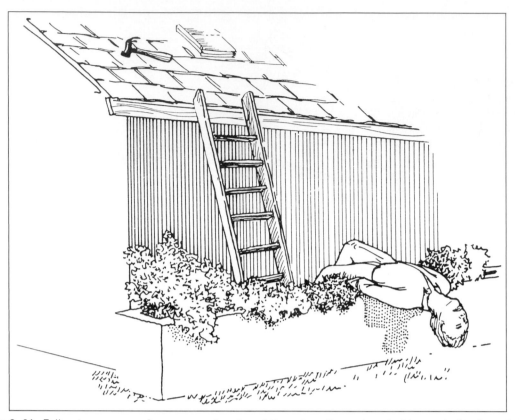

Figure 2–21. Fall onto uneven surface causes shearing of the spine. *(Reproduced with permission from Galli, R., Spaite, D., & Simon, R. [1989].* Emergency orthopedics: The spine *[p. 231]. Norwalk, CT: Appleton & Lange.)*

results in neurological damage (Cook, 1988). Associated abdominal injuries are common (Rieser et al., 1985).

Shear. A horizontally-directed force, such as occurs when a person is struck from behind by a heavy object or falls onto an uneven surface, causes shearing of the spine (Fig. 2–21). This force can cause total disruption of the ligaments with resulting dislocation of the vertebrae and severe neurological damage. Shear forces can also cause fractures of the vertebral body and the posterior arches (Cook, 1988).

Vertical Compression. As is true in more rostral regions of the vertebral column, violent force directed through the long axis of the lumbar spine can cause burst fractures. In this region burst fractures are usually caused by falls (Meyer, 1989). About 50% of people sustaining burst fractures in the thoracic or lumbar spine sustain neurological damage, usually incomplete (Denis, 1983).

NEUROPATHOLOGY

The spinal cord can be damaged by direct insult from a foreign body such as a bullet or knife. More often the cord sustains damage as a result of impingement by boney or soft tissue structures, such as occurs when vertebrae dislocate or a vertebral body explodes.

The spinal cord does not have to be severed for irreversible damage to occur. In fact, actual anatomical transsection of the cord is rare (Meyer, 1989). This is an important point to remember when educating people about their injuries. Often patients are told that their spinal cords were "bruised" instead of severed, and they interpret this fact to mean that they will recover from their paralysis. However, trauma that results in "bruising" or hemorrhaging in the spinal cord can (and *often* does) cause neurological damage that is just as complete and just as permanent as when the cord is severed.

Not all spinal cord damage occurs as the result of physical impingement on the cord itself. The spinal cord can also be damaged by interruption of its vascular supply. The cord's vascular supply can be disrupted by vertebral trauma, surgery, gunshot or knife wounds, or various other causes.

Although most spinal cord injuries occur as a result of trauma, the cord can be damaged by a variety of nontraumatic causes. Examples include spinal hematoma, infection, arachnoiditis, radiation, spondylosis, rheumatoid arthritis, neoplasm, and interruption of the cord's vascular supply due to surgery, cardiac arrest, or aortic aneurysm (Yashon, 1986).

Pathological Changes

Blunt trauma to the spinal cord results in some primary destruction of neurons at the level of injury. This neuronal damage is most severe in the cell bodies but can also occur in the axons (Hughes, 1988). The neurological damage that results from trauma to the spinal cord is due only in part to the initial trauma to the neurons themselves. Most of the damage to the cord is caused by secondary sequelae of the initial trauma[4] (Cotman & Nieto-Sampedro, 1985; Iizuka, Yamamoto, Iwasaki, Yamamoto, & Konno, 1987; Young & Ransohoff, 1989).

Typically the spinal cord sustains a contusion as the result of impingement by displaced bone, soft tissues, or both. Within hours following the initial trauma, a process of progressive tissue destruction is initiated within the cord. These secondary reactions lead to ischemia, edema, demyelination of axons, and necrosis of the spinal cord (Bohlman & Boada, 1989; Waxman, 1989).

The injured spinal cord may look undamaged upon visual examination soon after injury (Yashon, 1986). However, microscopic examination within the first few hours following injury reveals patchy hemorrhage, tissue laceration, edema, and necrosis, most prevalent in the central grey matter. In severe injuries, the central necrosis, hemorrhage, and edema spread outwardly as time passes, causing destruction in the white matter (Mackenzie & Ducker, 1986; Yashon, 1986). The extent of destruction that ultimately occurs is dependent on the severity of the initial trauma (Demediuk, Daly, & Faden, 1989).

The secondary tissue destruction initiated by trauma to the spinal cord can progress up and down the cord. The resulting area of cord necrosis is commonly spindle shaped, tapering in its rostral and caudal extensions (Hughes, 1988). The area of maximal cord damage usually spreads over 1 to 3 segments, with diminishing severity above and below. However, the tissue destruction can spread over several segments, leading to the formation of cystic cavities.

Gross edema of the spinal cord can also occur following trauma. As the cord swells, it becomes compressed within the meninges, and further damage to the cord occurs (Hughes, 1988).

As the primary and secondary reactions to trauma subside, the necrotic region of the spinal cord is gradually resorbed and replaced by scar tissue (Cotman & Nieto-Sampedro, 1985; Hughes, 1988).

Underlying Mechanisms of Secondary Tissue Destruction

There are a variety of possible mechanisms for the secondary process of tissue destruction that occurs after trauma to the spinal cord. These possible mechanisms include ischemia and disruption of ion concentrations in the injured tissues. These conditions have been found in traumatized spinal cord tissue, but it remains to be determined whether they are causes or results of tissue death (Young & Ransohoff, 1989).

Ischemia. Blood flow diminishes in the traumatized area of a spinal cord following injury. This reduction in circulation occurs rapidly in the grey matter. In severely traumatized cords, blood flow in the white matter falls after a 2- to 3-hour delay. It may not diminish at all in the white matter of less severely traumatized cords (Young & Ransohoff, 1989).

Ischemia may be due to the presence of substances such as norepinephrine, serotonin, histamine, and prostaglandins in the injured cord that induce vasoconstriction (Northrup & Alderman, 1989). Other possible causes of ischemia in the injured spinal cord include thromboses, metabolic disturbances, and elevated pressure due to edema (Young & Ransohoff, 1989).

Sodium and Potassium Ion Derangements. Disruption of cell membranes in the injured area of the spinal cord results in abnormal concentrations of sodium and potassium in the extracellular fluid. This derangement blocks the functioning of intact neurons in the area, since neurons require a normal ion balance to generate action potentials. The ion imbalance is probably also a significant cause of edema: the abnormally high concentration of sodium in the tissue following injury increases the osmotic pressure in the damaged area of the cord, encouraging the movement of water to the area (Young & Ransohoff, 1989).

Calcium. Calcium ions accumulate in injured cells after a spinal cord is traumatized, possibly due to the presence of neurotoxic neurotransmitters (Choi & Rothman, 1990; Demediuk et al., 1989; Faden & Simon, 1988). The abnormal concentration of calcium within the damaged cells disrupts their func-

---

[4] The following description of the pathological changes associated with spinal cord injury is based primarily on studies of blunt trauma to the cord as occurs when boney elements impinge on the cord as a result of vertebral injury. However, research indicates that the same process of secondary progressive tissue destruction occurs with any injury to the spinal cord, including cord damage from ischemia or slow compression (Young & Ransohoff, 1989).

tioning and causes breakdown of protein and phospholipids, with resulting demyelination and destruction of the cell membrane and axonal cytoskeleton (Balentine, 1988; Iizuka et al., 1987; Young & Ransohoff, 1989). The metabolic by-products of the deranged cell functioning and membrane destruction may contribute to further membrane destruction and the development of ischemia and edema (Young & Ransohoff, 1989).

Effect of Compression on Recovery of Function

Spinal cord trauma does not always result in complete disruption of the cord at the level of lesion. Incomplete lesions are common, with surviving neurons passing through the damaged portion of the cord. If this undamaged neural tissue is subjected to chronic compression, however, it may survive but not resume functioning while subjected to the compression (Bohlman & Boada, 1989).

Spinal Shock

Spinal shock is a transient phenomenon that occurs after trauma to the spinal cord. During spinal shock, the cord *temporarily* ceases to function below the lesion. Spinal reflexes, voluntary motor and sensory function, and autonomic control are absent below the level of lesion (deGroot & Chusid, 1988). The cause of spinal shock is unknown.

Spinal shock usually begins to resolve within 24 hours of injury. Resumed functioning in the spinal cord below the lesion is most often heralded by the return of the anal and bulbocavernosis reflexes (Illis, 1988). Absence of any sparing of sensation or voluntary motor function below the lesion when these reflexes return is considered to be an indication that the lesion is complete (Coogler, 1985; Stauffer, 1989).

Spinal shock usually resolves within a few weeks of injury (deGroot & Chusid, 1988; Coogler, 1985; Yashon, 1986). As spinal shock passes, the cord gradually resumes functioning below the level of lesion. This return of function is evidenced by (1) resumption of motor and sensory function below the level of the lesion if tracts are undamaged, or (2) return of reflex functioning of the cord below the level of the lesion, or (3) a combination of the two.

CLASSIFICATION OF SPINAL CORD INJURIES

Spinal cord injuries are named according to the level of neurological injury and are classified as complete or incomplete.

Chart 2–2. Key Muscles for Identification of Neurological Level of Injury[a]

Motor Level	Key Muscles
Cl-4	Sensory level and diaphragm
C-5	Biceps, brachialis, brachioradialis
C-6	Extensor carpi radialis longus and brevis
C-7	Triceps
C-8	Flexor digitorum profundus
T-1	Interossei
T2-L1	Sensory level and Beevor's sign
L-2	Iliopsoas
L-3	Quadriceps
L-4	Tibialis anterior
L-5	Extensor hallucis longus
S-1	Gastrocnemius, soleus
S2-S5	Sensory level and anal sphincter

[a] American Spinal Injury Association (1989)

Paraplegia versus Quadriplegia. When paralysis (complete or incomplete) involves all four extremities, the condition is called quadriplegia. "Paraplegia" refers to paralysis of the lower extremities. Sometimes the terms "quadriparesis" and "paraparesis" are used to denote weakness rather than total paralysis.

Neurological Level of Injury. The neurological level of injury is defined as the most caudal level of the spinal cord that exhibits intact sensory and motor functioning. To determine an individual's neurological level of injury, the clinician tests sensation in key areas (Fig. 2–22) and strength in key muscles (Chart 2–2) that are representative of specific cord segments.

The key sensory areas are well demarcated; each is innervated by a single spinal cord segment. As a result, the sensory ability in a key area provides a good representation of the functioning in the sensory portions of its corresponding cord segment. In contrast, muscles receive innervation from more than one spinal cord level. Thus the strength of a given muscle is a reflection of the functioning of two or more cord segments. A lesion in the caudal segment innervating a muscle will cause reduced strength in that muscle.[5] For the purposes of iden-

---

[5] For example, the biceps brachii receives C5 and C6 innervation, and normal functioning of this muscle requires intact innervation from both of these cord segments. A cord lesion that disrupts the functioning of the C6 level of the cord will result in a reduction of biceps strength.

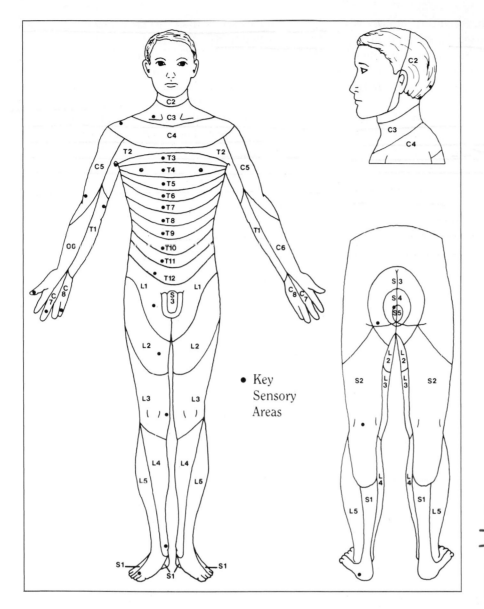

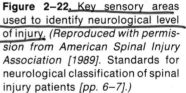

Figure 2–22. Key sensory areas used to identify neurological level of injury. *(Reproduced with permission from American Spinal Injury Association [1989]. Standards for neurological classification of spinal injury patients [pp. 6–7].)*

tifying the neurological level of injury, a key muscle is defined as demonstrating intact innervation from the cord segment that it represents[6] if (1) it exhibits 3/5 or greater strength, and (2) the next more rostral key muscle exhibits 4/5 or greater strength (American Spinal Injury Association, 1989).

Asymmetrical paralysis, sensory impairment, or both are common following spinal cord injury because lesions are often asymmetrical. When a person exhibits different levels of neurological injury on the right and left sides, the identified neurological level of injury should reflect this clinical picture

(ASIA, 1989). For example, a given person may have right C5, left C6 quadriplegia. Likewise, if there is a discrepancy between an individual's motor and sensory functioning, specification of the different motor and sensory neurological levels of injury will provide the most useful information.

Complete Versus Incomplete Lesion. A person is said to have a complete spinal cord injury if there is a total and permanent functional disruption of his cord. No sensory or voluntary motor function is present in areas innervated more than three segments below the neurological level of injury (ASIA, 1989).

With an incomplete lesion, the spinal cord is not totally disrupted at the level of injury. Some ascending or descending fibers or both remain intact

---

[6] Key muscles are identified with the more rostral of the spinal cord segments from which they receive innervation. For example, the biceps brachii, which is the C5 key muscle, receives innervation from both C5 and C6.

and continue to function. The resulting motor or sensory function is called sparing. A lesion is classified as incomplete if any sensation or voluntary motor function exists more than three segments below the neurological level of injury (ASIA, 1989).

Zone of Partial Preservation. Some people with spinal cord injuries exhibit partial preservation of sensory or motor function or both for 1 to 3 segments caudal to the neurological level of lesion. This area of partial innervation is called the zone of partial preservation (ASIA, 1989), or the zone of injury (Buchanan, 1987). As long as the preservation of function extends 3 or fewer segments caudal to the neurological level of injury, the lesion is still classified as complete (ASIA, 1989).

INCOMPLETE LESIONS

Incomplete lesions of the spinal cord can result in a variety of patterns of neurological deficit. The clinical presentation is determined by the exact area and extent of neurological damage. The three most prevalent syndromes are Brown-Séquard, anterior cord, and central cord.

Brown-Séquard Syndrome

When one side of the spinal cord is damaged, the resulting clinical picture is called Brown-Séquard syndrome (Fig. 2–23). The most common causes are stab and gunshot wounds. This syndrome is also often associated with unilateral facet locks or burst fractures (Rogers, 1989).

Damage to only one side of the cord results in motor paralysis and loss of proprioception, vibratory sense, and two-point discrimination ipsilaterally. At the level of the lesion, the skin is anesthetic ipsilaterally. Sensitivity to pain and temperature are lost contralaterally starting a few levels below the lesion. Spasticity is likely to be present below the lesion ipsilaterally (deGroot & Chusid, 1988; McLeod & Lance, 1989; Yashon, 1986).

The clinical presentation of Brown-Séquard syndrome makes sense when one recalls the course of the motor and sensory pathways. Most of the descending fibers of the corticospinal tract cross in the medulla and travel in the spinal cord on the same side of the body as the muscles that they innervate. The sensory fibers in the dorsal columns also travel in the cord on the same side as they innervate, crossing in the medulla. A lesion on one side of the spinal cord, then, disrupts motor functioning, proprioception, vibratory sense, and two-point discrimination on the side of the lesion.

Fibers carrying pain and temperature information cross soon after entry into the spinal cord, before ascending in the lateral spinothalamic tract. As a result they travel in the spinal cord on the side opposite the side of the body that they innervate. A lesion of one half of the cord results in contralateral loss of pain and temperature sensitivity.

True hemisection of the spinal cord is rare, but it is common in incomplete lesions for one side of the cord to sustain more damage than the other. The result is a Brown-Séquard–like clinical picture, with greater motor and proprioceptive deficit ipsilaterally and greater loss of pain and temperature contralaterally.

Anterior Cord Syndrome

Anterior cord syndrome (Fig. 2–24) results from trauma to the anterior cord itself or damage of the anterior spinal artery, or both (Yashon, 1986). This syndrome results most often from flexion teardrop fractures and burst fractures (Harris et al., 1986; Rogers, 1989).

Damage to the anterior and arterolateral aspects of the cord results in bilateral loss of motor function and pain/temperature sensation due to in-

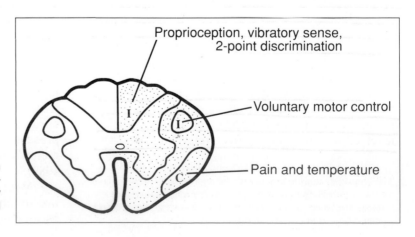

Figure 2–23. Area of spinal cord damage in Brown-Séquard syndrome. I: fiber tracts traveling ipsilateral to the side of the body that they innervate. C: fiber tracts traveling contralateral to the side of the body that they innervate.

Proprioception, vibratory sense, 2-point discrimination

Voluntary motor control

Pain and temperature

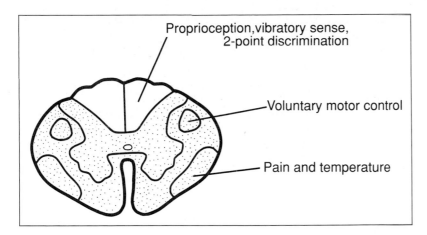

Proprioception, vibratory sense, 2-point discrimination

Voluntary motor control

Pain and temperature

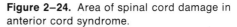

Figure 2–24. Area of spinal cord damage in anterior cord syndrome.

terruption of the anterior and lateral spinothalamic tracts and the corticospinal tract. The dorsal columns remain intact.

Central Cord Syndrome

Central cord syndrome (Fig. 2–25) results from damage to the central aspect of the spinal cord, with sparing of the peripheral portions of the cord. This syndrome is most common in older people, following extension injuries to the neck (Meyers, 1989; Rogers, 1989). However, it can occur at any age and can follow flexion injury. This syndrome often results from relatively minor trauma (especially in the elderly), with no evidence of vertebral trauma (Meyer, 1989).

Central cord syndrome results when the process of central hemorrhage and necrosis (secondary tissue destruction) described above does not progress to full destruction of the cord segment. Peripherally located fiber tracts are left intact. The seemingly unusual clinical picture that results is due to the spatial orientation of the fiber tracts in the

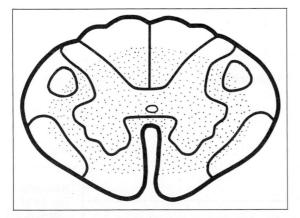

Figure 2–25. Area of spinal cord damage in central cord syndrome. The clinical picture resulting from central damage in the cord is due to the somatotopic organization of fibers within the tracts (see Fig. 2–5).

cord: fibers innervating cervical segments are located closer to the central gray matter. Fibers innervating thoracic, lumbar, and sacral segments are located progressively more peripherally in the cord.

The extent of neural damage in central cord syndrome varies. A "mild" case occurs when there is destruction of the central gray matter plus only the most centrally located nerve tracts. The result is paralysis and sensory loss in the upper extremities, with normal functioning in areas innervated by the thoracic, lumbar, and sacral cord. There is normal trunk and lower extremity function, bowel and bladder control, and genital functioning. A more severe case of central cord syndrome occurs when the process of central cord destruction progresses more peripherally, leaving only the most peripheral nerve fibers intact. A person with this extent of injury has total motor and sensory loss below the level of the lesion, with the exception of sacral sparing. Bowel, bladder, and sexual functioning remain intact.

PHYSICAL EFFECTS OF SPINAL CORD INJURIES

The location and extent of damage to neural tissue determines the symptoms produced by spinal cord injury. Complete spinal cord injury effectively disconnects the brain from the body below the lesion, disrupting control of all of the various systems innervated below the lesion (Fig. 2–26).

Primary Effects

Voluntary Motor Control. Paralysis of the voluntary musculature is the most obvious effect of a spinal cord injury. Damage of descending motor tracts, anterior horn cells, or spinal nerves leads to loss of control over the trunk and extremities. This loss affects an individual's ability to manipulate his environment and to move his body in space.

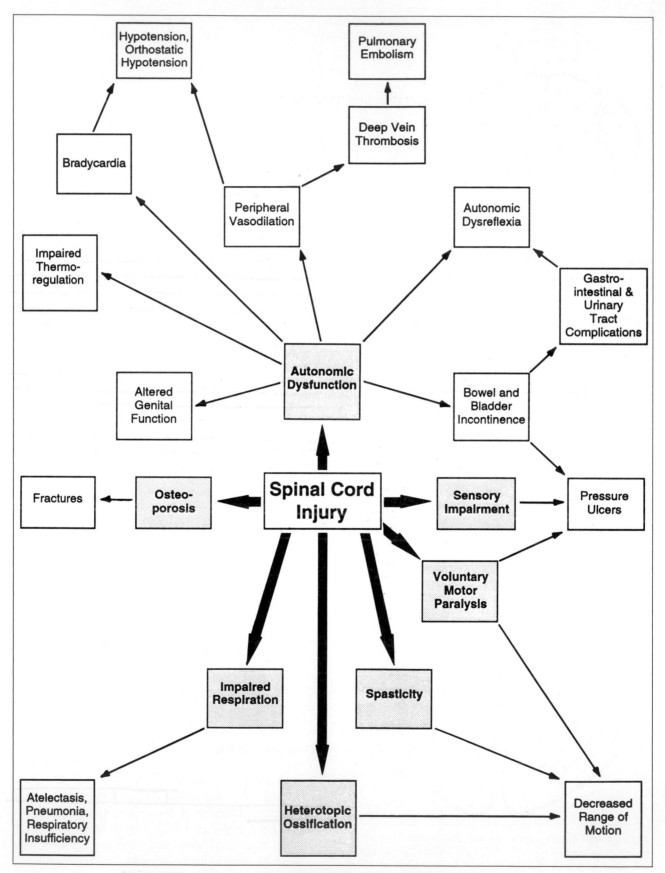

Figure 2–26. Schematic representation of the physical effects of spinal cord injury.

Damage that occurs at or peripheral to the anterior horn cell is a lower motor neuron lesion and results in flaccid paralysis of muscle innervated by that cord segment. Damage to descending tracts is an upper motor neuron lesion and results in spastic paralysis of muscle innervated by cord segments caudal to the lesion (deGroot & Chusid, 1988). Most spinal cord injuries are a combination of upper and lower motor neuron lesions, since both grey and white matter are disrupted at the level of the lesion (McLeod & Lance, 1989).

Fortunately most people with spinal cord injuries experience some recovery of motor function in the months and years after injury. The vast majority exhibit significant recovery in musculature innervated by cord segments one or more levels caudal to their neurological level of injury. The mechanism for this recovery is unknown. It is often attributed to nerve root recovery, but other factors may be involved (Ditunno, Sipski, Posuniak, Chen, Staas, & Herbison, 1987; Piepmeier & Jenkins, 1988; Young & Ransohoff, 1989).

Spasticity. During the period of spinal shock immediately following cord injury, muscles innervated below the lesion are areflexive. As time passes and spinal shock resolves, reflexes return. Reflexive functioning is weak at first but becomes stronger with time (Illis, 1988), commonly progressing to spasticity. Spasticity is more prevalent with higher lesions and with incomplete lesions (Little, Micklesen, Umlauf, & Britell, 1989; Robinson, Kett, & Bolam, 1988).

Spasticity following spinal cord injury is characterized by hypertonicity and hyperreflexia. Quick stretching of muscles elicits exaggerated reflexive responses. Cutaneous stimuli also evoke abnormal reflex responses (Illis, 1988; McQueen & Khan, 1989; Young & Shahani, 1986). Reflexive responses to cutaneous stimulation may appear to be spontaneous "spasms," since the stimuli by which they are elicited can be so subtle as to go unnoticed by the clinician (Young & Shahani, 1986).

The underlying neurological mechanism or mechanisms responsible for spasticity are as yet unknown. Possible causes include a loss of inhibition from higher centers, loss of descending facilitation of afferents from Golgi tendon organs, sprouting of new synaptic terminals within the spinal cord caudal to the lesion, and hypersensitivity of neurons caudal to the lesion in response to their reduced input (Illis, 1988; Yashon, 1986; Young & Shahani, 1986).

Sensation. Sensation is disrupted in most spinal cord injuries. A loss of sensation can lead to discoordination of body movements, vulnerability to trauma, and impaired body awareness. As is true with motor function, sensory ability usually improves as time passes after spinal cord injury (Young & Ransohoff, 1989).

Respiration. The diaphragm is the primary muscle of inspiration. Air enters the lungs when the diaphragm descends and lifts the rib cage, causing the thoracic cavity to expand (Morgan, Silver, & Williams, 1986). The diaphragm receives innervation from C3-5, with its greatest innervation from C4 (Meyer, 1989). Cord lesions above this level result in an inability to breathe without mechanical assistance.[7]

Although the diaphragm is the most critical respiratory muscle, it is not the only muscle involved in normal breathing. Both the external and internal intercostals (T1-12 innervation) aid in quiet inspiration by elevating the ribs and aid in expiration at high lung volumes (Morgan et al., 1986). The abdominals (T5-T12 innervation) are required for forced expiration such as occurs in coughing: the rectus abdominis, external and internal obliques, and transversus abdominis achieve forceful expiration by pulling the sternum caudally and pushing the abdominal contents and diaphragm rostrally into the thoracic cavity (Morgan et al., 1986).

Because the intercostals and abdominals assist in normal breathing, disruption of innervation to thoracic or to abdominal musculature or to both impairs respiration. Following spinal cord injury, tidal volume and vital capacity[8] are diminished due to the reduction of both inspiratory and expiratory ability (McCool, Pichurko, Slutsky, Sarkarati, Rossier, & Brown, 1986; Rinehart & Nawoczenski, 1987).

The secondary muscles of respiration include the trapezius (11th cranial nerve and C1-4 innervation), sternocleidomastoid (C1-3 innervation), scalenus (C3-5 innervation), and levator scapula (C3-5; Meyer, 1989; Morgan et al., 1986; Yashon, 1986). These accessory respiratory muscles work through elevation and expansion of the rib cage (Morgan et al., 1986; Rinehart & Nawoczenski, 1989; Wetzel, 1985). The accessory muscles of respiration are normally used during stressful inspiration, as occurs during strenuous aerobic exercise. They are also used to aid inspiration when normal

---

[7] With training, people can learn to breathe using their neck accessory musculature (neck breathing) or using mouth, throat, and pharynx musculature (glossopharyngeal breathing; Gilgoff, Barras, Jones, & Adkins, 1988).

[8] Tidal volume is the amount of air that is moved during quiet breathing. Vital capacity is the amount of air that can be expelled following full inspiration.

breathing is impaired and can be used to breathe in the absence of diaphragmatic innervation (Gilgoff et al., 1988).

The degree to which a spinal cord injury affects respiration depends upon the level of lesion. Cervical lesions result in the greatest impairment of respiration, with both inspiration and expiration affected. Among people with long-standing cervical lesions below C4, the average vital capacity is approximately 58% of normal. People with high thoracic lesions have the benefit of some intercostal function but lack the abdominal musculature required for effective coughing. Their average vital capacity is 73% of normal. Preservation of abdominal function in lumbar and low thoracic lesions results in improved expiratory ability proportional to the degree of abdominal function remaining (Morgan et al., 1986).

Following low cervical injury, breathing is most impaired initially. Vital capacity soon after injury averages approximately 30% of normal. Within a few weeks of injury, respiratory function begins to improve. Inspiratory ability continues to improve during the first year, with average vital capacity values almost doubling. Several factors may contribute to this improvement of respiratory status with the passage of time. Possible contributing factors include increasing strength in the accessory respiratory muscles, return of tone in the intercostals and abdominals with the passage of spinal shock, and stiffening of the joints of the rib cage (Morgan et al., 1986; Scanlon, Loring, Pichorko, McCool, Slutsky, Sarkarati, & Brown, 1989).

Bowel and Bladder Continence. Voluntary control of urination and defecation requires an intact sacral cord in communication with the brain. As a result, most spinal cord injuries lead to a loss of voluntary bowel and bladder control. Incontinence must be managed carefully to avoid a variety of physical and psychosocial problems.[9]

Genital Functioning. The genitals receive their innervation from the thoracolumbar and sacral regions of the spinal cord. Spinal cord injury alters the functioning of the genitals, disrupting sexual responses mediated by the brain and the spinal cord. Fertility is unchanged among women with cord injuries, but men are likely to be infertile.[10]

---

[9] Complete descriptions of bowel and bladder function, complications, and care following spinal cord injury are presented in Chapter 17.

[10] Sexuality, sexual functioning, and sexual rehabilitation strategies are addressed in Chapter 16.

Cardiovascular Function. The heart and peripheral vasculature are normally influenced by the autonomic nervous system. Sympathetic outflow, arising from spinal segments T1 to L2, causes an increase in heart rate, increased contractility of the cardiac musculature, and peripheral vasoconstriction. Parasympathetic outflow, transmitted through the vagus nerve from the brainstem, slows the heart rate and slightly reduces ventricular contractility (Bullock & Rosendahl, 1988).

When spinal cord injury blocks communication between the brainstem and the thoracolumbar cord, sympathetic input to the heart is lost and parasympathetic input remains. The result is bradycardia, or slowing of the heart. Loss of sympathetic outflow also causes dilation of the peripheral vasculature below the level of the lesion, resulting in hypotension (Cole, 1988; Lehmann, Lane, Piepmeier, & Batsford, 1987; McCagg, 1986; Meyer, 1989). Orthostatic hypotension also occurs following spinal cord injury: blood pressure drops when the individual moves to an upright position from horizontal. Symptoms of orthostatic hypotension include loss of vision, dizziness, ringing in the ears, and fainting (Cole, 1988; Yashon, 1986).

Bradycardia, hypotension, and orthostatic hypotension are usually significant only in people with lesions above T6 (Buchanan & Ditunno, 1987; Cole, 1988; Lehmann et al., 1987; Yashon, 1986). These cardiovascular effects are transient, resolving within a few weeks of injury (Cole, 1988; Lehmann et al., 1987; Yashon, 1986).

Thermoregulation. Normally when a person's core temperature falls, peripheral vasoconstriction and shivering serve to raise the temperature. When the core temperature rises above normal, peripheral vasodilation and sweating cause greater dissipation of heat with a fall in core temperature resulting (Bloch, 1986).

Thermoregulation involves both the autonomic and somatic nervous systems. The sympathetic nervous system (T1-L2 or L3) is involved in the regulation of body temperature through its influence on peripheral vascular tone and perspiration (Bullock & Rosendahl, 1988). The somatic system controls shivering.

Spinal cord injury that interrupts the cord's communication with the hypothalamus disrupts thermoregulation. Soon after injury, *hypo*thermia is likely to occur as a result of peripheral vasodilation, which allows loss of heat through the superficial vessels. When reflexive tone eventually returns in the peripheral vasculature, this problem resolves (Meyer, 1989). Although shivering remains absent below the level of lesion (Bloch, 1986), the tendency toward hypothermia is replaced by a tendency toward *hyper*thermia because sympathetic control of the apocrine (sweat) glands is lost. Below the level of lesion, sweating does not occur in response to a rise in body temperature (Meyer, 1989).

Complications

A variety of complications can result from spinal cord injury. With proper management, the incidence and severity of most of these complications can be minimized.

Decubiti. Decubitus ulcers, or pressure sores, are among the most common complications of spinal cord injury (Young, Burns, Bowen, & McCutchen, 1982). Decubiti are more prevalent among people with complete lesions and among people with quadriplegia (Berczeller & Bezkor, 1986; Lal, Hamilton, Heinemann, & Betts, 1989; Nawoczenski, 1987; Young et al., 1982). Pressure sores occur almost exclusively over bony prominences. The skin over the sacrum, heels, and ischium are the most common sites of skin breakdown (Kennedy et al., 1986).

A variety of factors are thought to make people with spinal cord injuries vulnerable to the formation of decubitus ulcers. Skin collagen degradation after spinal cord injury may make the skin more prone to decubiti (Rodriguez, Claus-Walker, Kent, & Garza, 1989). In addition, the circulatory sequelae of cord injury result in compromised peripheral blood flow, with resulting reduction in oxygen and nutrient supply to the tissues (Nawoczenski, 1987). Thus the skin and subcutaneous tissues are more vulnerable to normal trauma. This problem is compounded by the increased likelihood of trauma to the skin following spinal cord injury: combined paralysis and sensory impairment result in areas of the skin being subjected to pressure for prolonged periods.

Wherever external pressure on soft tissues is greater than capillary pressure,[11] ischemia results. This condition exists in tissues compressed between boney prominences and the supporting surface. (For example, over the ischial tuberosities when sitting.) The resulting ischemia does not present a problem for people with intact motor and sensory function because these people shift their positions frequently

during normal activities. These position changes redistribute pressure long before tissue damage occurs.

In contrast, people with spinal cord injuries lack the sensation that stimulates protective weight shifts. The tissue compressed between boney prominences and supporting surfaces or other objects (such as orthoses) is likely to be subjected to pressure for long periods of time. The resulting prolonged ischemia can lead to tissue necrosis and decubiti.

Prolonged pressure is not the only factor contributing to the development of decubiti (Fig. 2–27). High pressure applied for a short duration can also damage the skin and subcutaneous tissues, as can shear forces. Elevation in temperature, locally or systemically, can make the skin and subcutaneous tissue more prone to ischemia because temperature elevation increases the tissues' oxygen requirements. Prolonged exposure to moisture, as can occur with incontinence or excessive sweating, softens the skin and increases its vulnerability to trauma (Nawoczenski, 1987; Patterson & Fisher, 1986). Both low blood pressure and smoking can reduce peripheral circulation and increase the likelihood of breakdown (Yob, Wagner, Casson, & Leclerc, 1990).

Decubitus ulcers are of major concern because they can lead to osteomyelitis, sepsis, and even death (DeVivo, Kartus, Stover, Rutt, & Fine, 1989). (Hence the term "sitting suicide"). Additionally, a decubitus that heals leaves a scarred area that remains highly vulnerable to the development of decubiti in the future. Pressure sores are costly in terms of the expense of hospitalization and surgery, time lost from vocational and avocational activities, and postponement of physical rehabilitation and reintegration into the community (Buchanan & Ditunno, 1987; Kennedy et al., 1986). The prevalence of decubiti among people with spinal cord injuries is most tragic when one considers that this complication is preventable. With attention to positioning, equipment, nutrition, and skin care, pressure sores can be avoided.

Respiratory Complications. Respiratory complications are the most common cause of death following spinal cord injury (DeVivo, Kartus, Stover, Rutt, & Fine, 1989; Kennedy, Stover, & Fine, 1986). These complications occur as a result of a reduction in inspiratory and expiratory ability. Inadequate inspiration results in reduced ventilation of the lungs, leading to atelectasis. Ineffective coughing allows secretions to build in the lungs, with atelectasis, pneumonia, and respiratory insufficiency resulting

---

[11] It is generally accepted that prolonged uninterrupted pressure greater than 32 mm Hg produces ischemia, causing decubiti. However, research has demonstrated that tissue blood flow can occur despite significantly higher pressures (Patterson & Fisher, 1986).

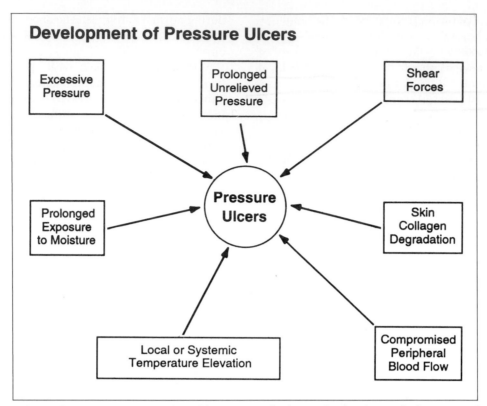

Figure 2–27. Schematic representation of factors contributing to the development of pressure ulcers.

(Buchanan & Ditunno, 1987; McCagg, 1986; Yashon, 1986).

Decreased Range of Motion. Any condition that causes joint immobilization can result in reduction of joint range of motion and muscle flexibility. A person with motor paralysis is vulnerable to contractures due to the simple fact that his or her muscles do not actively move the joints. Deformity is especially likely to develop when muscle strength imbalance, spasticity, gravity, or a habitual posture causes one or more joints to remain in a particular position for extended periods without intermittent motion out of the position.

Reduced range of motion can seriously impair a person's functional capacity and can create cosmetic problems. Moreover, deformity can increase vulnerability to decubitus ulcers by altering pressure distribution in sitting and by limiting the number of postures available for pressure relief when lying in bed.

This complication is completely preventable. Periodic motion of joints through their available range will preserve joint range of motion and muscle flexibility.

Osteoporosis. Following spinal cord injury, both calcium (Cole, 1988) and collagen (Rodriguez et al., 1989) are lost from the bones. The resulting osteo-porosis increases the likelihood of fractures. Osteo-porosis progresses gradually for five years after injury, at which time it reaches a plateau (Cole, 1988).

Deep Vein Thrombosis. Deep vein thrombosis occurs frequently following spinal cord injury, particularly in the acute phase after injury. Various studies have reached conflicting conclusions about the frequency of this complication, with deep vein thrombosis found in 15% to 100% of subjects tested (McCagg, 1986).

Several factors combine to promote the development of blood clots in the deep veins after spinal cord injury. Peripheral vasodilation, absent or reduced lower extremity muscular function, and immobility lead to venous stasis. Hypercoagulability, trauma, and sepsis may also play a role (Buchanan & Ditunno, 1987; McCagg, 1986; Morgan et al., 1986; Turpie, 1986; Yashon, 1986).

Thrombi in the deep veins are potentially life threatening. An estimated 2% to 16% of people with spinal cord injuries die of pulmonary emboli within the first three months of injury (Turpie, 1986). After that point, pulmonary embolization rarely occurs (Yashon, 1986).

Gastrointestinal Complications. From 5% to 22% of cord-injured people develop stress ulcers in the stomach or duodenum during the acute phase following injury (Berczeller & Bezkor, 1986; Seaton & Hollingworth, 1986). The cause of this complication is unknown. Possible contributing factors include shock, emotional stress, circulating catecholamines, steroid therapy, mechanical ventilation, and unopposed parasympathetic input to the stomach causing increased gastrin production (Berczeller & Bezkor, 1986; Buchanan & Ditunno, 1987; Cole, 1988; Seaton & Hollingworth, 1986).

Gastrointestinal (GI) bleeds are most likely to occur during the first month after injury (Yashon, 1986). This complication can be prevented with proper medical management (Buchanan & Ditunno, 1987).

Additional GI complications of spinal cord injury include paralytic ileus, gastric dilation, fecal impaction, and bowel obstruction (Cole, 1988; Seaton & Hollingworth, 1986; Yashon, 1986).

Urinary Tract Complications. Urinary tract complications were the leading cause of death after spinal cord injury until relatively recently. Advances in urological management practices have significantly reduced the mortality rate in recent years (DeVivo, Kartus, Stover, Rutt, & Fine, 1989; Kennedy et al., 1986).

Abnormal bladder function following spinal cord injury, combined with improper management, can lead to urinary retention, bladder infection, and reflux of urine into the ureters. Kidney and bladder stones, hydronephrosis, pyelonephritis, kidney failure, septicemia, and death can result (Achong, 1986; Buchanan & Ditunno, 1987; Hall, Hackler, Zampieri & Zampieri, 1989).

Autonomic Dysreflexia. People with spinal cord lesions above the T6 level can experience autonomic dysreflexia. This phenomenon, also called autonomic hyperreflexia, or crisis, is characterized by a sudden increase in blood pressure, bradycardia, a pounding headache, flushing, and profuse sweating, often accompanied by anxiety (Fig. 2–28). Autonomic dysreflexia is brought on by a noxious stimulus below the lesion that causes an increase in autonomic activity. Common origins of this noxious stimulus include bladder or rectal distension, bladder infection, and bowel impaction. A variety of other stimuli have been reported to trigger autonomic dysreflexia, including range of motion exercises, cutaneous stimulation, muscle spasm, decubiti, ingrown toenails, electroejaculation, labor, surgical and diagnostic procedures, and abdominal conditions such as appendicitis (Bloch, 1986; Cole, 1988; McCagg, 1986; McGuire & Kumar, 1986). The elevation in blood pressure that occurs with autonomic dysreflexia can lead to loss of consciousness, seizures, hypertensive encephalopathy, retinal hemorrhage, apnea, aphasia, cerebrovascular accidents, and renal failure (Bloch, 1986; McGuire & Kumar, 1986).

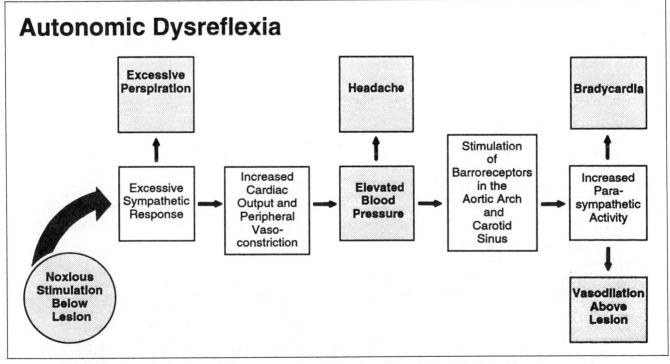

Autonomic Dysreflexia

Figure 2–28. Schematic representation of autonomic dysreflexia. Clinical signs and symptoms are in darkened boxes.

Autonomic dysreflexia occurs when a noxious stimulus below the lesion triggers an excessive sympathetic response. Possible causes of this exaggerated sympathetic response include loss of descending inhibition, sprouting of new synaptic terminals within the spinal cord caudal to the lesion, and hypersensitivity of the sympathetic neurons (Bloch, 1986). Hypertension results when increased sympathetic outflow causes an increase in cardiac output and peripheral vasoconstriction. The hypertension stimulates baroreceptors in the aortic arch and carotid sinus, triggering increased parasympathetic activity that slows the heart.[12] Vasodilation above the lesion also occurs as a compensatory mechanism in response to the elevated blood pressure (Bloch, 1986; Cole, 1988; Stjernberg, Blumberg, & Wallin, 1986).

Autonomic dysreflexia occurs after spinal shock has resolved, usually first appearing about six months after the injury. This complication is more prevalent among people with quadriplegia than among those with paraplegia (Bloch, 1986; Cole, 1988; McCagg, 1986).

Heterotopic Ossification. Heterotopic ossification, also called ectopic bone formation, is the formation of new bone within muscles or other connective tissue below the lesion. It occurs following 16% to 53% of all spinal cord injuries, usually appearing from 1 to 4 months after injury. Heterotopic ossification can restrict joint motion, which in turn can lead to impaired functional status and decubiti (Lal, Hamilton, Heinemann, & Betts, 1989; Yashon, 1986).

The cause of heterotopic ossification following spinal cord injury is unknown. Advanced age, complete lesions, and spasticity are risk factors (Lal et al., 1989).

SUMMARY

Most spinal cord injuries occur when direct or indirect forces applied to the vertebral column cause violent motion, resulting in failure of the vertebral or boney elements or both. With disruption of the vertebral column, the spinal cord is traumatized. Depending on the site and extent of the cord lesion, the injury may result in paralysis, spasticity, and sensory loss, as well as impaired control of the respiratory, GI, genitourinary, and thermoregulatory systems. A variety of complications can result.

---

[12] In some cases tachycardia (increased heart rate) occurs instead of bradycardia. The different clinical pictures occur because both parasympathetic and sympathetic stimulation to the heart is increased in autonomic dysreflexia (Bloch, 1986).

REFERENCES

Achong, M. (1986). Urinary tract infections in the patient with a neurogenic bladder. In R. Bloch & M. Basbaum (Eds.), *Management of spinal cord injuries* (pp. 164–179). Baltimore: Williams & Wilkins.

Allen, B. (1989). Recognition of injuries to the lower cervical spine. In H. Sherk, E. Dunn, F. Eismont (Eds.), *The cervical spine* (pp. 286–298). Philadelphia: J.B. Lippincott.

American Spinal Injury Association. (1989). *Standards for neurological classification of spinal injury patients.* (Available from the American Spinal Injury Association, 2020 Peachtree Road NW, Atlanta, GA 30309.)

Balentine, J. (1988). Spinal cord trauma: In search of the meaning of granular axoplasm and vesicular myelin. *Journal of Neuropathology and Experimental Neurology, 47*(2), 77–92.

Bedbrook, G. (1981). *The care and management of spinal cord injuries.* New York: Springer-Verlag.

Berczeller, P., & Bezkor, M. (1986). *Medical complications of quadriplegia.* Chicago: Year Book Medical Publishers.

Beric, A., Dimitrijevic, M., & Light, J. (1987). A clinical syndrome of rostral and caudal spinal injury: Neurological, neurophysiological and urodynamic evidence for occult sacral lesion. *Journal of Neurology, Neurosurgery, and Psychiatry, 50*, 600–606.

Bloch, R. (1986). Autonomic dysfunction. In R. Bloch & M. Basbaum (Eds.), *Management of spinal cord injuries* (pp. 149–163). Baltimore: Williams & Wilkins.

Bohlman, H., & Boada, E. (1989). Fractures and dislocations of the lower cervical spina. In Sherk, H., Dunn, F., & Eismont, J. (Eds.), *The cervical spine* (2nd ed.). Philadelphia: J.B. Lippincott.

Buchanan, L. (1987). An overview. In L. Buchanan & D. Nawoczenski (Eds.), *Spinal cord injury: Concepts and management approaches* (pp. 1–19). Baltimore: Williams & Wilkins.

Buchanan, L. (1987a). Emergency care. In L. Buchanan & D. Nawoczenski (Eds.), *Spinal cord injury: Concepts and management approaches* (pp. 21–34). Baltimore: Williams & Wilkins.

Buchanan, L., & Ditunno, J. (1987). Acute care: Medical/surgical management. In L. Buchanan & D. Nawoczenski (Eds.), *Spinal cord injury: Concepts and management approaches* (pp. 35–60). Baltimore: Williams & Wilkins.

Bullock, B., & Rosendahl, P. (1988). *Pathophysiology: Adaptations and alterations in function* (2nd ed.). Boston: Scott, Foresman & Company.

Choi, D., & Rothman, S. (1990). The role of glutamate neurotoxicity in hypoxic-ischemic neuronal death. *Annual Review of Neurosciences, 13*, 171–182.

Cole, J. (1988). The pathophysiology of the autonomic nervous system in spinal cord injury. In L. Illis (Ed.), *Spinal cord dysfunction: Assessment* (pp. 201–235). New York: Oxford University Press.

Coogler, C. (1985). Clinical decision making among neurologic patients: Spinal cord injury. In S. Wolf (Ed.),

Clinical decision making in physical therapy (pp. 149–170). Philadelphia: F.A. Davis.

Cook, P. (1988). Radiology of the spine and spinal cord injury. In L. Illis (Ed.), *Spinal cord dysfunction: Assessment* (pp. 41–103). New York: Oxford University Press.

• Cotman, C., & Nieto-Sampedro, M. (1985). Progress in facilitating the recovery of function after central nervous system trauma. *Annals of the New York Academy of Sciences, 457,* 83–104.

Crawford, P., & Shepherd, D. (1989). Hyperextension injuries to the cervical cord in the elderly. *British Medical Journal, 299*(6700), 669–670.

Crowell, R., Edwards, T., & White, A. (1989). Mechanisms of injury in the cervical spine: Experimental evidence and biomechanical modeling. In Sherk, H., Dunn, E., Eismont, F. (Eds.), *The cervical spine* (pp. 70–90). Philadelphia: J.B. Lippincott.

Davidoff, G., Roth, E., Guarrixini, M., Sliwa, J., & Yarkony, G. (1987). Function-limiting dysesthetic pain syndrome among traumatic spinal cord injury patients: A cross-sectional study. *Pain, 29*(1), 39–48.

deGroot, J., & Chusid, J. (1988). *Correlative neuroanatomy* (20th ed.). East Norwalk, CT: Appleton & Lange.

Demediuk, P., Daly, M., & Faden, A. (1989). Effect of impact trauma on neurotransmitter and nonneurotransmitter amino acids in rat spinal cord. *Journal of Neurochemestry, 52*(5), 1529–1536.

Denis, F. (1983). The three column spine and its significance in the classification of acute thoracolumbar spinal injuries. *Spine, 8*(8), 817–831.

DeVivo, M., Fine, P., Maetz, H., & Stover, S. (1980). Prevalence of spinal cord injury: A reestimation employing life table techniques. *Archives of Neurology, 37,* 707–708.

DeVivo, M., Kartus, P., Stover, S., Rutt, R., & Fine, P. (1989). Cause of death for patients with spinal cord injuries. *Archives of Internal Medicine, 149*(8), 1761–1766.

Ditunno, J., Sipski, M., Posuniak, E., Chen, Y., Staas, W., & Herbison, G. (1987). Wrist extensor recovery in traumatic quadriplegia. *Archives of Physical Medicine and Rehabilitation, 68*(5), 287–290.

Estenne, M., & De Troyer, A. (1987). Mechanism of the postural dependence of vital capacity in tetraplegic subjects. *American Review of Respiratory Disease, 135*(2), 367–371.

Faden, A., & Simon, R. (1987). A potential role for excitotoxins in the pathophysiology of spinal cord injury. *Annals of Neurology, 23*(6), 623–626.

Fine, P., Kuhlemeier, K., DeVivo, M., & Stover, S. (1979). Spinal cord injury: An epidemiological perspective. *Paraplegia, 17,* 237–250.

Galli, R., Spaite, D., & Simon, R. (1989). *Emergency orthopedics: The spine.* Norwalk, CT: Appleton & Lange.

Gilgoff, I., Barras, D., Jones, M., & Adkins, H. (1988). Neck breathing: A form of voluntary respiration for the spine-injured ventilator-dependent quadriplegic child. *Pediatrics, 82*(5), 741–745.

Grundy, D., Swain, A., & Russell, J. (1986). ABC of Spinal Cord Injury: Early Management and Complications—II. *British Medical Journal, 292*(6513), 123–125.

Hall, M., Hackler, R., Zampieri, T., & Zampieri, J. (1989). Renal calculi in spinal cord-injured patient: Association with reflux, bladder stones, and Foley catheter drainage. *Urology, 34*(4), 126–128.

Harris, J., Edeiken-Monroe, B., Kopaniky, D. (1986). A practical classification of acute cervical spine injuries. *Orthopedic Clinics of North America, 17*(1), 15–30.

Hughes, J. (1988). Pathological changes after spinal cord injury. In L. Illis (Ed.), *Spinal cord dysfunction: Assessment* (pp. 34–40). New York: Oxford University Press.

Iizuka, H., Yamamoto, H., Iwasaki, Y., Yamamoto, T., & Konno, H. (1987). Evolution of tissue damage in compressive spinal cord injury in rats. *Journal of Neurosurgery, 66*(4), 595–603.

Illis, L. (1988). Clinical evaluation and pathophysiology of the spinal cord in the chronic stage. In L. Illis (Ed.), *Spinal cord dysfunction: Assessment* (pp. 107–128). New York: Oxford University Press.

Kennedy, E., Stover, S., & Fine, P. (Eds.). (1986). *Spinal cord injury: The facts and figures.* Birmingham, AL: The University of Alabama Spinal Cord Injury Statistical Center.

Lal, S., Hamilton, B., Heinemann, A., & Betts, H. (1989). Risk factors for heterotopic ossification in spinal cord injury. *Archives of Physical Medicine and Rehabilitation, 70*(5), 387–390.

Lehmann, K., Lane, J., Piepmeier, J., & Batsford, W. (91987). Cardiovascular abnormalities accompanying acute spinal cord injury in humans: Incidence, time course and severity. *JACC, 10*(1), 46–52.

Little, J., Micklesen, P., Umlauf, R., & Britell, C. (1989). Lower extremity manifestations of spasticity in chronic spinal cord injury. *American Journal of Physical Medicine and Rehabilitation, 68*(1), 32–36.

Mackenzie, C., & Ducker, T. (1986). Cervical spinal cord injury. In J. Matjasko & J. Katz (Eds.), *Clinical controversies in neuroanesthesia and neurosurgery* (pp. 77–134). New York: Grune & Stratton.

Martin, J. (1989). *Neuroanatomy: Text and Atlas.* New York: Elsevier.

McCagg, C. (1986). Postoperative management and acute rehabilitation of patients with spinal cord injuries. *Orthopedic Clinics of North America, 17*(1), 171–182.

McCool, F., Pichurko, B., Slutsky, A., Sarkarati, M., Rossier, A., & Brown, R. (1986). Changes in lung volume and rib cage configuration with abdominal binding in quadriplegia. *Journal of Applied Physiology, 60*(4), 1198–1202.

McGuire, T., & Kumar, N. (1986). Autonomic dysreflexia in the spinal cord-injured: What the physician should know about this medical emergency. *Postgraduate Medicine, 80*(2), 81–89.

McLeod, J., & Lance, J. (1989). *Introductory neurology* (3rd ed.). Boston: Blackwell Scientific Publications.

McQueen, J., & Khan, M. (1989). Evaluation of patients

with cervical spine lesions. In Sherk, H., Dunn, E., & Eismont, F. (Eds.), *The cervical spine* (pp. 199–211). Philadelphia: J.B. Lippincott.

Meyer, P. (Ed.). (1989). *Surgery of Spine Trauma*. New York: Churchill Livingstone.

Meyer, P., & Heim, S. (1989). Surgical Stabilization of the Cervical Spine. In P. Meyer (Ed.), *Surgery of spine trauma* (pp. 397–523). New York: Churchill Livingstone.

Morgan, M., Silver, J., & Williams, S. (1986). The Respiratory System of the Spinal Cord Patient. In R. Bloch & M. Basbaum (Eds.), *Management of spinal cord injuries* (pp. 78–116). Baltimore: Williams & Wilkins.

National Spinal Cord Injury Association. (1988). *Fact sheet #2: spinal cord injury statistical information.* (Available from the National Spinal Cord Injury Association, 600 West Cummings Park, Suite 2000, Woburn, MA.)

Nawoczenski, D. (1987). Pressure sores: Prevention and management. In L. Buchanan & D. Nawoczenski (Eds.), *Spinal cord injury: Concepts and management approaches* (pp. 99–121). Baltimore: Williams & Wilkins.

Netter, F. (1989). *Atlas of Human Anatomy*. Summit, NJ: Ciba-Geigy Corporation.

Northrup, B., & Alderman, J. (1989). Nonsurgical treatment. In Sherk, H., Dunn, E., & Eismont, F. (Eds.), *The cervical spine* (2nd ed.). Philadelphia: J.B. Lippincott.

Pang, D., & Pollack, I. (1989). Spinal cord injury without radiologic abnormality in children—the SCIWORA syndrome. *Journal of Trauma, 29*(5), 654–664.

Patterson, R., & Fisher, S. (1986). Sitting pressure-time patterns in patients with quadriplegia. *Archives of Physical Medicine and Rehabilitation, 67*(11), 812–814.

Peterson, D., & Altman, K. (1989). Central cervical spinal cord syndrome due to minor hyperextension injury. *Western Journal of Medicine, 150*(6), 691–694.

Piepmeier, J., & Jenkins, R. (1988). Late neurological changes following traumatic spinal cord injury. *Journal of Neurosurgery, 69,* 399–402.

Rieser, T., Mudiyam, R., & Waters, R. (1985). Orthopedic evaluation of spinal cord injury and management of vertebral fractures. In H. Adkins (Ed.), *Spinal cord injury* (pp. 1–35). New York: Churchill Livingstone.

Rinehart, M., & Nawoczenski, D. (1987). Respiratory care. In L. Buchanan & D. Nawoczenski (Eds.), *Spinal cord injury: Concepts and management approaches* (pp. 61–79). Baltimore: Williams & Wilkins.

Robinson, C., Kett, N., & Bolam, J. (1988). Spasticity in spinal cord injured patients: 2. Initial measures and long-term effects of surface electrical stimulation. *Archives of Physical Medicine and Rehabilitation, 69*(10), 862–868.

Rodriguez, G., Claus-Walker, J., Kent, M., & Garza, H. (1989). Collagen metabolite excretion as a predictor of bone- and skin-related complications in spinal cord injury. *Archives of Physical Medicine and Rehabilitation, 70*(6), 442–444.

Rogers, L. (1989). Radiologic assessment of acute neurologic and vertebral injuries. In P. Meyer (Ed.), *Surgery of Spine Trauma* (pp. 185–263). New York: Churchill Livingstone.

Scanlon, P., Loring, S., Pichurko, B., McCool, F., Slutsky, A., Sarkarati, M., & Brown, R. (1989). Respiratory mechanics in acute quadriplegia: Lung and chest wall compliance and dimensional changes during respiratory maneuvers. *American Review of Respiratory Disease, 139*(3), 615–620.

Seaton, T., & Hollingworth, R. (1986). Gastrointestinal complications in spinal cord injuries. In R. Bloch & M. Basbaum (Eds.), *Management of spinal cord injuries* (pp. 134–148). Baltimore: Williams & Wilkins.

Stauffer, E. (1989). Rehabilitation of posttraumatic cervical spinal cord quadriplegia and pentaplegia. In Sherk, H., Dunn, F., & Eismont, F. (Eds.), *The cervical spine* (2nd ed.). Philadelphia: J.B. Lippincott.

Stjernberg, L., Blumberg, H., & Wallin, G. (1986). Sympathetic Activity in Man After Spinal Cord Injury. *Brain, 109,* 695–715.

Thelan, L., Davie, J., & Urden, L. (1990). *Textbook of critical care nursing: Diagnosis and management.* Baltimore: C.V. Mosby.

Turpie, A. (1986). Thrombosis prevention and treatment in spinal cord injured patients. In R. Bloch & M. Basbaum (Eds.), *Management of spinal cord injuries* (pp. 212–240). Baltimore: Williams & Wilkins.

Waxman, S. (1989). Demyelination in spinal cord injury. *Journal of Neurological Sciences, 91*(1–2), 1–14.

Wetzel, J. (1985). Respiratory evaluation and treatment. In H. Adkins (Ed.), *Spinal cord injury* (pp. 75–98). New York: Churchill Livingstone.

Yashon, D. (1986). *Spinal injury* (2nd ed.). Norwalk, CT: Appleton, Century, Crofts.

Yob, S., Wagner, D., Casson, H., & Leclerc, J. (1990). Skin management of the SCI patient. In *Dawn of a new decade: spinal cord injury in the 1990's.* Symposium sponsored by National Rehabilitation Hospital, Washington, DC.

Young, J., Burns, P., Bowen, A., & McCutchen, R. (1982). *Spinal cord injury statistics: Experience of the regional spinal cord injury systems.* Phoenix, AZ: Good Samaritan Medical Center.

Young, R., & Shahani, B. (1986). Spasticity in spinal cord injured patients. In R. Bloch & M. Basbaum (Eds.), *Management of spinal cord injuries* (pp. 241–283). Baltimore: Williams & Wilkins.

Young, W., & Ransohoff, J. (1989). Acute spinal cord injuries: Experimental therapy, pathophysiological mechanisms, and recovery of function. In Sherk, H., Dunn, E., & Eismont, F. (Eds.), *The cervical spine* (2nd ed., pp. 464–495). Philadelphia: J.B. Lippincott.

3

Medical and Surgical Management

Following injury to the vertebral column or spinal cord, specialized management is imperative. The effects of spinal trauma can be lessened or worsened by the first aid and subsequent medical and surgical management provided. At the accident site, care must be taken to avoid causing additional neurological damage. At the hospital, operative or nonoperative measures or both are taken to stabilize the spine to preserve neurological functioning. From the time of spinal cord injury on, proper medical management is required to prevent a host of secondary complications.

EMERGENCY MANAGEMENT

Prehospital Care
The first aid treatment that a person receives following spinal cord injury is crucial to his health and neurological integrity. Stabilization of the injured spine is of particular importance: if the vertebral column is allowed to move, the cord can sustain additional damage. Improper handling causes up to 25% of all neurological damage that occurs following trauma to the spinal column (Karbi, Caspari, & Tator, 1988; Soderstrom & Brumback, 1986). Probably most rehabilitation personnel have had cord-injured patients tell them of being pulled out of cars or dragged up beaches by friends immediately after their accidents. Some neurological damage is even caused by Emergency Medical Service (EMS) personnel, but that problem is decreasing as training and techniques improve (Castillo & Bell, 1988; Soderstrom & Brumback, 1986).

Unless an individual has received specialized training in the emergency handling of people with spinal cord injuries, he should not attempt to move someone who might have sustained a cord injury.[1] The only exception to this rule is when trained personnel are not available and failure to move the injured person would lead to death, as when he is in a burning car or is lying with his face under water.

In an emergency situation, a person should be treated as though he has a spinal cord injury if there is *any* reason to believe that there is a *possibility* of an injury of the spinal cord or spinal column. Signs of possible vertebral or spinal cord injury include neck or back pain; motor or sensory deficits, however minor; paresthesias, especially in dermatomal patterns; and head injury or unconsciousness. Proper handling of people displaying any of these characteristics will prevent much unnecessary neurological damage.

Proper emergency management involves measures to enhance both survival and neurological integrity. The emergency medical personnel must first ensure that ventilation and circulation are adequate, avoiding unnecessary motion of the spine while doing so (Barker & Higgins, 1989; Barker & Higgins, 1989a; Maher, 1985). Intubation or ventilation with an air-mask bag unit may be necessary if cord damage above C5 or associated injuries significantly impair breathing (Castillo & Bell, 1988; Nikas, 1986).

The spine must be immobilized before the injured person is moved and must remain immobilized during transport and emergency treatment until spinal column injury has been ruled out. Possible spinal injury necessitates stabilization from the head to below the buttocks (Marshall, Marshall, Vos, & Chesnut, 1990). A variety of devices are available

---

[1] Health professionals are no exception (Soderstrom & Brumback, 1986).

for vertebral immobilization (Barker & Higgins, 1989; Castillo & Bell, 1988; Graziano, Scheidel, Cline, & Baer, 1987; Karbi et al., 1988; Lehman, 1987; Nikas, 1986; Soderstrom & Brumback, 1986).

Once the patient's spinal column has been stabilized and adequate ventilation and circulation have been assured, the injured person can be taken by ambulance or helicopter to a trauma center. Ideally he is taken to a center that specializes in spinal cord injury care (Soderstrom & Brumback, 1986).

Hospital Care

When someone with a known or suspected spinal injury arrives at the hospital, the trauma team works to discover and treat any life-threatening conditions and to preserve neurological function. All noncritical associated injuries[2] are given lower priority (Soderstrom & Brumback, 1986). During all procedures, care is taken to avoid motion in the spine.

The establishment of adequate ventilation, oxygenation, and circulation are of highest priority. Respiratory status is evaluated and arterial blood gasses are monitored. Intubation and ventilation are performed if indicated (Nikas, 1986; Soderstrom & Brumback, 1986). The trauma team controls hemorrhaging from associated injuries and monitors for cardiac arrhythmias or severe hypotension (Romeo, 1988; Soderstrom & Brumback, 1986).

Once the priority survival needs have been addressed, a neurological examination can be performed. The neurological evaluation should include assessment of level of consciousness and brainstem function (pupillary reactions), since the patient may have sustained a head injury during the accident. Sensation, voluntary motor function, and reflexes should also be evaluated thoroughly (Buchanan & Ditunno, 1987; Marshall, Marshall, Vos, & Chesnut, 1990; Soderstrom & Brumback, 1986; Swain, Grundy, & Russell, 1985a). This baseline data will influence decisions regarding fracture management and will make it possible to detect any future improvement or deterioration in neurological status.

Radiologic investigation is performed to detect spinal column damage, to determine whether these injuries are stable, and to determine the extent to which the spinal canal is compromised (Cook, 1988). Standard x-rays are typically performed initially, while the spine is still immobilized (Castillo & Bell, 1988; Karbi, Caspari, & Tator, 1988; Leh-

man, 1987; Nikas, 1986). Radiologic examination of the entire spine will make it possible to detect multiple spinal injuries (Meyer, 1989). Computerized tomography (CT) scan and magnetic resonance imaging (MRI) can be performed when additional information is required (Johnston, 1989; Karbi et al., 1988). These techniques, particularly MRI, provide superior visualization of morphological changes in ligamentous, hematological, intervertebral disc, and spinal cord tissue following trauma to the vertebral column (Castillo & Bell, 1988; Kulkarni, McArdle, Kopanicky, Miner, Cotter, Lee, & Harris, 1987; Mirvis, Geisler, Jelinek, Joslyn, & Gellad, 1988).

Additional emergency procedures include obtaining a complete medical history, evaluation and initial management of gastrointestinal and urinary systems,[3] and a complete evaluation for associated injuries (Buchanan & Ditunno, 1987; Swain, Grundy, & Russell, 1985a).

Probably the greatest recent breakthrough in the medical management of people with spinal cord injuries has been the demonstration that methylprednisolone can enhance neurological recovery following spinal cord injury. Treatment with high doses of methylprednisolone, initiated within eight hours of injury, apparently minimizes the secondary tissue destruction that occurs within the cord following trauma. Recovery of both motor and sensory function is enhanced whether the lesion is clinically complete or incomplete (Bracken et al., 1990).

FRACTURE MANAGEMENT

The primary goal of spinal fracture management is the minimization of the neurological damage caused by vertebral injury. This process begins at the site of the accident, with careful handling and stabilization of the spine when injury is suspected. At the scene, during transport, and in the emergency room, extreme care is taken to avoid moving the spine while evaluations and treatments are being administered. The spine is evaluated by x-ray as soon as is feasible in the hospital, and any vertebral column injuries found are reduced and stabilized. This early detection, reduction, and stabilization of vertebral injuries serve to optimize the ultimate neurological outcome of the injured person.

In addition to the initial preservation of neurological function, fracture management inter-

---

[2] An estimated 28% to 67% of people who sustain spinal cord injuries have additional injuries at the time of the initial trauma (Nikas, 1986).

[3] Gastrointestinal and urinary management are addressed in Chapter 17.

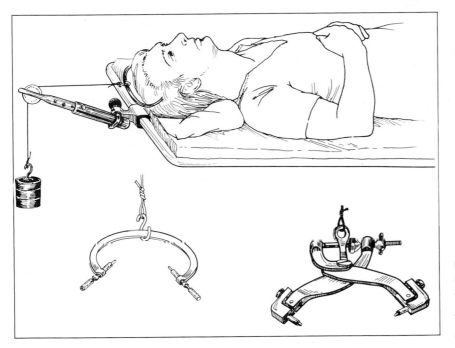

Figure 3–1. Cervical skeletal traction using tongs. *Reproduced with permission from Galli, R., Spaite, D., & Simon, R. (1989). Emergency Orthopedics: The Spine [p.115]. Norwalk, CT: Appleton & Lange.*

ventions are aimed at minimizing deformity and stabilizing the injured spine to prevent the late development of spinal deformity. Fracture management regimens include the use of traction, positioning, surgery, or orthoses, or any combination thereof for restoration of vertebral alignment, stabilization of the injured spine, and elimination of impingement upon neural tissue.

Nonsurgical Management

When radiologic investigation reveals vertebral displacement in the cervical region, the spine is realigned as soon as possible using skeletal traction. Since this alignment decompresses the spinal cord (Meyer, 1989), it may increase the patient's chances of neurological recovery (Brunette & Rockswold, 1987; Meyer, 1989).

In the cervical region, skeletal traction is achieved with a halo device or tongs that are affixed to the skull (Fig. 3–1). The halo or tongs are attached through a pulley system to weights that apply traction to the cervical vertebrae. Reduction is confirmed by x-ray. Failure to achieve optimal alignment through traction may make surgery necessary (Brunette & Rockswold, 1987; Castillo & Bell, 1988; Hansebout, 1986; Meyer, 1989). In some instances, a cervical spine that will not reduce with traction can be realigned through nonsurgical manipulation (Meyer & Heim, 1989).

In the treatment of thoracic and lumbar injuries, initial conservative (nonoperative) management generally involves careful positioning in a bed

(either standard or rotating bed, described below) or Stryker frame[4] (Fig. 3–2). Pillows placed under the patient can position the spine in slight extension or flexion. The nature of the spinal column injury determines the optimal position. With some high thoracic injuries, reduction can be achieved through skeletal traction applied through the skull (Meyer, 1989).

In some cases nonsurgical reduction and stabilization of the spine is the definitive management approach. Conservative management is particularly appropriate in instances of either stable or multiple-level vertebral injuries. Surgical stabilization of multiple-level injuries results in severe restriction of spinal motion, potentially interfering with functional status (Meyer, 1989).

When nonsurgical management techniques are used as the definitive treatment, the patient is immobilized initially in traction or with bed positioning for several weeks. This treatment is followed by immobilization of the vertebral column in a spinal orthosis for a period of weeks or months. The length of time that a patient spends in traction, positioned in bed, or immobilized in an orthosis varies with the nature of the injury and the philosophy of his

---

[4] Use of a Stryker frame is controversial due to its ineffectiveness in stabilizing the spine and its potential for compromised respiratory function during prone positioning (Marshall et al., 1990; McGuire, Green, Eismont, & Watts, 1988; Slabaugh & Nickel, 1978). Positioning in a standard bed is also controversial, as significant vertebral motion can occur during log rolling (McGuire, Neville, Green, & Watts, 1987).

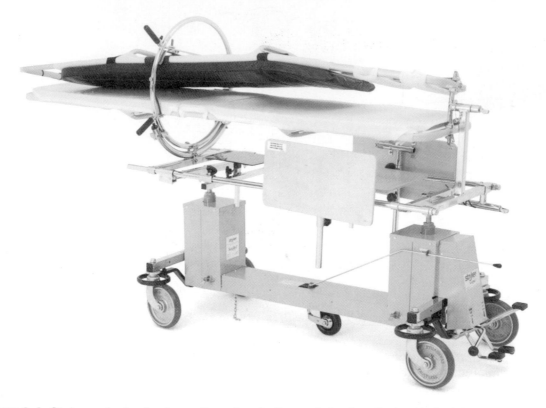

Figure 3–2. Stryker wedge turning frame. *Reproduced with permission from Stryker Medical, 6300 Sprinkle Road, Kalamazoo, MI 49001–9799.*

physician (Donovon, Kopaniky, Stolzmann, & Carter, 1987; Meyer, 1989).

At the end of the period of orthotic stabilization, the injured region of the patient's spine is evaluated radiologically. Persistent instability may make surgical stabilization necessary (Castillo & Bell, 1988; Meyer, 1989).

Surgical Management

Spinal column injury may be managed surgically, either immediately following admission to the hospital, following a two- to three-week period of skeletal traction or positioning in bed, or after several weeks or months have passed. Indications for surgical intervention include an unstable fracture, a fracture that will not reduce without surgery, gross spinal malalignment, evidence of continued cord compression in the presence of an incomplete injury, deteriorating neurological status, and continued instability following conservative management (Fig. 3–3). Open reduction and internal fixation may be done to restore optimal vertebral alignment and to stabilize the injured portion of the spine. Surgery may also be performed for decompression of neural tissue through removal of any boney fragments, soft-tissue structures, or foreign bodies impinging

on the cord. Finally, surgery is often performed to enable the patient to get out of bed earlier, thus avoiding the physical and psychological deterioration that can come from prolonged bedrest. (Bradford & McBride, 1987; Castillo & Bell, 1988; Denis, 1983; Lehman, 1987; Meyer, 1989).

Bone fragments, soft-tissue structures, or foreign bodies that are impinging on the cord are removed during surgery, and the spinal column is aligned and stabilized. Depending on the type of surgery performed, wires or other devices may be used to enhance stability. A bone graft is often done, usually with bone harvested from an iliac crest (Meyer, 1989; Meyer & Heim, 1989). The spine is generally immobilized with an orthosis for several months postoperatively to allow boney fusion to occur (Bradford & McBride, 1987; Lehman, 1987; Meyer, 1989; Meyer & Heim, 1989).

A variety of surgical procedures are available for achieving decompression, reduction, and stabilization. An anterior, posterior, or combined anterior and posterior approach may be used. The divers instruments used to stabilize the spine include devices that distract or compress the spine while immobilizing it. Other internal fixation devices immobilize the spine without distraction or

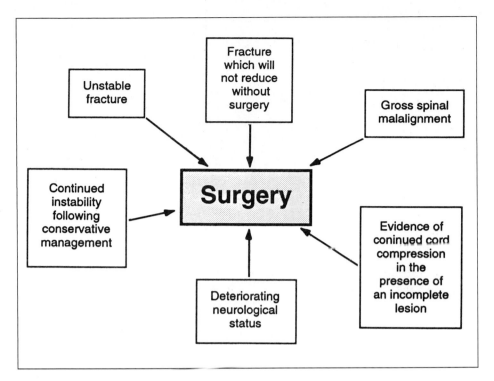

Figure 3-3. Indications for surgical management of spinal injury.

compression. Factors influencing the surgical approach and internal stabilization device chosen include the level and type of spinal column injury, extent of spinal instability present, number of vertebral levels requiring stabilization, location of boney or soft tissue encroaching on the spinal canal, extent of neurological impairment, and length of time that has passed since the injury (Bradford & McBride, 1987; Castillo & Bell, 1988; Donovon et al., 1987; Meyer, 1989; Meyer & Heim, 1989).

Management Controversy
There is no generally agreed-upon protocol for the management of spinal column injuries. Decisions regarding surgical versus nonsurgical management, surgical procedure, and timing of surgery and orthotic management are largely based on the philosophy of the institution or the surgeon involved (Bradford & McBride, 1987; Donovon et al., 1987; Hardcastle, Bedbrook, & Curtis, 1987; Meyer, 1989).

MEDICAL MANAGEMENT

Spinal cord injury can affect the functioning of virtually every system in the body. A variety of debilitating and potentially lethal complications can result. With proper medical management involving the coordinated efforts of a multidisciplinary team, many of these complications can be prevented.

Without proper management, unnecessary morbidity and mortality are virtually inevitable. For this reason, specialized care is essential.

During the first few days following spinal cord injury, a person's neurological status may deteriorate due to progression of the cord lesion. For this reason neurological status should be assessed frequently (Marshall et al., 1990). Deterioration may indicate the need for a change in surgical or nonsurgical interventions.

Proper medical management following spinal cord injury also involves measures to ensure that patients do not develop secondary medical problems as a result of the cord injury. Appropriate bladder, gastrointestinal, skin, respiratory, and cardiovascular care is imperative.

Bladder Care
During the period of spinal shock, the bladder will not empty spontaneously. Bladder distention, urinary reflux, and kidney failure can result if the bladder is not drained by catheterization. An indwelling catheter is usually inserted upon admission to the hospital. In many centers, the indwelling catheter is removed within a few days, and the bladder is drained using intermittent catheterization. This practice reduces the risk of infection.[5]

---

[5] Chapter 17 addresses bladder function and management strategies following spinal cord injury.

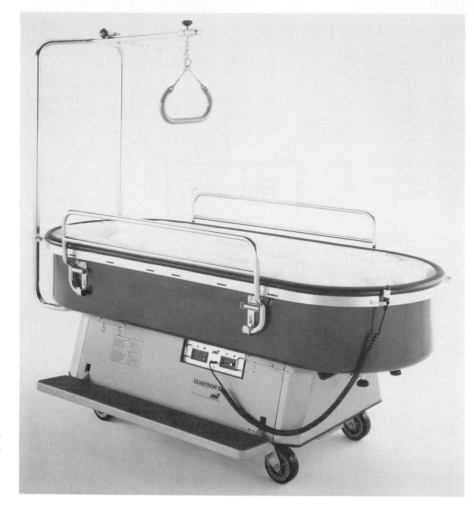

Figure 3–4. Air-fluidized bed. *Reproduced with permission from Support Systems International, 4349 Corporate Road, Charleston, SC 29405.*

Gastrointestinal Care

During spinal shock, gastric dilation and paralytic ileus may develop. This is of particular concern because of the potential threat to the patient's already compromised respiratory system: diaphragmatic movements are inhibited by this distention, and vomiting and aspiration may occur. To avoid these complications, the stomach can be decompressed using a nasogastric tube (Nikas, 1986).[6]

Stress ulcers may also occur during the acute stage following spinal cord injury. Prophylactic treatment with cimetidine, which inhibits gastric secretions, significantly reduces the incidence of GI bleeding (Buchanan & Ditunno, 1987).

Skin Care

People with spinal cord injuries are vulnerable to the development of decubitus ulcers. This complication can be avoided with proper care.

Prevention of Ducubiti. Pressure sore prevention involves avoidance of prolonged pressure on the skin, particularly over boney prominences. Acutely following spinal cord injury, the patient on a standard hospital bed must be turned *every two hours* around the clock to avoid the development of decubiti[7] (Grundy, Swain, & Russell, 1986a; McCagg, 1986; Nawoczenski, 1987; Nikas, 1986; Shenaq & Dinh, 1990). Some may require more frequent turning (Maklebust, 1987). The time spent in each position can be increased gradually as skin tolerance allows. Specially designed foam or water mattresses or mattress overlays can help to maintain the skin's integrity by reducing pressure over boney prominences. These devices should be used in addition to, not in place of, regular position changes (Goode & Allman, 1989; Knight, 1988; Maklebust, 1987; Willey, 1989). Ring-shaped donut cushions are *not* appropriate for either prevention or management of de-

---

[6] Chapter 17 addresses bowel function and management strategies following spinal cord injury.

[7] Bed positions are presented in Chapter 8.

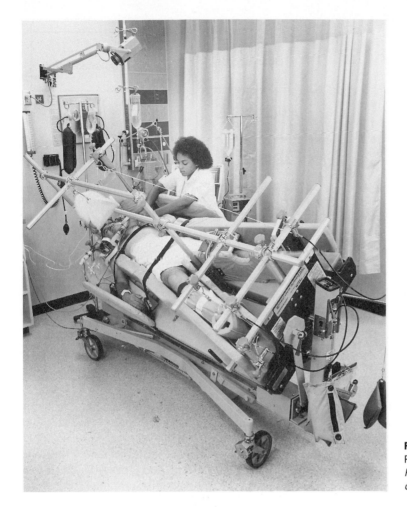

Figure 3–5. Patient with multiple trauma in Roto-Rest bed with traction apparatus attached. *Reproduced with permission from Kinetic Concepts, P.O. Box 8588, San Antonio, TX 78208.*

cubiti, as they create ischemia in tissues encircled by the donut (Goode & Allman, 1989).

As an alternative to a rigid turning schedule, a specialized pressure-reducing bed may be used. Low-air-loss beds, oscillating low-air-loss beds, or air-fluidized beds (Fig. 3–4) may be used by people with stable spines (Willey, 1989). A patient with an unstable spine may be placed on a rotating bed (oscillating support surface, or kinetic treatment table) to prevent decubiti[8] (Fig. 3–5). These beds rock slowly side to side in a continuous motion. A rotating bed must be adjusted properly. Otherwise it will allow the patient to slide back and forth as the bed rocks. This sliding subjects the skin to shear forces, *causing* skin breakdown instead of preventing it (Willey, 1989). These beds are most practical for patients who are confined to bed, as transfers in and out are difficult.

When out-of-bed activities are initiated, a properly fitting and adjusted wheelchair, a good sitting posture, and an appropriate wheelchair cushion are required to protect the skin over the buttocks and sacrum.[9] At first, pressure reliefs should be performed every 15 to 20 minutes when sitting[10] (McCagg, 1986; Nawoczenski, 1987; Shenaq & Dinh, 1990). The time between pressure reliefs can be increased gradually as skin tolerance allows.

Periodic relief of pressure is important after spinal cord injury, but it is only one facet of the preventive skin-care program. Measures must also be taken to minimize other factors that cause skin breakdown (Fig. 3–6). The patient and rehabilitation team should protect the patient's skin from shear

[8] The Roto-Rest bed effectively immobilizes the spine while providing constant turning. This constant motion reduces the risk of decubitus ulcers, enhances pulmonary status, and reduces the risk of pulmonary emboli (McGuire, Green, Eismont, & Watts, 1988; Willey, 1989).

[9] Wheelchair and cushion considerations are addressed in Chapter 19.

[10] Dependent and independent techniques for pressure reliefs are presented in Chapters 8 and 13, respectively.

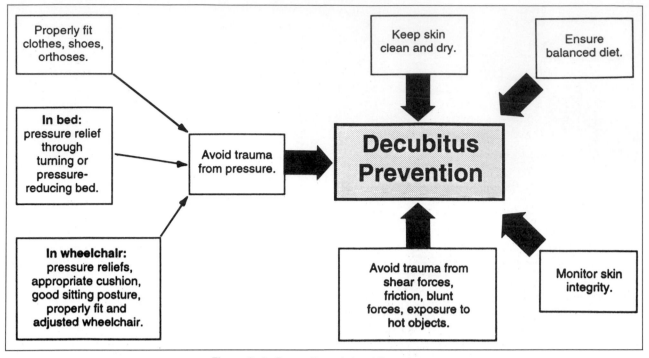

Figure 3–6. Prevention of decubitus ulcers.

forces, friction, blunt trauma, and exposure to hot objects. Clothes, shoes, and orthoses should fit properly; if too tight, they exert prolonged pressure on the skin. The cord-injured person's skin should be kept clean and dry, with special attention given to preventing prolonged contact with urine, feces, or excessive perspiration (Goode & Allman, 1989; Gosnell, 1987; Knight, 1988; Maklebust, 1987; Nawoczenski, 1987). Additionally, a balanced diet must be ensured, as nutritional deficiencies are important contributors to skin breakdown (Gosnell, 1987; Maklebust, 1987).

Following spinal cord injury, insensitive areas of the skin should be checked frequently for signs of skin damage. Special attention should be directed to skin overlying boney prominences. The skin's status provides feedback on the effectiveness of the skin care program. Additionally, early detection of imminent or actual breakdown makes it possible to intervene before undue damage occurs.

Treatment of Decubiti. The treatment indicated for pressure sores depends on their severity. Chart 3–1 presents a classification system that grades pressure ulcers by their severity.

When a decubitus develops, the source of the problem must be identified: did the skin breakdown occur as the result of trauma to the skin[11] sustained while lying in bed, during functional training, while

sitting in a wheelchair, or while wearing an orthosis? Did skin maceration from incontinence or excessive sweating contribute to the problem? Was the skin subjected to friction as a result of repeated motions caused by spasticity? Identification of the causative factors may make it possible to eliminate or reduce them.

First and foremost, pressure over the affected area must be avoided. A grade I pressure sore may heal without any intervention other than this relief of pressure (Knight, 1988). Depending on the source of trauma to the skin, pressure relief may be as simple as adjusting an orthosis or avoiding a certain posture such as supine or sitting. With severe or multiple decubiti, an air-fluidized or low-air-loss bed may promote healing by reducing pressure over boney prominences (Black & Black, 1987; Bristow,

Chart 3–1. Classification of Pressure Ulcers[a]

Grade I:	Nonblanchable erythema of intact skin
Grade II:	Partial thickness skin loss involving epidermis or dermis
Grade III:	Full-thickness skin loss involving subcutaneous tissue that may extend to, but not through, the underlying fascia
Grade IV:	Deeper, full-thickness lesions extending into muscle or bone

[a] Uniform classification system proposed by the National Pressure Ulcer Advisory Council, 1989. (Goode & Allman, 1989)

---

[11] Here, "trauma" can refer to prolonged, unrelieved pressure, friction, shear, or blunt force.

Goldfarb, & Green, 1987; Goode & Allman, 1989; Willey, 1989).

In the presence of an open wound (grades II through IV), prevention or elimination of infection will facilitate healing. Topical antiseptics and antibiotics can be used to achieve this end, although their use remains controversial. Some substances may even impede healing (Abramowicz, 1990; Fowler, 1987; Goode & Allman, 1989; Knight, 1988). Careful cleaning of the wound with nonirritating wound cleansers may promote wound healing as or more effectively than topical antibiotics (Fowler, 1987; Knight, 1988).

Wound management also involves the removal of eschar and necrotic tissue, as this tissue promotes bacterial growth and interferes with healing. Debridement can be achieved with hydrophylic polymers, enzymatic agents, wet-to-dry dressings, forceful wound irrigation, whirlpool baths, occlusive dressings, or surgery (Abramowicz, 1990; Black & Black, 1987; Fowler, 1987; Goode & Allman, 1989; Knight, 1988; Shenaq & Dinh, 1990). Enzymatic agents, wet-to-dry dressings, irrigation, whirlpool baths, and surgery can damage epithelial or granulation tissue (Cassell, 1986; Gorse & Messner, 1987; Goode & Allman, 1989; Knight, 1988).

Once a decubitus is clean (lacking infection), occlusive dressings can facilitate healing of grades I, II, and superficial grade III pressure ulcers (Gorse & Messner, 1987; Goode & Allman, 1989; Knight, 1988). Deeper ulcers should be packed with moist gauze (Goode & Allman, 1989).

Ultrasound (Cassell, 1986; Knight, 1988), hyperbaric oxygen therapy[12] (Cassell, 1986; Nawoczenski, 1987), or high-voltage electrical stimulation (HVS) may be used to promote wound healing. High voltage electrical stimulation in particular has been shown to increase the rate of pressure-ulcer healing dramatically (Akers & Gabrielson, 1984; Kloth & Feedar, 1988).

Although pressure sores can heal without surgical closure, this process can take weeks or months when the ulcer is large and deep. For this reason surgical closure may be considered for full-thickness pressure ulcers (grades III and IV) greater than 2 cm in diameter (Black & Black, 1987; Knight, 1988). For surgical closure of large wounds, a myocutaneous flap procedure has the advantage of creating a well-vascularized and padded area (Black & Black, 1987; Shenaq & Dinh, 1990). Postoperative care includes avoidance of pressure on the grafted area through positioning and use of a pressure-re-

ducing bed. In addition, care should be taken to avoid shearing or tension on the grafted tissue until adequate healing has occurred. Range of motion exercises must be suspended (Black & Black, 1987), and antispasmodic drugs may be administered to prevent excessive motion caused by spasticity (Shenaq & Dinh, 1990).

In addition to treatment of the decubitus itself, optimal pressure-sore management addresses the patient's general health. Treatment of anemia, hypoalbuminemia, and edema may promote pressure-ulcer healing (Knight, 1988). Systemic antibiotics are indicated for patients who develop cellulitis, abscesses, osteomyelitis, or septicemia (Abramowicz, 1990; Black & Black, 1987; Knight, 1988; Shenaq & Dinh, 1990). The patient's nutritional status is also important. Wound healing requires an adequate intake of proteins, carbohydrates, fats, vitamins, minerals, and fluids (Bobel, 1987; Cassell, 1986; Maklebust, 1987). Supplemental vitamin C and a high-calorie, high-protein diet may facilitate wound healing. Zinc, iron, magnesium, and vitamin A supplements may be indicated, particularly for people with deficiencies of these nutrients (Abramowicz, 1990; Cassell, 1986; Goode & Allman, 1989; Knight, 1988; Shenaq & Dinh, 1990).

Respiratory Care

When spinal cord injury disrupts the functioning of the diaphragm, intercostals, or abdominals, the resulting impaired ability to breathe and cough effectively can lead to atelectasis, pneumonia, and death. The clinical picture is further complicated if the cord-injured person sustained trauma to the thorax during the initial accident or if he has a history of respiratory disease, aspiration, or smoking (Buchanan & Ditunno, 1987; Grundy, Swain, & Russell, 1986; Marshall et al., 1990).

A thorough respiratory evaluation should be performed as soon as possible after injury and repeated periodically thereafter. This early evaluation will make it possible to formulate an appropriate plan of care and to monitor progress or deterioration in respiratory status. The evaluation should include assessment of arterial blood gases, tidal volume, vital capacity,[13] respiratory rate, adequacy of cough, strength in respiratory musculature, mobility of the chest wall, chest expansion, chest and abdominal motion during respiration, and posture. The evaluation should also investigate the presence of complicating conditions such as chest injury or a

---

[12] Oxygen may also be administered to the wound using a face mask or similar device (Cassell, 1986; Miller, 1986).

[13] Tidal volume is the amount of air that is moved during quiet breathing. Vital capacity is the amount of air that can be expelled following full inspiration.

history of smoking or preexisting pulmonary disease (Brownlee & Williams, 1987; McCagg, 1986; Morgan, Silver, & Williams, 1986; Nikas, 1986; Rinehart & Nawoczenski, 1987; Wetzel, 1985).

A high cervical lesion that results in seriously impaired respiratory ability may make it necessary to initiate mechanical ventilation during the emergency phase of management. Even if unassisted ventilation is adequate initially, respiratory ability can deteriorate in the first few days after spinal cord injury. For this reason respiratory function should be monitored closely during the initial phase following injury. Frequent checks of arterial blood gasses and vital capacity will provide information on the patient's status and will allow prompt response if needed. Mechanical ventilation may be necessary if vital capacity falls too low[14] or in the presence of complicating factors such as advanced age, preexisting respiratory disease, or fever (Brownlee & Williams, 1987; Grundy, Swain, & Russell, 1986; McCagg, 1986; Meyer, 1989; Rinehart & Nawoczenski, 1987). Fortunately, respiratory function usually improves significantly with the passage of time after spinal cord injury (Brownlee & Williams, 1987; Morgan et al., 1986; Scanlon et al., 1989).

The respiratory component of a comprehensive rehabilitation program following spinal cord injury is directed toward the prevention of pulmonary complications and the maximization of respiratory ability. It should be initiated soon after injury and continue throughout acute and postacute rehabilitation. Respiratory rehabilitation includes measures to mobilize secretions, enhance breathing ability, and provide the cord-injured person with the knowledge and skills required to avoid complications after discharge.

Clearing Secretions. An inability to cough effectively leads to the accumulation of secretions within the lungs. Enforced recumbency after spinal cord injury compounds the problem. Retention of secretions can lead to atelectasis, infection, and respiratory insufficiency. These complications can be avoided with appropriate management. Acutely following injury, all patients with impaired respiratory ability should be treated prophylactically with postural drainage, percussion and vibration of the chest, and assisted coughing (Grundy, Swain, & Russell, 1986; McCagg, 1986; Nikas, 1986; Rinehart & Nawoczenski, 1987). Intermittent positive pressure breath-

ing (IPPB) may also be used prophylactically or as an adjunct to these treatments when patients exhibit retention of secretions and atelectasis (Brownlee & Williams, 1987).

Postural drainage, percussion, vibration, and IPPB are standard respiratory physical therapy techniques. They can be adapted to the medical and orthopedic needs of individual cord-injured patients as needed. Assisted coughing is a technique used to help cord-injured people achieve forceful expiration while coughing. To assist in a cough, the health professional pushes up and in on the patient's abdomen, just below the xiphoid process.[15] This maneuver must be coordinated with the patient's voluntary efforts at coughing after maximal inhalation. Some cord-injured people are able to learn to "assist" their own coughs (self-cough) by pushing up and in on their abdomens while coughing after a maximal inhalation. Forward flexion of the trunk can enhance the cough (Rinehart & Nawoczenski, 1987; Wetzel, 1985).

A regular turning schedule is also helpful in mobilizing secretions. When a person lies in bed in one position for prolonged periods, fluid accumulates in dependent portions of his or her lungs. Regular changes in position help alleviate this problem by preventing each area of the lung from being dependent for too long (Brownlee & Williams, 1987; Morgan et al., 1986; Rinehart & Nawoczenski, 1987). As an alternative to regular turning on standard hospital beds, patients are often placed on rotating beds (described above) that keep them in constant motion. These beds may prevent the build-up of secretions within the lungs. Additionally, early activity out of bed can help. As soon as it is medically and orthopedically feasible, patients should begin participating in out-of-bed activities.

Breathing Capacity. Respiratory rehabilitation following spinal cord injury goes beyond the clearing of secretions from the lungs. It also involves maximizing the patient's ability to breathe. This is accomplished by strengthening the patient's respiratory musculature and preserving the mobility of the thoracic cage.

Breathing exercises should be initiated soon after injury. These exercises can increase the strength and endurance of innervated respiratory musculature and can improve ventilation of the lungs (Brownlee & Williams, 1987; Clough, Lin-

---

[14] There is no generalized agreement regarding the vital capacity values that may necessitate the initiation of mechanical ventilation. The cut-off values range from 500 to 600 mL (Grundy, Swain, & Russell, 1986) to 1,000 to 1,200 mL (McCagg, 1986).

[15] If medical conditions such as abdominal trauma or paralytic ileus preclude the use of force on the abdomen, the health professional can apply force to the chest wall instead (Brownlee & Williams, 1987).

denauer, Hayes, & Zekany, 1986; Rinehart & Na-woczenski, 1987). If greater inspiratory capacity is achieved, a more effective cough may be possible (Morgan et al., 1986). During initial diaphragmatic exercises, the patient can breathe deeply without resistance. As inspiratory ability increases, he can practice breathing deeply while the therapist applies manual resistance and finally progress to breathing with weights placed on the upper abdomen (Rinehart & Nawoczenski, 1987; Wetzel, 1985). The therapist and patient can also work to improve ventilation of isolated lobes, with the therapist providing manual, visual, or verbal feedback, or a combination thereof on chest motions during inspiration (Brownlee & Williams, 1987; Voss, Ionta, & Myers, 1985). These exercises are most likely to be of benefit when the intercostals are innervated (Rinehart & Nawoczenski, 1987).

Chest mobility is also important for breathing capacity. Range of motion in the chest wall can be preserved or improved through deep-breathing exercises, passive stretching, joint mobilization, IPPB, glossopharyngeal breathing, and airshift maneuvers. Glossopharyngeal breathing involves forcing air into the lungs using the tongue, mouth, and throat musculature. An airshift maneuver involves inhaling deeply, closing the glottis, and relaxing the diaphragm to move air into the upper chest (Clough et al., 1986; Rinehart & Nawoczenski, 1987; Wetzel, 1985).

Posture is another factor that affects breathing ability; a thoracic kyphosis or scoliosis will impair respiration. During rehabilitation after spinal cord injury, posture should be optimized through exercise, functional training, and the acquisition of appropriate seating equipment (Rinehart & Nawoczenski, 1987).

Following spinal cord injury that results in paralysis of the abdominal musculature, vital capacity is greater in supine than in upright positions (Estenne & De Troyer, 1987). Inspiration is more difficult in upright positions because the paralyzed abdominal musculature allows the abdominal contents to protrude and descend, with resulting descent of the diaphragm. During early out-of-bed activities, an abdominal binder can improve vital capacity and tidal volume by containing the abdominal contents and thus placing the diaphragm in a more efficient position for inspiration (Brownlee & Williams, 1987; Clough et al., 1986; McCool et al., 1986; Rinehart & Nawoczenski, 1987; Wetzel, 1985). Abdominal binders should be used temporarily to ease the transition to upright activities. As a cord-injured person's breathing capacity improves, the binder should be discontinued. The binder can be loosened

gradually over a period of days to allow the patient to accommodate to breathing without it.

Ventilator-Dependent Program. The respiratory care program for ventilator-dependent, cord-injured people includes mobilization of secretions through postural drainage, vibration and percussion, and suctioning. When possible, the program should also work toward developing the capacity to breathe without mechanical assistance. Some ventilator-dependent people who lack diaphragm function are able to learn to breathe without mechanical assistance for at least brief periods using glossopharyngeal breathing (Clough et al., 1986; Rinehart & Nawoczenski, 1987). Others with at least partial innervation of their diaphragms can undergo gradual weaning from their ventilators. During the weaning process, a patient practices breathing with assistance from a ventilator, progresses to breathing unassisted for brief periods, and increases the independent breathing time as tolerated. As breathing ability improves, breathing exercises can help strengthen the diaphragm and reduce dependence on neck musculature for breathing (Rinehart & Nawoczenski, 1987; Wetzel, 1985).

Diaphragmatic pacing is an alternative to mechanical ventilation for people who have permanently paralyzed diaphragms. With this procedure breathing is accomplished through the use of surgically implanted electrodes that stimulate the phrenic nerve (Brownlee & Williams, 1987; Morgan et al., 1986; Rinehart & Nawoczenski, 1987; Vincken & Corne, 1987). Diaphragmatic pacing frees the individual from a ventilator and achieves superior arterial oxygenation (Vincken & Corne, 1987).

Cardiovascular Care

When spinal cord injury interrupts sympathetic innervation, peripheral vasodilation and bradycardia result. These effects are usually significant only in people with lesions above T6 and resolve within a few weeks of injury. During the initial days following spinal cord injury, however, continuous cardiac monitoring is advisable for all patients (Buchanan & Ditunno, 1987; Meyer, 1989). Vasopressor medication or intravenous (IV) fluids may be indicated to maintain an adequate blood pressure (Meyer, 1989; Thelan, Davie, & Urden, 1990). IV fluids should be administered judiciously; pulmonary edema is likely to result if large volumes are given (Grundy, Swain, & Russell, 1986; McCagg, 1986; Nikas, 1986). Placement of a temporary pacemaker or treatment with atropine (parasympatholytic agent) or inotropic medication may be indicated for severe bradycardia (Buchanan & Ditunno, 1987; Grundy, Swain, & Russell, 1986; Nikas, 1986; Thelan et al., 1990).

Vasovagal Response. Acutely after spinal cord injury, tracheal suctioning or endotracheal intubation can cause a precipitous fall in heart rate and cardiac arrest. This problem may be avoided by administration of oxygen prior to and after these procedures. Atropine may be given prophylactically or to correct the problem if it develops (Bloch, 1986; Grundy, Swain, & Russell, 1986; McCagg, 1986).

Orthostatic Hypotension. Orthostatic hypotension is commonly exhibited by people with recent spinal cord injuries when upright activities are first initiated. Strategies for developing tolerance to upright sitting are presented in Chapter 8.

Autonomic Dysreflexia. Autonomic dysreflexia is a potentially life-threatening, exaggerated, sympathetic response to noxious stimulation below the lesion. This complication occurs only among people with cervical and high thoracic lesions, usually first appearing six or more months after the injury.

When autonomic dysreflexia occurs, the patient should be positioned with his head and torso elevated and the lower extremities lowered. This positioning will decrease blood pressure and promote cerebral venous return (Matthews & Carlson, 1987; Thelan et al., 1990). The underlying source of the noxious sensation causing the dysreflexia should be investigated and eliminated as quickly as possible. Since bowel and bladder distention are common stimuli for autonomic crisis, draining the bladder or removing a bowel impaction may stop the crisis. If these measures do not stop the dysreflexic response, other possible sources of the dysreflexia should be investigated. If the patient's blood pressure remains elevated after the underlying cause has been removed, it can be controlled using antihypertensive medication (Bloch, 1986; McCagg, 1986; Matthews & Carlson, 1987; Thelan et al., 1990).

Prevention of Deep Venous Thrombosis. Deep venous thrombi (DVT) are common in the early months after spinal cord injury and can lead to pulmonary emboli and death. For this reason patients should be monitored for signs of DVT. Swelling, discoloration, and local or systemic temperature elevation are indications of possible deep vein thrombosis. However, these symptoms are often present without DVT, and thrombus formation often occurs without clinically recognizable symptoms (Turpie,

1986). The diagnosis of DVT requires more sophisticated diagnostic procedures, such as venography, impedance plethysmography, Doppler ultrasound, and I-fibrinogen scans (Buchanan & Ditunno, 1987; McCagg, 1986; Turpie, 1986). When venous thromboembolism is detected, anticoagulant therapy is indicated.

There is no generally accepted approach to the prevention of deep venous thrombosis following spinal cord injury. Antiembolic stockings, lower extremity range of motion exercises, alternating pressure devices, and low-dose prophylactic anticoagulation therapy are commonly employed (Buchanan & Ditunno, 1987; Grundy, Swain, & Russell, 1986a; Marshall et al., 1990; Matthews & Carlson, 1987; McCagg, 1986; Meyer, 1989; Morgan et al., 1986; Nikas, 1986; Turpie, 1986).

EDUCATION

Following spinal cord injury, the threats of pressure ulcers, respiratory complications, bowel and urinary tract complications, and autonomic dysreflexia never go away. These complications can be avoided but only with meticulous care. For people with spinal cord injuries, health maintenance is an active and never-ending process.

During rehabilitation, a cord-injured person must acquire the knowledge and skills needed to stay healthy. The patient should learn about how his body functions, the complications that can result, how to avoid these complications, and what to do if they occur. The patient should also gain the self-reliance and communication skills required to take control of his care. Unfortunately many members of the general medical community are ignorant about the special health needs of people with spinal cord injuries. As a result, someone who places total trust in the system may not get adequate care. If he is to stay healthy through the years, a cord-injured person needs to learn to manage his own health care.

> Our people are really obnoxious when they leave here. Our goal is that when these people leave here, since they have to live with their injury all their lives, is for them to know more about their body than most doctors know. Indeed, most doctors don't know much about spinal cord injury. We want our patients to recognize when they need a urine culture, when they should take antibiotics, when they should not, when they should call a doctor, and what

they should tell the doctor they need. We want them to be able to take charge of their own care.

Julie Botvin Madorski (Maddox, 1987)

SUMMARY

The early medical and surgical management that a spinal cord-injured person receives has a tremendous impact on his health and function. When someone first sustains a spinal column injury, motion of the spine may result in trauma to previously undamaged neural tissue; appropriate fracture management is required to preserve neurological function. In addition, spinal cord injury leaves an individual susceptible to a variety of serious complications. During acute care and rehabilitation, a cord-injured person must receive specialized medical management to avoid these complications. As importantly, the patient must acquire the knowledge and skills needed to take care of his medical care.

REFERENCES

Abramowicz, M. (Ed.). (1990). Treatment of pressure ulcers. *Medical Letter on Drugs and Therapeutics, 32,* 17–18.

Akers, T., & Gabrielson, A. (1984). The effect of high voltage galvanic stimulation on the rate of healing of decubitus ulcers. *Biomedical Science Instrumentation, 20,* 99–100.

Barker, E., & Higgins, R. (1989). Managing a suspected spinal cord injury. *Nursing, 19*(4), 52–59.

Barker, E., & Higgins, R. (1989a). Rescuing an SCI victim from a pool. *Nursing, 19*(5), 58–64.

Black, J., & Black, S. (1987). Surgical management of pressure ulcers. *Nursing Clinics of North America, 22*(2), 429–438.

Bloch, R. (1986). Autonomic dysfunction. In R. Bloch & M. Basbaum (Eds.), *Management of spinal cord injuries* (pp. 149–163). Baltimore: Williams & Wilkins.

Bobel, L. (1987). Nutritional implications in the patient with pressure sores. *Nursing Clinics of North America, 22*(2), 379–390.

Bracken, M., Shepard, M., Collins, W., Holford, T., Young, W., Baskin, D., Eisenberg, H., Flamm, E., Leo-Summers, L., Maroon, J., Marshall, L., Perot, P., Piepmeyer, J., Sonntag, V., Wagner, F., Wilberger, J., & Winn, H. (1990). A randomized, controlled trial of methylprednisolone or naloxone in the treatment of acute spinal-cord injury. *New England Journal of Medicine, 322*(20), 1405–1411.

Bradford, D., & McBride, G. (1987). Surgical management of thoracolumbar spine fractures with incomplete neurologic deficits. *Clinical Orthopaedics and Related Research, 218,* 201–216.

Bristow, J., Goldfarb, E., & Green, M. (1987). Clinitron therapy: Is it effective? *Geriatric Nursing, 8*(3), 120–124.

Brownlee, S., & Williams, S. (1987). Physiotherapy in the respiratory care of patients with high spinal injury. *Physiotherapy, 73*(3), 148–152.

Brunette, D., & Rockswold, G. (1987). Neurologic recovery following rapid spinal realignment for complete cervical spinal cord injury. *Journal of Trauma, 27*(4), 445–447.

Buchanan, L., & Ditunno, J. (1987). Acute care: Medical/surgical management. In L. Buchanan & D. Nawoczenski (Eds.), *Spinal cord injury: Concepts and management approaches* (pp. 35–60). Baltimore: Williams & Wilkins.

Cassell, B. (1986). Treating pressure sores stage by stage. *RN, 49,* 36–40.

Castillo, R., & Bell, J. (1988). Cervical spine injury: Stabilization and management. *Postgraduate Medicine, 83*(7), 131–138.

Clough, P., Lindenauer, D., Hayes, M., & Zekany, B. (1986). Guidelines for routine respiratory care of patients with spinal cord injury. *Physical Therapy, 66*(9), 1395–1402.

Cook, P. (1988). Radiology of spine and spinal cord injury. In L. Illis (Ed.), *Spinal cord dysfunction: Assessment* (pp. 41–103). New York: Oxford University Press.

Denis, F. (1983). The three column spine and its significance in the classification of acute thoracolumbar spinal injuries. *Spine, 8*(8), 817–831.

Donovon, W., Kopaniky, D., Stolzmann, E., & Carter, R. (1987). The neurological and skeletal outcome in patients with closed cervical spinal cord injury. *Journal of Neurosurgery, 66*(5), 690–694.

Estenne, M., & De Troyer, A. (1987). Mechanism of the postural dependence of vital capacity in tetraplegic subjects. *American Review of Respiratory Disease, 135*(2), 367–371.

Fowler, E. (1987). Equipment and products used in management and treatment of pressure ulcers. *Nursing Clinics of North America, 22*(2), 449–460.

Goode, P., & Allman, R. (1989). The prevention and management of pressure ulcers. *Medical Clinics of North America, 73*(6), 1511–1524.

Gorse, G., & Messner, R. (1987). Improved pressure sore healing with hydrocolloid dressings. *Archives of Dermatology, 123*(6), 766–771.

Gosnell, D. (1987). Assessment and evaluation of pressure sores. *Nursing Clinics of North America, 22*(2), 399–416.

Graziano, A., Scheidel, E., Cline, J., & Baer, L. (1987). A radiographic comparison of prehospital cervical immobilization methods. *Annals of Emergency Medicine, 16*(10), 1127–1131.

Grundy, D., Swain, A., & Russell, J. (1986). ABC of spinal cord injury: Early management and complications I. *British Medical Journal, 292*(6512), 44–47.

Grundy, D., Swain, A., & Russell, J. (1986a). ABC of spinal cord injury: Early management and complications II. *British Medical Journal, 292*(6513), 123–125.

Hansebout, R. (1986). The neurosurgical management of cord injuries. In R. Bloch & M. Basbaum (Eds.), *Management of spinal cord injuries* (pp. 1–27). Baltimore: Williams & Wilkins.

Hardcastle, P., Bedbrook G., & Curtis K. (1987). Long-term results of conservative and operative management in complete paraplegics with spinal cord injuries between T10 and L2 with respect to function. *Clin Ortho and Rel Res, 224*, 88–96.

Johnston, R. (1989). Management of old people with neck trauma. *British Medical Journal, 299*(6700), 633–634.

Karbi, O., Caspari, D., & Tator, C. (1988). Extrication, immobilization, and radiologic investigation of patients with cervical spine injuries. *Canadian Medical Association Journal, 139*(7), 617–621.

Kloth, L., & Feedar, J. (1988). Acceleration of wound healing with high voltage, monophasic, pulsed current. *Physical Therapy, 68*(4), 503–508. {Erratum: *Physical Therapy, 69*(8), 702.}

Knight, A. (1988). Medical management of pressure sores. *Journal of Family Practice, 27*(1), 95–100.

Kulkarni, M., McArdle, C., Kopanicky, D., Miner, M., Cotler, H., Lee, K., & Harris, J. (1987). Acute spinal cord injury: MR imaging at 1.5 T. *Radiology, 164*(3), 837–843.

Lehman, L. (1987). Injury of the cervical spine: Some fundamentals of management. *Postgraduate Medicine, 82*(2), 193–200.

Maddox, S. (1987). *Spinal network.* Boulder, CO: Spinal Network.

Maher, A. (1985). Dealing with head and neck injuries. *RN, 48*(3), 43–46.

Maklebust, J. (1987). Pressure ulcers: Etiology and prevention. *Nursing Clinics of North America, 22*(2), 359–377.

Marshall, S., Marshall, L., Vos, H., & Chesnut, R. (1990). *Neuroscience critical care: Pathophysiology and patient management.* Philadelphia: W.B. Saunders Company.

Matthews, P., & Carlson, C. (1987). *Spinal cord injury: A guide to rehabilitation nursing.* Rockville, MD: Aspen Publishers.

McCagg, C. (1986). Postoperative management and acute rehabilitation of patients with spinal cord injuries. *Orthopedic Clinics of North America, 17*(1), 171–182.

McCool, F., Pichurko, B., Slutsky, A., Sarkarati, M., Rossier, A., & Brown, R. (1986). Changes in lung volume and rib cage configuration with abdominal binding in quadriplegia. *Journal of Applied Physiology, 60*(4), 1198–1202.

McGuire, R., Green, B., Eismont, F., & Watts, C. (1988). Comparison of stability provided to the unstable spine by the kinetic therapy table and Stryker frame. *Neurosurgery, 22*(5), 842–845.

McGuire, R., Neville, S., Green, B., & Watts, C. (1987). Spinal instability and the log-rolling maneuver. *Journal of Trauma, 27*(5), 525–531.

Meyer, P. (1989). *Surgery of Spine Trauma.* New York: Churchill Livingstone.

Meyer, P., & Heim, S. (1989). Surgical stabilization of the cervical spine. In P. Meyer (Ed.), *Surgery of Spine Trauma* (pp. 397–523). New York: Churchill Livingstone.

Miller, B. (1986). Procedures for stage 4 pressure sores. *RN, 49*, 40–41.

Mirvis, S., Geisler, F., Jelinek, J., Joslyn, J., & Gellad, F. (1988). Acute cervical spine trauma: Evaluation with 1.5-T imaging. *Radiology, 166*(3), 807–816.

Morgan, M., Silver, J., & Williams, S. (1986). The respiratory system of the spinal cord patient. In R. Bloch & M. Basbaum (Eds.), *Management of spinal cord injuries* (pp. 78–116). Baltimore: Williams & Wilkins.

Nawoczenski, D. (1987). Pressure sores: Prevention and management. In L. Buchanan & D. Nawoczenski (Eds.), *Spinal cord injury: Concepts and management approaches* (pp. 99–121). Baltimore: Williams & Wilkins.

Nikas, D. (1986). Resuscitation of patients with central nervous system trauma. *Nursing Clinics of North America, 21*(4), 693–704.

Rinehart, M., & Nawoczenski, D. (1987). Respiratory care. In L. Buchanan & D. Nawoczenski (Eds.), *Spinal cord injury: Concepts and management approaches* (pp. 61–79). Baltimore: Williams & Wilkins.

Romeo, J. (1988). The critical minutes after spinal cord injury. *RN, 51*(4), 61–67.

Scanlon, P., Loring, S., Pichurko, B., McCool, F., Slutsky, A., Sarkarati, M., & Brown, R. (1989). Respiratory mechanics in acute quadriplegia: Lung and chest wall compliance and dimensional changes during respiratory maneuvers. *American Review of Respiratory Disease, 139*(3), 615–620.

Shenaq, S., & Dinh, T. (1990). Decubitus ulcers: How to prevent them—and intervene should prevention fail. *Postgraduate Medicine, 87*(4), 91–95.

Simpson, R., Venger, B., & Narayan, R. (1989). Treatment of acute penetrating injuries of the spine: A retrospective analysis. *Journal of Trauma, 29*(1), 42–46.

Slabaugh, P., & Nickel, V. (1978). Complications with use of the Stryker frame. *Journal of Bone and Joint Surgery, 60-A*(8), 1111–1112.

Soderstrom, C., & Brumback, R. (1986). Early care of the patient with cervical spine injury. *Orthopedic Clinics of North America, 17*(1), 3–13.

Swain, A., Grundy, D., & Russell, J. (1985). ABC of spinal cord injury: At the accident. *British Medical Journal, 291*(6508), 1558–1560.

Swain, A., Grundy, D., & Russell, J. (1985a). ABC of spinal cord injury: Evacuation and initial management at the hospital. *British Medical Journal, 291*(6509), 1623–1625.

Thelan, L., Davie, J., & Urden, L. (1990). *Textbook of critical care nursing: Diagnosis and management.* Baltimore: C.V. Mosby.

Turpie, A. (1986). Thrombosis prevention and treatment in spinal cord injured patients. In R. Bloch & M. Basbaum (Eds.), *Management of spinal cord injuries* (pp.

212–240). Baltimore: Williams & Wilkins.

Vincken, W., & Corne, L. (1987). Improved arterial oxygenation by diaphragmatic pacing in quadriplegia. *Critical Care Medicine, 15*(9), 872–873.

Voss, D., Ionta, M., & Meyers, B. (1985). *Proprioceptive neuromuscular facilitation* (3rd ed.). Philadelphia: Harper & Row.

Wetzel, J. (1985). Respiratory evaluation and treatment. In H. Adkins (Ed.), *Spinal cord injury* (pp. 75–98). New York: Churchill Livingstone.

Willey, T. (1989). High-tech beds and mattress overlays: A decision guide. *American Journal of Nursing*, (89)9:1142–1145.

4

Psychosocial Issues

Spinal cord injury brings sudden and profound life changes. The cord-injured person, often an active male in his adolescence or early adulthood, may be swimming, playing football, driving, or earning a living one minute, and the next minute he is incapable of moving his extremities. Over the next days and weeks he finds himself paralyzed, incontinent, immobile, dependent, and isolated. As his rehabilitation progresses and he ventures out from the rehabilitation center, he is faced with a social and physical environment that seems almost hostile in its inaccessibility.

Despite the magnitude and scope of the problems that spinal cord injury can cause, most who sustain a cord injury are able to adjust. For some people, the injury ultimately results in psychological and spiritual growth. Others never fully recover psychologically from their loss. The outcome depends partly upon the individual and partly upon the psychosocial support that he receives. To maximize a person's potential for adaptation and growth following spinal cord injury, the rehabilitation team must address itself to his psychosocial needs.

PSYCHOSOCIAL IMPACT OF SPINAL CORD INJURY

Losses Associated With Spinal Cord Injury

The physical losses engendered by spinal cord injury are perhaps the most obvious. Depending on the completeness and level of his injury, a person can lose control of some or all of his limb and trunk musculature. His physique changes dramatically as his muscles atrophy. Where his sensation is affected, he loses the ability to perceive the presence, position, and motion of his limbs or to experience the myriad pleasant and unpleasant sensations from his environment. He is likely to lose bowel and bladder control, and his sexual functioning will be altered.[1]

The cord-injured person loses the ability to care for himself and to move from place to place. Dependent on others to care for him and placed in an environment where all power and self-direction are taken from him, he loses his autonomy. Additionally he is unable to participate in the recreational, social, and vocational activities that previously filled his days. With rehabilitation he may regain the capacity to do some of these things, but his manner of doing them will be altered.

Spinal cord injury also threatens financial security and disrupts plans for the future. Approximately 50% of people who sustain spinal cord injuries remain unemployed following injury (DeVivo & Fine, 1982), and those who do work make less money on the average than nondisabled people (Trieschmann, 1988). Financial security is also threatened by the expenses of medical care, attendant care, and equipment.

During his acute hospitalization and rehabilitation, a cord-injured person is likely to experience separation from loved ones. Even after discharge, his friendship and family relationships are likely to be altered. Old friends tend to drift away (Trieschmann, 1986 & 1988). Roles may be altered within the family, and patterns of communication and levels of intimacy are likely to change (McGowan & Roth, 1987; Urey & Henggeler, 1987).

Faced with the changes in his physique, physical functioning, functional capacities, accustomed activities, financial status, relationships, and plans for the future, a person's previous concept of himself no longer fits. Thus personal identity can be

---

[1]Chapter 16 addresses the impact of spinal cord injury on sexuality and sexual functioning and presents strategies for promoting adjustment in this area.

added to the list of losses brought on by spinal cord injury (Krueger, 1984; Trieschmann, 1988).

Finally, spinal cord injury challenges a person's notions about how the world functions. Each of us has illusions about the world and our place in it. These irrational beliefs, left over from early childhood, may include feelings of invulnerability, immortality, or a sense of total control over one's life (Moses, 1989; Schneider, 1984). Spinal cord injury can make these and other illusions untenable.

> I think with a spinal cord injury, one realizes that one is not going to live forever, that you are mortal.
>
> Don Rugg (Maddox, 1987)

Social Impact of Spinal Cord Injury

People with disabilities are devalued in our society. As a group, they are seen as substantially different from and less desirable than able-bodied people. As a result, they are subject to discrimination (English, 1977; Gilliland & James, 1988; Stubbins, 1988; Tunks, Bahry, & Basbaum, 1986).

> Most of us know by now that our physical limitations cut less keenly than the needless limitations placed upon us by an unwittingly hostile society. We should let the world in on that secret.
>
> Barry Corbet (1987)

Discrimination against people with disabilities manifests itself in many ways. Architectural and transportation barriers serve to handicap those with mobility impairments. A disabled person is likely to encounter discriminatory treatment when seeking education, employment, medical insurance, and housing (Chesler & Chesney, 1988; Gellman, 1977; McCarthy, 1988; Stubbins, 1988). Financial disincentives within public assistance programs can make it extremely difficult to break out of a cycle of unemployment and poverty: because employment can result in a loss of medical insurance[2] and funding for attendant care, a disabled person may not be able to afford to work (DeJong, Branch, & Corcoran, 1984; Trieschmann, 1988).

Disabled people are also subject to discrimination in their interpersonal relationships. When meeting someone with a disability, an able-bodied person's perception of the individual is likely to be dominated by the disability; people focus on the disabling characteristics rather than on the person's other qualities. Likewise, the media tends to focus on a person's disability rather than other, usually more relevant, characteristics. For example, a few years ago a woman was in the local news. Although her disability had no bearing on why she was in the news, it was *always* mentioned when she was discussed. The wording progressed (deteriorated) from "Lucy Jones,[3] the wheelchair athlete," to "Lucy Jones, the woman in a wheelchair," and finally to "Lucy Jones, a 33-year-old wheelchair."

People with disabilities are viewed as fundamentally different from "normal" people and are afforded less esteem and status (Wolfensberger & Tullman, 1982). They are often perceived as dependent and helpless (Fichten, 1988; Lindemann, 1981), tragic victims who remain bitter about their misfortune (Weinberg, 1988).

Because of this devaluation and stereotyping of people with disabilities, able-bodied people are likely to be uncomfortable talking with them and tend to avoid contact (Fichten, 1988; Haney & Rabin, 1984). As a result, social isolation is common following spinal cord injury (Trieschmann, 1988).

After sustaining a spinal cord injury, a person soon discovers that he is a member of a disadvantaged minority, "the disabled." The demoralizing effects of the stereotyping and discrimination that he inevitably experiences are likely to be compounded by his own preexisting prejudices regarding people with disabilities (Tunks, Bahry, & Basbaum, 1986).

> I have never felt despised for being in a wheelchair. I have felt pitied; I have despised myself.
>
> Barry Corbet (1980)

Additional Factors Affecting Behavior

Immediately after sustaining a spinal cord injury, a person is likely to be whisked away in an ambulance to an emergency room from which he will proceed to an intensive care unit. Once in the unit he will be bombarded by a constant stream of monotonous noises from monitors and other equipment. He will have few meaningful sights or sounds to attend to, despite the constant noise, and at the same time he will have an absence of tactile and proprioceptive sensations as a result of his injury. Health care workers will come and go to minister to his needs, but he will not have prolonged periods of social con-

---

[2] Upon losing Medicare coverage, private insurance may be prohibitively expensive. In addition, policies are likely to exclude any conditions related to the disabling condition. With spinal cord injury, this could result in exclusion of coverage of medical problems associated with the skin, urinary, pulmonary, and musculoskeletal systems.

---

[3] Fictitious name.

tact. As the activity, noise, and lighting remains fairly constant through the day and night, his sleep will be disrupted and he will have few cues to orient him to the passage of time.

> It is too easy to lie in bed just counting spots on the ceiling and allowing the mind to wander and sleep. I know. That's exactly what I did for months; but in my case, as I lay, being turned from side to side, it was the colorful parrots printed on the material covering the screens. I counted them so many times they eventually started flying.
>
> Michael Rogers (1986)

During the acute phase following spinal cord injury, a person is likely to experience sensory deprivation, social isolation, lack of time cues, sleep deprivation, and pain. He is likely to be on medications that have psychoactive effects. He may undergo surgery with general anesthesia. Any of these conditions *alone* can have a profound impact on cognitive functioning, emotions, and behavior (Brown & Hughson, 1987; Richards, Seitz, & Eisele, 1986; Trieschmann, 1986 & 1988). When faced with a recently injured person, it is difficult, if not impossible, for the health professional to determine which behaviors are the result of psychological reaction to spinal cord injury and which are due to other circumstances and physical variables.

Many of the conditions described above, particularly medication and sleep deprivation, may persist throughout and beyond rehabilitation. Additionally, during inpatient rehabilitation the cord-injured person may be bored (French, McDowell, & Keith, 1977) and is likely to find himself in an environment that encourages complacency and inactivity.

Cautionary Note. Many health professionals are quick to interpret any of a variety of behaviors as psychological reaction to spinal cord injury. Before making this judgment, health professionals should keep in mind the multiple factors that can impact on a recently injured person's cognitive functioning, emotions, and behavior. If someone who has recently sustained a spinal cord injury seems confused, is it the result of a psychological response to overwhelming loss? Is it a result of pain, medication, social isolation, or sensory deprivation? If he expresses anger, is this a manifestation of inner turmoil brought on by his injury, or could it be a reaction to demeaning treatment? Before dismissing behavior as "denial," "anger," "depression," or other psychological response to a spinal cord injury,

health professionals should consider other possible explanations for the behavior. Most importantly, they should attempt to discern whether anything in the physical or social environment could be contributing to the behavior in question.

Health professionals should also keep in mind the following humbling fact: research has demonstrated that as a group, we are not very good at determining our patients' moods. There is a strong tendency to view cord-injured patients as more depressed than they actually are (Howell, Fullerton, Harvey, & Klein, 1981; Lawson, 1978). Many people with spinal cord injuries report that they do not view their injuries as tragic or even as the worst thing that ever happened to them (Corbet, 1980; Trieschmann, 1986). Health professionals who view spinal cord injury in an overly catastrophic light are more likely to convey a defeatist and pitying attitude.

Psychological Adjustment/Adaptation Following Injury

Spinal cord injury causes significant losses in many areas: physical, functional, social, financial, personal identity, and world view. In general, the process of adjustment to these losses takes years (McGowan & Roth, 1987; Schneider, 1984; Trieschmann, 1988).

Until recently it was believed that people who sustained spinal cord injuries went through a specific series of mood states as they adjusted. Typically each patient was expected to experience shock, denial, depression, anger, dependency, and, finally, adjustment (Krueger, 1984a; Trieschmann, 1986). Although various theorists described slightly different stages of adjustment, it was generally agreed that adjustment required progression through these stages. Anyone who did not fit the pattern was not "doing it right."

Research in recent years has shown the stage theory of adjustment to be inaccurate (DeJong, Branch, & Corcoran, 1984; Trieschmann, 1986 & 1988). People do not progress through a neat series of mood states in a lock-step fashion as they adapt to life following spinal cord injury. Each adapts in his own way.

If people do not pass through a predictable and universal series of stages, what do they do? After spinal cord injury, as after any significant loss, people grieve. Each grieves, however, in his own way and at his own pace. A variety of factors influence the manner in which an individual handles the losses engendered by spinal cord injury. These include personal characteristics such as personality; cognitive style; values, attitudes, and psychological health prior to the injury; prior loss experiences; and age (Auvenshine & Noffsinger, 1984; Bracken, Shepard, & Webb, 1981; Carlson, 1979; Frank, Elliott, Buckelew, & Haut, 1988; Green, Pratt, & Grigsby, 1984; Servoss & Krueger, 1984; Trieschmann, 1988). The nature of the social support provided by loved ones and health professionals also has a strong influence on adaptation following cord injury (Auvenshine & Noffsinger, 1984; Green, Pratt, & Grigsby, 1984; Trieschmann, 1988). Finally, such factors as financial security,[4] education, and access to transportation impact on adjustment (Brown, Gordon, & Ragnarsson, 1987; Green, Pratt, & Grigsby, 1984; Trieschmann, 1988). Contrary to common assumptions, level of injury is not a significant factor; people with quadriplegia adjust as successfully as those with paraplegia (Goldberg & Freed, 1982; Green, Pratt, & Grigsby, 1984; Malec & Neimeyer, 1983).

Tasks of Grieving. Grieving involves more than a passive acceptance, "getting used to" a loss. It is an active process by which a person lets go of what has been lost and formulates a life without it.

Following spinal cord injury, a person may feel that he has literally lost everything. It may seem that all aspects of his life, his relationships, himself, and his future have been destroyed. But in grieving, he gradually gains perspective on his loss. One task of grieving involves sorting through his losses, identifying what aspects of his life and himself he has truly lost, and what remains. He can then let go of what he has lost and reclaim what remains (Servoss & Krueger, 1984).

In response to the loss of his old self-image, a cord-injured person forges a new identity (Gilliland & James, 1988; Tunks, Bahry, & Basbaum, 1986). This identity is "an amalgamation of all of the 'I am's' from pre-injury that are still relevant with the new 'I am's' that are consonant with the physical disability." (Trieschmann, 1988).

In a like manner, the cord-injured person discovers and develops a new lifestyle, with new goals and sources of satisfaction (Ducharme & Ducharme, 1984). By creating a new existence rather than holding onto the old, the person with a spinal cord injury can feel good about himself and his life.

Early Reactions to Spinal Cord Injury. After spinal cord injury, people commonly go through a period of confusion and forgetfulness. Often a newly in-

jured person appears to have difficulty processing information. For example, he may ask a question that he has already asked on several occasions and seem to have no memory of discussing the topic.[5] A newly injured health professional may ask questions or express beliefs that are inconsistent with his medical expertise.

In the past, the period of confusion that often follows spinal cord injury has been assumed to be a sign of denial. Lately, however, this assumption has been challenged. Sensory deprivation, social isolation, lack of time cues, sleep deprivation, pain, and medications are other possible explanations (Brown & Hughson, 1987; Richards, Seitz, & Eisele, 1986; Trieschmann, 1986 & 1988).

Research has not demonstrated that denial is the cause of the confused behavior commonly seen after injury. By the same token, research has not ruled out the occurrence of denial following spinal cord injury. If people do, in fact, grieve after sustaining spinal cord injuries, denial remains a possibility. Certainly the losses associated with spinal cord injury are on the magnitude of the loss of a loved one. When grieving such a loss, denial serves a purpose: it allows a person to rally his psychological and social resources and prepare himself for the loss. Denial is *not* a sign of pathology. It is a normal, healthy psychological response that makes it possible for the reality of a loss to sink in gradually as the person becomes able to cope (Krueger, 1984; Lindemann, 1981; Moses, 1989; Schneider, 1984).

Whether the confusion commonly seen following spinal cord injury is due to denial, other factors, or a combination remains to be determined. Whatever the source of the confused behavior, health professionals should recognize that recently injured people process information and deal with their losses as best they can. There is no benefit in attempting to force them to face reality (Decker, 1984).

Grief. After an initial period of confusion, whatever the source, people tend to grieve following spinal cord injury. Grief is a natural, healthy process by which a person adapts to a significant loss. It is not a linear process, with the person plodding through a series of stages one by one. People vary in the order, intensity, and length of time experiencing the various emotions associated with grieving. An in-

---

[4] Research has provided conflicting information on financial security. Green, Pratt, and Grigsby (1984) found that income and employment had no relation to self-concept following cord injury.

[5] At one time this author was incensed by the apparent fact that nobody was explaining to newly injured people anything about their injuries or prognoses. People who had been injured for months would ask, "Why can't I move my legs? Nobody has explained this to me." Eventually, however, I began hearing the same question from people to whom *I* had provided careful explanations in the early weeks following injury.

dividual may alternate rapidly between moods or "move past" a particular mood state, only to return at a later time[6] (Schneider, 1984).

A variety of emotions and behaviors are associated with grief. During normal grief following spinal cord injury, a person may experience any of the following: sadness, anger, hostility, anxiety, panic, and feelings of inadequacy, shame, helplessness, and vulnerability (Bracken, Shepard, & Webb, 1981; Ducharme & Ducharme, 1984). He may have periods of regression and self-neglect (Ducharme & Ducharme, 1984; Macleod, 1988). Many consider suicide, although few actually attempt it (Pinkerton & Griffin, 1983; Tunks, Bahry, & Basbaum, 1986). In normal grief after the death of a loved one, which is analogous to grief following spinal cord injury (Servoss & Krueger, 1984), a person may experience hallucinations, changes in sleep and appetite, forgetfulness, and social withdrawal (Worden, 1982).

It is important to make the distinction between grief, which is a normal and healthy response to loss, and clinical depression, which is pathological. True depression involves a specific, fairly global, and persistent pattern of emotions and behaviors.[7] Whereas most grieve after spinal cord injury, the majority do not exhibit true depression[8] (Howell, Fullerton, Harvey, & Klein, 1981; Malec & Neimeyer, 1983; Trieschmann, 1986 & 1988). Among those who become depressed, the depression is usually brief and mild and tends to occur within the first few months of injury (Howell, Fullerton, Harvey, & Klein, 1981; Richards, 1986; Trieschmann, 1986 & 1988).

Outcomes. Most people adapt well following spinal cord injury. After a period of adjustment, they tend to have positive self-concepts (Green, Pratt, & Grigsby, 1984) and in general are satisfied with life, neither more anxious (Carlson, 1979) nor more depressed (Richards, 1986) than noninjured people.

---

[6] This is true for denial, as well as for the various mood states of grieving (Moses, 1989).

[7] A person who is clinically depressed will exhibit at least four of the following almost every day for at least two weeks: (1) increase or decrease in appetite, (2) insomnia or hypersomnia, (3) psychomotor retardation or agitation, (4) loss of interest or pleasure in usual activities or decreased sex drive, (5) decreased energy or fatigue, (6) decreased ability to think or concentrate, or (7) recurrent thoughts of death or suicidal ideation (Trieschmann, 1988).

[8] The estimated frequency of true depression following spinal cord injury is 10% to 30% (Trieschmann, 1988). Interestingly, this frequency is comparable to the estimated incidence (10% to 20%) of clinical depression among widows one year following their husbands' deaths (Osterweis, Solomon, & Green, 1984).

We are the living demonstration that even if life circumstances become tough, life satisfaction can remain high. We're proof that things can be Hard, but Good. People need to know that.

Barry Corbet (1987)

Spinal cord injury is not a devastating catastrophe that leaves its victims forever bitter and psychologically impaired. In fact, for many it is a powerful stimulus for growth. Because it brings such profound losses, a spinal cord injury can shatter a person's identity and basic assumptions about himself and his world. In the aftermath of this disruption, it is possible for him to examine and alter his self-image and world view. Thus he has an opportunity to grow in ways in which he may otherwise never have grown, as these assumptions are rarely questioned except during times of crisis (Noyes, 1984).

It really changes your perspective. The one thing I really come back to is that I've gained an incredible sense of perspective—different people's realities, how relative the whole bit is. For that, I'm grateful.

John Galland (Corbet, 1980)

People often report that they have grown as a result of spinal cord injury. Some even state that they would not opt for a cure if it were available.

I'm happier now than I was before I broke my neck. I love my wife and my family more. I have a better rapport with people. I wasn't exactly a jerk when I was still walking, but I'm a better person now than I was before my disability. . . . if nothing else, this experience we have come to call disability has caused me to take a closer look at myself—at the nature of my existence.

I realize that it's not the physical impressions we make in life that endure, but the mental ones. I roll away knowing that I don't need a cure. I survived. And I'm proud of who I've become.

Ed Hooper (1989)

Although most adapt well after spinal cord injury and many grow from the experience, some do not fare so well. Depression, though not universal, is more prevalent among cord-injured people than in the general population (MacDonald, Nielson, &

Cameron, 1987). A small percentage exhibits self-neglect, even years following injury (MacLeod, 1988). A few find themselves unable to adapt to their disability and never regain a sense of happiness and satisfaction with their lives.

STRATEGIES FOR GROWTH

The purpose of rehabilitation after spinal cord injury is to enable a person to return to a lifestyle as near normal as possible. Teaching the physical skills needed to function independently is not enough to meet this end; living is more than getting in and out of bed and regulating bowels. These activities are not life—they are things that we do to live. To prepare a person to *live* with his disability, the rehabilitation team must focus beyond mere functional training and promote his psychosocial adaptation as well. This involves providing the needed support as he grieves his losses and develops a new identity, lifestyle, future, and world view. It also involves preparing him to function in a society that views him as less than he used to be.

The development of self-advocacy skills is a critical task of social adjustment after spinal cord injury. Disabled people are protected by law against discrimination in housing, transportation, and employment. Unfortunately these laws are not always enforced. If he is to function in society, a cord-injured person must be aware of his rights and know how to ensure that they are not violated.

Social adaptation after spinal cord injury involves more than the injured individual; the members of his family have significant adjustments of their own to make. When someone becomes disabled, there is disruption of his family's usual mode of functioning. Major changes are likely to occur in lifestyles, roles, communication patterns, and finances. The rehabilitation team can support the family as they learn to cope with these changes. In turn, the family will be better able to provide needed social support to the injured person as he adjusts to his disability.

Destructive Practices in Rehabilitation

Most, if not all, rehabilitation professionals would agree that they should (and do) work to prepare disabled people to live as independently as possible and to develop positive attitudes toward themselves and their lives. In practice, however, this is all too often not the case. While we teach the physical skills needed for independent functioning, we also teach people that they are second-class citizens, incapable or unworthy of self-direction or independence.

Dependence. From the moment a person sustains a spinal cord injury, he loses control of his life. He is handled, poked, prodded, examined, treated, and "done to" by an endless stream of health professionals as they care for his physical needs. Even once he reaches a rehabilitation unit, he is not likely to be treated in ways that enable him to regain control of his life. He is not given any real choices, being expected to conform to the goals and practices of the rehabilitation team. If his desires do not coincide with those of the team, and if he asserts himself, he is likely to be labeled "noncompliant" and a "difficult patient." Passive, compliant behavior is expected and rewarded (Lindemann, 1981; Tunks, Bahry, & Basbaum, 1986; Trieschmann, 1988).

Another harmful practice involves assisting people who are capable of performing an activity independently. This is often done for the sake of expedience. ("Yes, you worked hard in OT to learn how to dress yourself, but I'm going to dress you so that you won't be late for your appointment.") The underlying message is that the person can do the activity in therapy, but in *real life* he needs others to help him. In addition to receiving this negative message, the person is deprived of practice of the activity. His skill then does not develop as it should, he ultimately cannot perform the task as well or as quickly as he should, and he in fact ends up needing assistance.

Negative Attitudes. Many health professionals, being products of society at large, have negative attitudes about people with disabilities (Wright, 1988). These attitudes influence their behavior as they interact with their patients. By talking to a disabled adult as though he were a child or by talking about him in his presence as though he couldn't hear, the health professional dehumanizes and infantalizes him.

Labeling people by their disabilities is another way in which we dehumanize our patients. This practice is so accepted and widespread among health professionals that for many, it is hard to comprehend that there could be any harm in it. But language is very powerful. Anyone who has ever cringed at hearing a black person called "nigger" or a woman called "girl" knows this. The words we use express and perpetuate our values and attitudes. When we call a disabled person "patient" even when he is no longer a patient, we communicate the notion that he remains dependent on health professionals. When we label someone by his disabling condition, we focus attention on the disability rather than on the person. It then becomes easier to lose sight of the person himself.

Medical Model. The practices described above are symptomatic of the medical model of health care. In systems operating according to this model, there is a rigid hierarchy of power with physicians at the top, other health professionals in the middle, and patients and family members at the bottom. The job of the staff is to "fix" patients, and the patients are expected to accept that treatment passively (Chesler & Chesney, 1988; DeJong, 1979; Trieschmann, 1988). Health professionals are firmly in control. Even the clothes that they wear, laboratory coats and uniforms, express their authority (Gilliland & James, 1988). Rounds are likely to be conducted either in the patient's absence or at bedside, with the patient lying down (Halstead et al., 1986). Clearly a unit functioning according to the medical model does not provide an atmosphere that encourages those undergoing rehabilitation to exercise their autonomy.

Inherent in the medical model is the inferior, powerless status of the patient. Health professionals dominate all interactions. These practices and values are so ingrained in the medical community that the demeaning domination/subjugation inherent in these interactions is seen by many as appropriate professional/patient relations.

> The submissive and devaluing aspects of the role of patient are so frequently accepted by both patient and staff that some curious phenomena become apparent only when a person in a wheelchair enters a medical institution as a professional. On countless occasions, I have been wheeling along in treatment settings in various parts of the country, attending to my business as a teacher, researcher, or clinical psychologist, when an attendant or nurse would hustle alongside and challengingly or sarcastically say, "Hey, where do you think you're going?" or sometimes "You're not supposed to be out here—go to your room." On one occasion, solely on the basis of my occupancy of a wheelchair, a nurse tried physically to put me in bed! More than once my wheelchair has been hijacked by an attendant who, without comment, wheeled me to the dining room of his institution.
>
> Although I have no objection to consuming a free meal, in general, following one of the "You can't come here" comments or "You must go there" actions, I tactfully explain my business. Invariably the response is, "Oh, I'm sorry, I thought you were a patient!" There is immediate recognition by the staff member that his behavior toward me was inappropriate. But there does not seem to be the slightest trace of awareness that the same ordering, grabbing, and shoving would be inappropriate even if I were a patient.
>
> Nancy Kerr (1977)

A facility operating according to the medical model, with its emphasis on "treatments," "patients," and hospital attire, conveys the idea that the people receiving services are sick. This use of the medical model "serves the function of differentiating devalued clients from staff and society and imaging clients as diseased, contagious, impaired, incompetent, passive, and so on" (Wolfensberger & Tullman, 1982).

During rehabilitation, people are often exposed to practices and attitudes that convey to them that they are dependent, sick, incapable of running their own lives, and less than fully human. These messages of dependence and dehumanization may be particularly destructive to a newly injured person. At a time when he is piecing together a new identity, he is likely to be more vulnerable to feedback from others about who he is now that he is disabled. This may be especially true when the feedback comes from health professionals, "experts" on disabled people.

Constructive Practices in Rehabilitation

Within the social environment of a hospital or rehabilitation center, there is a massive potential for breaking anyone's spirit. There is also great potential for healing and growth. For the latter to occur, the health care team must consciously and consistently pursue this goal. From day 1, from the scene of the accident on, the cord-injured person must be treated as the thinking, feeling, autonomous person that he is. Instead of relentlessly stripping him of his power and dignity, all members of the team must treat him with respect and support his right to self-determination.

Normalization. Normalization (also called social role valorization) is a philosophy of human service delivery that is highly applicable to physical rehabilitation. It is based on the recognition that certain groups of people are devalued in our society, that these groups are subject to discriminatory treatment, and that service delivery systems often perpetuate and reinforce the devaluation of and discrimination against those whom they serve. The normalization movement focuses on rectifying these problems, using "culturally valued means in order to enable, establish, and/or maintain valued social roles for people" (Wolfensberger & Tullman, 1982).

One facet of normalization addresses the characteristics of the individuals receiving services. Assisting a person to attain or maintain socially valued roles includes enhancing both his image and level of competence. If a member of a devalued group (in this case, someone who has a visible physical disability) projects an image and displays skills (social, intellectual, vocational, etc.) that are valued in our society, he will be afforded greater value. Enhancement of image and competencies can create a positive cycle: someone who projects a valued image is likely to be perceived by others as more competent, and someone who exhibits competence is likely to be seen in a more positive light (Wolfensberger & Tullman, 1982; Yuker, 1988).

Although normalization principles include addressing individuals' characteristics, this is not the main focus of the movement. Normalization is unique among human service philosophies in that it focuses on "fixing" service delivery systems. The manner in which services are delivered, and the characteristics of the service delivery organizations themselves, affect the image of the people receiving those services (Flynn, 1981; Wolfensberger & Tullman, 1982). For example, a vocational training program for people with disabilities that labels them "patients" and segregates them from able-bodied trainees will have a negative impact on the social value of those being "served" by the program.

Often unconscious motivations can taint services that are well meaning and, on the surface, good (Wolfensberger & Tullman, 1982). For example, a rehabilitation unit sponsored a race that included both able-bodied runners and disabled athletes using wheelchairs. (So far so good.) At the awards ceremony after the race, the able-bodied runners received such prizes as athletic equipment and gift certificates from athletic stores. The disabled athlete received a lap blanket. On the surface, the race would seem to be an event that could work to enhance the image of the disabled participants and of disabled people in general. However, one seemingly minor detail in the event, the nature of the awards, could cause the opposite to occur.

Being members of a society in which people with physical disabilities are devalued, rehabilitation personnel are likely to have some negative attitudes about disabled people. Though these attitudes tend to remain beneath the surface, unconscious motivations can sabotage good intentions. For this reason, careful and honest self-scrutiny is required if we wish to provide services in a manner that will enhance rather than depreciate the social value of those served. Normalization-based evaluation tools such as PASS (Wolfensberger & Glenn, 1978) and PASSING[9] (Wolfensberger & Thomas, 1983) can provide guidance for this self-evaluation and for program planning.

Independence/Autonomy. To adapt successfully after spinal cord injury, a person must gain (or retain) a sense of personal effectiveness and control over his life. For this to occur, he must be provided with the opportunity to make choices throughout his acute care and rehabilitation. He should be given true control, not just the opportunity to choose between compliance and noncompliance. From the day of his injury onward, he should be provided with information about his condition and treatment options and should be given a voice in setting goals, scheduling activities, and making decisions about his care.

To promote independence, the rehabilitation team should include the cord-injured person in problem solving. With guidance and encouragement, he can participate in analyzing problems, coming up with possible solutions, and evaluating outcomes. This can be done while learning functional skills, deciding on bowel and bladder management practices, choosing between equipment options, and determining virtually any aspect of his care. By participating in problem solving in this manner, the cord-injured person can develop his ability to problem solve on his own. This skill will prove invaluable to his independent functioning during and subsequent to rehabilitation.

Independent functioning also requires a sense of personal responsibility. To live independently, a person must know what to do and when to do it and must take the initiative to get things done. For this sense of responsibility to develop during rehabilitation, the cord-injured person should be given as much responsibility as possible for his rehabilitation. He should know his schedule and be accountable for getting to his various activities, either under his own power or by asking for assistance when needed. Once in therapy, he should be encouraged to initiate exercises or functional practice without waiting to be told what to do. The same kind of initiative can be encouraged in his personal care, such as pressure reliefs, morning hygiene, and bowel and bladder programs. From the time of his initial hospitalization onward, he should be ex-

---

[9] These manuals and information about training in their use are available from the Person to Person Citizen Advocacy Association, 501 E. Fayette Street, Syracuse, NY; (315) 472-9190.

pected to take as much responsibility for himself as he can, with increasing expectations of independent functioning as he progresses in his rehabilitation.

Positive Atmosphere. While a person is forging a new identity following spinal cord injury, the physical and social environment of the rehabilitation center can have a powerful impact. A prevailing climate of gloom and tragedy conveys a sense of hopelessness and despair to all involved: those undergoing rehabilitation, family members, friends, and health professionals. A more positive atmosphere will encourage the development of a more optimistic outlook.

The physical environment in a rehabilitation setting is important. Dark corridors and institutional decor convey a feel of sickness and debilitation. At the other extreme, a saccharine and childlike atmosphere communicates a sense of dependence and childishness. Upbeat, age-appropriate decor and music will provide a more positive environment for rehabilitation.

Staff attire also contributes to the atmosphere of a rehabilitation center. Uniforms and laboratory coats help create a hospital-like atmosphere, with all of its connotations of illness and power hierarchies. Likewise, the dress of those undergoing rehabilitation is important. Pajamas are appropriate attire for people who are either sick or asleep. Certainly they are inappropriate for conferences, therapies, or any other activities that take place outside of an individual's room.

Another element in a rehabilitation setting's atmosphere is the activity level of those undergoing rehabilitation. Long, empty hours in the days and evenings can deaden the spirit. Meaningful activity can provide a sense of purpose and personal control (Gilliland & James, 1988). Active participation in therapies and recreational activities can also reduce boredom, promote better sleep at night (Trieschmann, 1986), and facilitate the grieving process (Schneider, 1984).

In working to create a positive atmosphere, the rehabilitation team should focus on abilities rather than on impairments. Too often health practitioners concern themselves with the problems while ignoring the strengths of those whom they serve (Wright, 1988). To convey a greater sense of optimism, the rehabilitation team should emphasize what a person *can* do rather than dwelling on what he *cannot* do. In discussions during conferences, problem-solving sessions, and informal interactions, the focus can be placed on abilities and accomplishments. During therapies and other activities, the cord-injured person should be provided with activities that are structured in such a way that he can experience success and see his accomplishments. Success experiences can go far to improve motivation (Gilliland & James, 1988) and develop a sense of mastery and control (Tunks, Bahry, & Basbaum, 1986).

At the same time, people undergoing rehabilitation should be encouraged to take risks (Park, 1977). If an individual's goals and activities are limited to those in which he is certain to succeed, functional progress will be limited. Perhaps more importantly, this overprotectiveness communicates to him and others that he is not capable of coping with possible failure. A person who is "protected" from risk may never develop the self-confidence and experience the psychological growth that comes from challenging one's limits.

> There is human dignity in risk. There can be dehumanizing indignity in safety.
> Irving Zola (1982)

Interactions With Staff. Interactions with the staff are critical in rehabilitation. The values and attitudes that health professionals communicate can serve to demean or to support growth. To foster the development of a positive self-image, all members of the rehabilitation team must treat the cord-injured person as an equal, worthy of respect.[10] This respect should be evident in formal interactions, such as in conferences, as well as in informal daily communication.

Demeaning language should be avoided at all times, even when only health professionals are present. Referring to groups or individuals by their diagnoses serves to reinforce a negative attitude among those present.

Finally, it is imperative for rehabilitation personnel to maintain appropriate "professional" relations with people undergoing rehabilitation. This does not mean that interactions should be cold and formal or patterned on the dominance/submission relations inherent in the medical model. Rather the relationship should have clearly defined and mutually understood boundaries. A newly injured person who becomes too attached to a health professional may grow dependent on that person. Likewise, a health professional who becomes overly involved with someone undergoing rehabilitation may not act in that person's best interests, pro-

---

[10] In addition to benefiting those undergoing rehabilitation, equal-status interactions can benefit the staff by promoting the development of more positive attitudes. Equal-status contact is necessary for the development of positive attitudes toward those with disabilities (Geskie & Salasek, 1988).

longing rehabilitation unnecessarily and encouraging dependence (Ducharme & Ducharme, 1984). In an appropriate professional relationship, mutual respect, caring, and enjoyment can coexist with an understanding of the relationship's limits.

Social Support. Social support can enhance a person's capacity to cope and recover following loss (Cobb, 1976; Osterweis, Solomon, & Green, 1984; Schneider, 1984). The rehabilitation team can promote emotional recovery and growth after spinal cord injury by providing this support. Health professionals should listen to people as they air their feelings, helping them to clarify their emotions and reassuring them that their feelings are normal. Staff should listen with empathy, not pity, and avoid judging what they hear (Gilliland & James, 1988; Hoff, 1989; Schneider, 1984; Tunks, Bahry, & Basbaum, 1986). This support should be available from all members of the team, not just from the psychiatric or counseling staff.

Each individual should be allowed to grieve in his own way; staff members must not impose their own notions of how people should feel and act following spinal cord injury. The cord-injured person should neither be required to mourn nor be rushed to complete his grieving prematurely.

Hope. Health professionals have conflicting attitudes about hope. On the one hand, expressions of hope may be labeled as "denial" and seen as signs of failure to cope with reality. On the other hand, health professionals are often reluctant to provide newly injured people with information in the fear that the truth will crush all hope.

Neither hope nor denial are necessarily bad, as long as they do not interfere with an individual's progress in psychosocial and functional adaptation after injury. In fact, hope can help a person cope with his disability.

> Hope is the most potent of medicines, one that can heal and rejuvenate. Referenced in the future, grounded in the past, and experienced in the present, it involves the expectation that life will be a little more meaningful tomorrow. Hope is essential in any struggle with a major disability or catastrophic illness.
>
> Joan Mader (1988)

While hope has its benefits, information is critical to adjustment after a spinal cord injury. Knowledge, even if unpleasant, can help a person with an illness or disability regain a sense of control of his

life (Brockopp, Hayko, Davenport, & Winscott, 1989; Northouse & Northouse, 1985). Anyone who asks a question has the right to get an honest answer; feigned ignorance and vague or inaccurate answers are not helpful responses.

> The truth is better than telling a patient that he will be fine tomorrow. For tomorrow never comes, and the long-term depressive effect will be greater if the truth is withheld.
>
> Michael Rogers (1986)

Although health professionals should provide honest information, they should do so in a way that does not destroy all hope (Decker, 1984; Trieschmann, 1986). Perhaps it is best to speak in terms of probabilities rather than absolutes. In truth, we rarely have definitive answers anyway. Who can predict with certainty whether a particular individual will get neurological return, father a child, or walk again?

Educational Model. Many of the growth-enhancing practices described above are inherent in an educational model of rehabilitation. Using this model, health professionals and people undergoing rehabilitation work as partners in pursuit of mutually agreed-upon goals. The model relationship is one of teacher–student[11] rather than healer–patient. This nonmedical orientation conveys the attitude that those undergoing rehabilitation are not sick. This understanding is crucial to coping with a disabling condition (Judd & Brown, 1987).

In the educational model, people undergoing rehabilitation are expected to be active participants in designing, carrying out, and evaluating their programs. Respect for the individual is inherent in this model. Emphasis is placed on consumerism and autonomous functioning rather than on compliance. Clearly this approach is superior to the medical model in fostering independence and growth (Trieschmann, 1986 & 1988).

A rehabilitation team attempting to implement a program structured on the educational model should keep in mind the fact that it is likely to run counter to their natural tendencies. Having grown up in society in which disabilities are strongly stigmatized, health professionals are likely to hold negative attitudes about people undergoing rehabilitation. In addition, most of their professional training and practice is likely to have been in delivery systems based on the medical model. Thus many prac-

---

[11] Teacher–*Adult* student.

tices inherent in the medical model (and contrary to the educational model) may go unquestioned.

Because the educational model is likely to run counter to the natural tendencies of health professionals, its implementation requires careful scrutiny and vigilance. All members of the team, and the team as a whole, must take a close look at their own behavior and practices. In *all* formal and informal interactions, health professionals must approach the individuals undergoing rehabilitation with an attitude of respect and equality. All aspects of the social and physical environment must be examined for consistency with the educational model.

Formal Strategies

Personal control, a positive atmosphere, and supportive and respectful interaction provide the necessary foundation for rehabilitation. Additional strategies that can be used to promote growth and adaptation after spinal cord injury are presented below. These include various approaches to dealing with the personal loss and changes in family dynamics, as well as strategies aimed at successful reintegration into society.

Evaluation. Individuals and their families are highly variable in their responses to the life changes brought on by spinal cord injury. Thus the psychosocial interventions that are most appropriate will vary. For this reason, evaluation is the logical starting point of planning the psychosocial component of a rehabilitation program (Judd & Brown, 1987 & 1988; Malec & Neimeyer, 1983). An initial evaluation should be performed soon after injury, since many may benefit from intervention during their acute hospitalization (Bracken, Shepard, & Webb, 1981). Once an evaluation has been completed, a program can be designed that best meets the needs of a particular individual and his family. Subsequent evaluations will make it possible to alter the program as the needs change.

The psychosocial evaluation can address the cord-injured person's personality structure, coping styles and ability to cope with the cord injury, current level of distress and depression, and past history of interpersonal relations, loss, psychiatric illness, and substance abuse. The assessment can also include an investigation of the family's communication patterns, coping styles, and level of distress (Heinemann, Donohue, & Schnoll, 1988; Judd & Brown, 1987 & 1988; Malec & Neimeyer, 1983).

The evaluation results can provide the cord-injured person, his family, and health professionals with a better understanding of the individual's and family's reactions to the injury and its sequelae. It can also alert them to potential areas of future difficulty. The cord-injured person, his family, and rehabilitation professionals can then work together to identify problems, set goals, and develop a plan of action.

Education. Education provides a critical foundation for psychosocial rehabilitation. To maintain or regain control of his life following spinal cord injury, a person must first have an understanding of his body's altered functioning and of strategies for avoiding complications and promoting health. Without this understanding, he will be unable to participate fully in his rehabilitation program planning or to take responsibility for his self-care.

Education regarding the physical sequelae of spinal cord injury is just a start. Instruction (forewarning) regarding what social problems may arise at home or in the community after discharge can better prepare a person and his family for this transition. To function in society, a disabled person needs to know about his legal rights and available resources in the community. He will also require financial management skills. Those who require attendant care must know how to obtain and manage attendants (Gilliland & James, 1988; Trieschmann, 1988).

Education can take the form of lectures, discussions, audiovisual presentations, and printed material. Inclusion of family members can enhance their capacity to provide constructive support to the cord-injured person during and following rehabilitation (Rohrer et al., 1980).

Counseling. Recovering, adapting, and growing after spinal cord injury involves coming to terms with a host of losses, developing a new self-concept, and often redefining roles within a family. Social support can facilitate this process. For many, counseling is an important source of this support.

Group counseling provides an arena for people to discuss their experiences with others who have sustained spinal cord injuries. In this exchange there is opportunity for the expression of emotions, enhancement of self-awareness, mutual encouragement, exchange of information, role modeling, examination and expansion of values and perceptions, feedback, and problem solving. Participation in group work may enhance motivation, normal grief resolution, and overall adjustment to the spinal cord injury (Gilliland & James, 1988; Lasky, Dell Orto, & Marinelli, 1977; Moeller & Hartman, 1984; Worden, 1982).

Family members can be included in group counseling, either in "family groups" with other families or in family or marital therapy. Family adjustment is important not only for the benefit of the family members but for the adaptation of the cord-injured person himself. In a group setting, families of people with spinal cord injuries can gain information, express and come to grips with their emotions, give and receive support, grow in their attitudes regarding disability, develop more constructive communication patterns, and learn new coping strategies (Gilliland & James, 1988; Judd & Brown, 1988; McGowan & Roth, 1987; Moeller & Hartman, 1984; Tunks, Bahry, & Basbaum, 1986). Group counseling need not be limited to disabled people and their families; other members of a disabled person's social support system may be included (Hoff, 1989).

Some cord-injured people and their family members also benefit from individual counseling. In one-on-one counseling, a person may receive more individualized support and more assistance with grieving, clarification of intrapsychic and interpersonal conflicts, and the development of new coping skills. Individual counseling is especially (but not exclusively) indicated when a person feels overwhelmed by his emotions, exhibits signs of pathology, or has a personal or family history of early or unresolved loss, psychiatric illness, substance abuse, or difficulty with interpersonal relations (Decker, 1984; Hoff, 1989; Judd & Brown, 1988; Macleod, 1988; Osterweis, Solomon, & Green, 1984; Servoss & Krueger, 1984; Worden, 1982).

Social Skills Training. Reintegration into society is an important aspect of psychosocial adaptation after spinal cord injury. The social devaluation of disabled people can present a formidable barrier to this reintegration. Following spinal cord injury, an individual is likely to find that people are uncomfortable around him. As a result, he may find it difficult to meet people or to maintain old friendships.

Fortunately there are things that a disabled person can do to lessen the negative impact of his disability on interactions with others. By projecting a positive self-image and putting others at ease, he can enhance the quality of his interactions with non-disabled people and facilitate a positive change in their attitudes (Cogswell, 1977; Haney & Rabin, 1984; Trieschmann, 1988; Yuker, 1988). These behaviors can be acquired in social skills training.

Social skills training involves learning stigma management strategies: verbal and nonverbal behaviors that can improve the quality of interactions with others. These communication techniques center primarily around putting others at ease and establishing rapport during initial encounters. Typical strategies include acknowledging the disability, legitimizing curiosity, providing information, answering questions, behaving assertively, and projecting a positive self-image and acceptance of the disability (Cogswell, 1977; Fichten, 1988; Horne, 1988; Trieschmann, 1988; Yuker, 1988).

A variety of approaches can be used for social skills training. Through videotapes, lectures, and discussions, people can be introduced to the concept of stigma management and can gain some ideas on behavior that will help or hinder their interactions with others. Actual practice of communication techniques is helpful in the development of these skills. Feedback from others can alert people to behaviors that they display that may impede interactions and can help them to hone their communication skills (English, 1977; Trieschmann, 1988).

Recreation Training. Many people who become disabled find themselves unable to participate in the recreational activities to which they were previously accustomed. This represents a significant loss; leisure activities are an important source of pleasure, personal pride, relaxation, physical wellness, and social support. Through recreation training, a person can learn ways to resume many of his previous activities or find alternative leisure activities. Resumption of an active leisure life can promote physical and psychological health and can provide an avenue for reintegration into society (Brown & Hughson, 1987). By including spouses in leisure training, the team can assist couples in finding activities that they can enjoy together. This may in turn have a beneficial effect on marital relations (Urey & Henggeler, 1987).

Pharmaceutical Treatment. People exhibit a variety of emotions as they grieve their losses following spinal cord injury. Often these emotions are unpleasant, both to experience and to witness. For this reason, it can be tempting to medicate people to lessen their (and our) discomfort (Decker, 1984). Although pharmaceutical treatment can be beneficial in cases of clinical depression or psychosis (Macleod, 1988; Trieschmann, 1988), it is not indicated for normal grief reactions. Medication aimed at ameliorating emotional pain can impede a person's ability to work through his loss (Morgan, 1980; Schneider, 1984).

Postdischarge Strategies. When a recently disabled person leaves a rehabilitation center, his adjustment has just begun. During rehabilitation he has gained knowledge and skills required for living in the community. Upon returning home, however, he finds that he has more to learn. In addition, he is faced with the challenging task of applying his new knowledge and skills in his daily life at home and in the community.

Because adaptation and growth after spinal cord injury do not end at discharge, people can benefit from continued psychosocial support after completing their initial rehabilitation. Any of the strategies described above can be used either during inpatient rehabilitation or following discharge. Additional strategies specific to people living in the community are presented below.

One approach that can be beneficial is to put a recently disabled person in contact with an individual who lives in his community and has adjusted successfully following spinal cord injury. The "veteran" can share information and coping strategies and can provide support to the recently injured person and his family (Trieschmann, 1988). This approach has been shown to facilitate adjustment of recently widowed women (Vachon, Lyall, Rogers, Freedman-Letofsky, & Freeman, 1980).

Self-help groups can also facilitate adjustment and growth after spinal cord injury. True self-help groups are comprised of *and run by* people with common experiences (Jaques & Patterson, 1977), in this case spinal cord injuries. The focus and structure of self-help groups vary, depending on the needs and priorities of the membership. Groups may concern themselves with any or all of the following: education (of members, health professionals, or society at large), fund raising, sharing emotions, mutual social support, recreation, or social action. Individuals participating in self-help groups can gain information, new coping skills, and an increased sense of personal responsibility for their health and social well-being. Self-help groups can also be a source of affirmation, foster a sense of belonging, and provide motivation and reinforcement for successful coping. Perhaps most importantly, self-help groups are empowering for the participants as individuals and as a group (Chesler & Chesney, 1988; Hoff, 1989; Jaques & Patterson, 1977; Osterweis, Solomon, & Green, 1984).

> I think the group support lets you be strong together; the group gives you that real sense of strength and optimism and resilience that most people don't have by themselves . . .
>
> Judy Heumann (Maddox, 1987)

Independent living centers located (sparsely) throughout the United States provide a variety of services to people with disabilities. These services can include logistical assistance with equipment repair, home modification, attendant services, and financial counseling. Independent living centers can also provide legal advocacy and peer counseling (DeJong, 1979; Trieschmann, 1988). Many centers engage in disability rights activism (Maddox, 1987). The independent living movement focuses on improving the quality of life of disabled people by increasing architectural and transportation accessibility and by obtaining services that enable people to function independently in the community (DeJong, 1979).

Vocational rehabilitation and formal education can also facilitate psychosocial adjustment after spinal cord injury. Education and vocational training can enhance a person's self-confidence, increase his chances of obtaining gainful employment, and promote social interaction (El Ghatit & Hanson, 1979). Since education and employment are valued characteristics in our society, they can serve to increase an individual's social status, facilitating his reintegration into society.

Psychological healing and growth and social adaptation to life with a disability can continue for years. In essence, they continue for the remainder of a person's life (Trieschmann, 1988) as new issues and challenges continue to surface through the years. Rehabilitation professionals can aid the process following discharge by including a psychosocial evaluation in routine follow-up visits (Judd & Brown, 1988) and by referring people to appropriate services and resources available in the community.

THE BIGGER PICTURE: OUR IMPACT ON THE COMMUNITY

As rehabilitation professionals, our function is to facilitate adjustment and reentry into society after the acquisition of a disabling condition. Traditionally, to reach this end we have placed our focus exclusively on disabled people themselves, teaching them various physical and social skills needed for living with a disability. The other side of the equation, society, has been largely ignored. The assumption underlying this approach is that the problem of disability lies in those who are disabled rather than in society itself. In recent years, however, the disability rights movement has asserted that people are handicapped not by their physical conditions but by negative attitudes and barriers in transportation, architecture, employment, and public assistance programs (Brown, Gordon, & Ragnarsson, 1987; DeJong, 1979; DeJong, Branch, & Corcoran, 1984). When disablement is seen in this light, it follows that we should direct attention to our impact on society rather than solely concerning ourselves with disabled individuals.

One area with which we must concern ourselves is the devalued status of disabled people in our society. Our attention in this area is imperative because of the powerful impact that rehabilitation professionals have on society's attitudes. By our actions and inactions, by what we say and do, and by the nature of our service delivery systems, we can strengthen or weaken the stigmatizing attitudes of those around us and of society at large.

As health care professionals, we are seen as experts on people with spinal cord injuries and other disabling conditions. How we portray these people can influence others' attitudes. Our communication about people with spinal cord injuries occurs in a variety of situations, from casual social encounters ("You work with cripples? You must be soooo patient.") to interviews with television or newspaper reporters. Any discussion relating to people with disabilities presents an opportunity to either reinforce devaluing attitudes and beliefs or to portray a more positive picture.

The characteristics of the services that we provide can also impact positively or negatively society's attitudes. Such details as an agency's physical setting, name, logo, and funding sources convey messages about those receiving services (Wolfensberger & Tullman, 1982). Normalization-based evaluation tools such as PASS (Wolfensberger & Glenn, 1978) and PASSING (Wolfensberger & Thomas, 1983) can provide guidance for programs attempting to convey positive images of their clientele.

Professional responsibility dictates that rehabilitation professionals direct attention to their impact on society's perceptions of people with disabilities. Additionally, some may choose to promote change through political action. Much work is needed in the areas of architectural barriers in the community, accessible housing, accessible transportation, and discriminatory practices and legislation (English, 1977; Trieschmann, 1988; Wright, 1978).

SUMMARY

Anyone who sustains a spinal cord injury is faced with major losses, ranging from changes in his physique and functional ability to disruption of his relationships, financial security, and future plans. His former self-image no longer fits. He has become a member of a devalued and disadvantaged minority, "the disabled." Psychosocial adjustment after spinal cord injury involves coming to terms with these losses, formulating a new identity, and learning communication skills needed for returning to life in his family and in society.

Most people with spinal cord injuries are able to adjust satisfactorily, and many even grow from the experience. A minority remains unable to adapt. Whether an individual grows from or succumbs to his disability can be influenced by the support that he receives during and after rehabilitation. To promote growth and adaptation following spinal cord injury, the rehabilitation team must support the cord-injured person as he comes to terms with his disability. Attention must also be directed to empowering him; *all* interactions must be based on respect, equality, and mutuality. Additional formal strategies for enhancing psychosocial adaptation include education, counseling, social skills training, recreation training, pharmaceutical treatment, and a variety of postdischarge strategies.

REFERENCES

Auvenshine, C., & Noffsinger, A. (1984). *Counseling: An introduction for the health and human services*. Baltimore: University Park Press.

Bracken, M., Shepard, M., & Webb, S. (1981). Psychological response to acute spinal cord injury: An epidemiological study. *Paraplegia, 19*, 271–283.

Brockopp, D., Hayko, D., Davenport, W., & Winscott, S. (1989). Personal control and the needs for hope and information among adults diagnosed with cancer. *Cancer Nursing, 12*(2), 112–116.

Brown, M., Gordon, W., & Ragnarsson, K. (1987). Unhandicapping the disabled: What is possible? *Archives of Physical Medicine and Rehabilitation, 68*, 206–209.

Brown, R., & Hughson, E. (1987). *Behavioral and social rehabilitation and training*. New York: Wiley.

Carlson, C. (1979). Conceptual style and life satisfaction following spinal cord injury. *Archives of Physical Medicine and Rehabilitation, 60*, 346–352.

Chesler, M., & Chesney, B. (1988). Self-help groups: Empowerment attitudes and behaviors of disabled or chronically ill persons. In H. Yuker (Ed.), *Attitudes toward persons with disabilities* (pp. 230–245). New York: Springer Publishing.

Cobb, S. (1976). Social support as a moderator of life stress. *Psychosomatic Medicine, 38*(5), 300–313.

Cogswell, B. (1977). Self-socialization: Readjustment of paraplegics in the community. In R. Marinelli & A. Dell Orto (Eds.), *The psychological and social impact of physical disability* (pp. 151–159). New York: Springer Publishing.

Corbet, B. (1987). Options revisited. In S. Maddox (Ed.), *Spinal network*. Boulder, CO: Spinal Network.

Corbet, B. (1980). *Options: Spinal cord injury and the future*. Denver, CO: A. B. Hirschfeld Press.

Decker, N. (1984). Brief psychotherapy of chronic illness. In D. Krueger (Ed.), *Emotional rehabilitation of physical trauma and disability* (pp. 195–218). New York: SP Medical & Scientific Books.

DeJong, G. (1979). Independent living: From social movement to analytic paradigm. *Archives of Physical Medicine and Rehabilitation, 60,* 435–446.

DeJong, G., Branch, L., & Corcoran, P. (1984). Independent living outcomes in spinal cord injury: Multivariate analyses. *Archives of Physical Medicine and Rehabilitation, 65,* 66–73.

DeVivo, M., & Fine, P. (1982). Employment status of spinal cord injured patients 3 years after injury. *Archives of Physical Medicine and Rehabilitation, 63,* 200–203.

Ducharme, S. & Ducharme, J. (1984). Psychological adjustment to spinal cord injury. In D. Krueger (Ed.), *Emotional rehabilitation of physical trauma and disability* (pp. 149–156). New York: SP Medical & Scientific Books.

El Ghatit, A., & Hanson, R. (1979). Educational and training levels and employment of the spinal cord injured patient. *Archives of Physical Medicine and Rehabilitation, 60,* 405–406.

English, R. (1977). Combating stigma toward physically disabled persons. In R. Marinelli & A. Dell Orto (Eds.), *The psychological and social impact of physical disability* (pp. 183–193). New York: Springer Publishing.

Fichten, C. (1988). Students with physical disabilities in higher education: Attitudes and beliefs that affect integration. In H. Yuker (Ed.), *Attitudes toward persons with disabilities* (pp. 171–186). New York: Springer Publishing.

Flynn, R. (1981). Normalization, social integration, and sex behavior: A service approach and evaluation method for improving rehabilitation programs. In A. Sha'ked (Ed.), *Human sexuality and rehabilitation medicine: Sexual functioning following spinal cord injury* (pp. 37–66). Baltimore: Williams & Wilkins.

Frank, R., Elliott, T., Buckelew, S., & Haut, A. (1988). Age as a factor in response to spinal cord injury. *American Journal of Physical Medicine and Rehabilitation, 67*(3), 128–131.

French, D., McDowell, R., & Keith, R. (1977). Participant observation as a patient in a rehabilitation hospital. In R. Marinelli & A. Dell Orto (Eds.), *The psychological and social impact of physical disability* (pp. 289–296). New York: Springer Publishing.

Gellman, W. (1977). Projections in the field of physical disability. In R. Marinelli & A. Dell Orto (Eds.), *The psychological and social impact of physical disability* (pp. 34–48). New York: Springer Publishing.

Geskie, M., & Salasek, J. (1988). Attitudes of health care personnel toward persons with disabilities. In H. Yuker (Ed.), *Attitudes toward persons with disabilities* (pp. 187–200). New York: Springer Publishing.

Gilliland, B., & James, R. (1988). *Crisis intervention strategies*. Pacific Grove, CA: Brooks/Cole Publishing.

Goldberg, R., & Freed, M. (1982). Vocational development of spinal cord injury patients: An 8-year follow-up. *Archives of Physical Medicine and Rehabilitation, 63,* 207–210.

Green, B., Pratt, C., & Grigsby, T. (1984). Self-concept among persons with long-term spinal cord injury. *Archives of Physical Medicine and Rehabilitation, 65,* 751–754.

Halstead, L., Rintala, D., Kanellos, M., Griffin, B., Higgins, L., Rheinecker, S., Whiteside, W., & Healy, J. (1986). The innovative rehabilitation team: An experiment in team building. *Archives of Physical Medicine and Rehabilitation, 67,* 357–361.

Haney, M., & Rabin, B. (1984). Modifying attitudes toward disabled persons while resocializing spinal cord injured patients. *Archives of Physical Medicine and Rehabilitation, 65,* 431–436.

Heinemann, A., Donohue, R., & Schnoll, S. (1988). Alcohol use by persons with recent spinal cord injury. *Archives of Physical Medicine and Rehabilitation, 69,* 619–624.

Hoff, L. (1989). *People in crisis: Understanding and helping*. Redwood City, CA: Addison-Wesley Publishing.

Hooper, E. (1989). If the cure came tomorrow, would I want it? *Spinal Network, Spring 1989,* 50–52.

Horne, M. (1988). Modifying peer attitudes toward the handicapped: Procedures and research issues. In H. Yuker (Ed.), *Attitudes toward persons with disabilities* (pp. 203–222). New York: Springer Publishing.

Howell, T., Fullerton, D., Harvey, R., & Klein, M. (1981). Depression in spinal cord injured patients. *Paraplegia, 19,* 284–288.

Jaques, M., & Patterson, K. (1977). The self-help group model: A review. In R. Marinelli & A. Dell Orto (Eds.), *The psychological and social impact of physical disability* (pp. 270–281). New York: Springer Publishing.

Judd, F., & Brown, D. (1988). The psychosocial approach to rehabilitation of the spinal cord injured patient. *Paraplegia, 26,* 419–424.

Judd, F., & Brown, D. (1987). Psychiatry in the spinal injuries unit. *Paraplegia, 25,* 254–257.

Kerr, N. (1977). Staff expectations for disabled persons: Helpful or harmful. In R. Marinelli & A. Dell Orto (Eds.), *The psychological and social impact of physical disability* (pp. 342–350). New York: Springer Publishing.

Krueger, D. (1984). Emotional rehabilitation: An overview. In D. Krueger (Ed.), *Emotional rehabilitation of physical trauma and disability* (pp. 3–12). New York: SP Medical & Scientific Books.

Krueger, D. (1984a). Psychological rehabilitation of physical trauma and disability. In D. Krueger (Ed.), *Rehabilitation psychology: A comprehensive textbook* (pp. 3–13). Rockville, MD: Aspen Publishers.

Lasky, R., Dell Orto, A., & Marinelli, R. (1977). Structured experimental therapy: A group approach to rehabilitation. In R. Marinelli & A. Dell Orto (Eds.), *The psychological and social impact of physical disability* (pp. 319–333). New York: Springer Publishing.

Lawson, N. (1978). Significant events in the rehabilitation process: The spinal cord patient's point of view. *Archives of Physical Medicine and Rehabilitation, 59,* 573–579.

Lindemann, J. (1981). *Psychological and behavioral aspects of physical disability: A manual for health practitioners.* New York: Plenum Press.

MacDonald, M., Nielson, W., & Cameron, M. (1987). Depression and activity patterns of spinal cord injured persons living in the community. *Archives of Physical Medicine and Rehabilitation, 68,* 339–342.

Macleod, A. (1988). Self-neglect of spinal injured patients. *Paraplegia, 26,* 340–349.

Mader, J. (1988). The importance of hope. *RN, 51*(12), 17–18.

Maddox, S. (1987). *Spinal network.* Boulder, CO: Spinal Network.

Malec, J., & Neimeyer, R. (1983). Psychological prediction of duration of inpatient spinal cord injury rehabilitation and performance of self-care. *Archives of Physical Medicine and Rehabilitation, 64,* 359–363.

McCarthy, H. (1988). Attitudes that affect employment opportunities for persons with disabilities. In H. Yuker (Ed.), *Attitudes toward persons with disabilities* (pp. 246–261). New York: Springer Publishing.

McGowan, M., & Roth, S. (1987). Family functioning and functional independence in spinal cord injury adjustment. *Paraplegia, 25,* 357–365.

Moeller, T., & Hartman, D. (1984). The group psychotherapy process in rehabilitation settings. In D. Krueger (Ed.), *Emotional rehabilitation of physical trauma and disability* (pp. 219–233). New York: SP Medical & Scientific Books.

Morgan, D. (1980). Not all sadness can be treated with antidepressants. *West Virginia Medical Journal, 76*(6), 136–137.

Moses, K. (Speaker). (1989). *Shattered dreams and growth: A workshop on helping and being helped* (Cassette Recording). Evanston, IL: Resource Networks, Inc.

Northouse, P., & Northouse, L. (1985). *Health communication: A handbook for health professionals.* Englewood Cliffs, NJ: Prentice-Hall.

Noyes, R. (1984). The existential crisis of serious illness. In D. Krueger (Ed.), *Emotional rehabilitation of physical trauma and disability* (pp. 51–61). New York: SP Medical & Scientific Books.

Osterweis, M., Solomon, F., & Green, M. (1984). *Bereavement: reactions, consequences, and care.* Washington, DC: National Academy Press.

Park, L. (1977). Barriers to normality for the handicapped adult in the United States. In R. Marinelli & A. Dell Orto (Eds.), *The psychological and social impact of physical disability* (pp. 25–33). New York: Springer Publishing.

Pinkerton, A., & Griffin, M. (1983). Rehabilitation outcomes in females with spinal cord injury: A follow-up study. *Paraplegia, 21,* 166–175.

Richards, J., Seitz, M., & Eisele, W. (1986). Auditory processing in spinal cord injury: A preliminary investigation from a sensory deprivation perspective. *Archives of Physical Medicine and Rehabilitation, 67,* 115–117.

Richards, J. (1986). Psychologic adjustment to spinal cord injury during first postdischarge year. *Archives of Physical Medicine and Rehabilitation, 67,* 362–365.

Rogers, M. (1986). *Living with paraplegia.* Boston: Faber & Faber.

Rohrer, K., Adelman, B., Puckett, J., Toomey, B., Talbert, D., & Johnson, E. (1980). Rehabilitation in spinal cord injury: Use of a patient–family group. *Archives of Physical Medicine and Rehabilitation, 61,* 225–229.

Schneider, J. (1984). Stress, loss, and grief: Understanding their origins and growth potential. Baltimore: University Park Press.

Servoss, A., & Krueger, D. (1984). Normal vs. pathological grief and mourning: Some precursors. In D. Krueger (Ed.), *Emotional rehabilitation of physical trauma and disability* (pp. 45–49). New York: SP Medical & Scientific Books.

Stubbins, J. (1988). The politics of disability. In H. Yuker (Ed.), *Attitudes toward persons with disabilities* (pp. 22–32). New York: Springer Publishing.

Trieschmann, R. (1988). *Spinal cord injuries: Psychological, social, and vocational rehabilitation.* New York: Demos.

Trieschmann, R. (1986). The psychosocial adjustment to spinal cord injury. In R. Bloch & M. Basbaum (Eds.), *Management of spinal cord injuries* (pp. 302–319). Baltimore: Williams & Wilkins.

Tunks, E., Bahry, N., & Basbaum, M. (1986). The resocialization process after spinal cord injury. In R. Bloch & M. Basbaum (Eds.), *Management of spinal cord injuries* (pp. 387–409). Baltimore: Williams & Wilkins.

Urey, J., & Henggeler, S. (1987). Marital adjustment following spinal cord injury. *Archives of Physical Medicine and Rehabilitation, 68,* 69–74.

Vachon, M., Lyall, W., Rogers, J., Freedman-Letofsky, K., & Freeman, S. (1980). A controlled study of self-help intervention for widows. *American Journal of Psychiatry, 137*(11), 1380–1384.

Weinberg, N. (1988). Another perspective: Attitudes of persons with disabilities. In H. Yuker (Ed.), *Attitudes toward persons with disabilities* (pp. 141–153). New York: Springer Publishing.

Wolfensberger, W., & Glenn, L. (1978). *PASS (program analysis of service systems: A method for the quantitative evaluation of human services—field manual)* (3rd ed.). Toronto: National Institute on Mental Retardation.

Wolfensberger, W., & Thomas, S. (1983). *PASSING (program analysis of service systems' implementation of normalization goals)* (2nd ed.). Toronto: National Institute on Mental Retardation.

Wolfensberger, W., & Tullman, S. (1982). A brief outline of the principle of normalization. *Rehabilitation Psychology, 27*(3), 131–145.

Worden, J. (1982). *Grief counseling and grief therapy: A handbook for the mental health practitioner.* New York: Springer Publishing.

Wright, B. (1988). Attitudes and the fundamental negative bias: Conditions and corrections. In H. Yuker (Ed.), *Attitudes toward persons with disabilities* (pp. 3–21). New York: Springer Publishing.

Yuker, H. (1988). The effects of contact on attitudes toward disabled persons: Some empirical generalizations. In H. Yuker (Ed.), *Attitudes toward persons with disabilities* (pp. 262–274). New York: Springer Publishing.

Zola, I. (1982). Social and cultural disincentives to independent living. *Archives of Physical Medicine and Rehabilitation, 63,* 394–397.

5

Physical Therapy Evaluation

Evaluation is the foundation of any physical therapy program. A thorough and accurate understanding of the patient's initial status is required for the therapist to identify areas of weakness and strength and potential roadblocks to progress. This knowledge makes it possible to make an informed estimation of the person's ultimate potential and provides the basis for the development of goals and a plan of action tailored to the individual involved. Documentation of initial status is also needed for later comparison, facilitating the detection of any improvement or deterioration in the patient's condition.

During the early days and weeks after spinal cord injury, evaluation has an even greater than usual significance. During this initial period following injury, improvement or deterioration in neurological status can occur rapidly. If a good baseline is not available for comparison, these changes are more likely to be missed.

The evaluation process should continue throughout the program. This is not to say that complete, formal evaluations should be performed continually. Rather the therapist should remain aware of the patient's changing status. By monitoring any significant changes in physical and functional status, the therapist obtains feedback on the program's effectiveness. This feedback allows for adjustments to be made as appropriate.

Periodically a more complete reevaluation should be performed. These repeat evaluations provide the opportunity for the therapist and patient to evaluate progress, reassess goals, and update the program. They can also redirect attention to areas that may have been neglected inadvertently.

A thorough evaluation at discharge is also important. A complete record of physical and functional status at the end of the program will be useful for health professionals with whom the cord-injured person will come in contact in the future. The final evaluation is also an important source of feedback for the patient, who should be given a clear explanation of his status and the potential areas for future

progress. Finally, the discharge evaluation provides another opportunity to judge the therapeutic program's effectiveness. With this feedback on the program, the clinician can evaluate the therapeutic strategies employed and alter his approach with future patients when indicated.

COOPERATIVE APPROACH TO EVALUATION

The initial evaluation often constitutes the first contact between a health professional and a patient and thus sets the stage for future interactions. Unfortunately this evaluation often involves the pokings and proddings of an "expert" who approaches the patient as an object rather than as another person who happens to be a patient at the moment. The health professional dominates the interaction, issuing commands and noting responses.

Another unfortunate practice that is common during evaluations is dishonesty. Health professionals often "protect" their patients from evaluation results, providing them with incomplete or even inaccurate information. This protection may stem from a belief that the information will somehow damage the patient. It may also be due to health professionals' own discomfort regarding communicating bad news to their patients.

Whatever the reason behind these approaches to evaluation, they have a negative impact. By assuming total command of the situation, treating the cord-injured person as less than equal, and by concealing information from him, the health professional communicates to the patient that he is helpless and should assume a passive role.

To provide a more constructive experience, the therapist should include the patient as an active participant in the evaluation. (After all, the person being evaluated has a vested interest in the findings!) As an active participant, the cord-injured person is encouraged to express concerns, provide information, and share in any evaluation findings. The evaluation then becomes a positive learning experience in which both parties achieve a better understanding of the patient's status. As importantly, the cord-injured person becomes an active participant in his program from the outset. The stage is set for active participation throughout the program.

CONTENT

Any complete physical therapy evaluation includes subjective statements and a history. The evaluation of someone who has had a spinal cord injury should also include an assessment of the areas of physical functioning that are directly affected by trauma to the cord and areas in which any complications are likely to occur. The therapist should also evaluate functional capabilities, equipment needs, and home environment.

Subjective Statements
The therapist should document any significant statements that provide information on such matters as the patient's emotional status, concerns, or understanding of the injury. The patient's stated goals should also be included, as they give insight into his priorities.

History
Information for the history should be gathered by reading the medical record and interviewing the patient. The history should contain any background information relevant to the individual's physical or psychosocial status and prognosis. This information will affect goal-setting and the therapeutic strategies employed.

A history should include the date, level, extent, and etiology of the damage to the spinal cord and any complications or additional injuries sustained at or since the time of the cord injury. It should note any changes in neurological status that have occurred since the injury. Any other medical conditions that could impact on the person's health or functional status should be documented. The history should also include a brief summary of the medical/surgical management received following the injury, with particular attention given to fracture management techniques.

The therapist should also investigate social issues, getting a sense of the patient's lifestyle prior to and since the injury. This knowledge is essential when establishing meaningful goals, since the overall purpose of a rehabilitation program is to enable a person to return to a lifestyle as near as possible to that experienced prior to the cord injury. Perti-

nent areas to investigate include vocation and avocations, as well as living arrangements.

If the patient has had previous hospitalizations, the history should include a brief summary of any rehabilitation that he has undergone since the time of the initial injury. It should also include a description of his functioning since the injury.

Finally, the history should note any restrictions that have been placed upon the patient's activities. For example, the therapist should document any limitations such as confinement to bed, skeletal traction, or respirator dependence.

Motor Function
An accurate evaluation of voluntary motor function is of vital importance because it will provide a starting point for the therapeutic program. Motor function is one of the most important factors that affects a person's abilities following spinal cord injury; his ultimate potential for physical activities is largely dependent upon what musculature remains functioning. The muscle test is used to prognosticate on the level of function that an individual can expect to achieve. In addition, the findings of the muscle test will indicate areas of weakness that should be addressed in the strengthening program.

Motor function is also significant in that it is a reflection of neurological status. A cord-injured person's neurological level of injury is in part defined by the strength that he exhibits in key muscles representative of specific cord segments.[1] These key muscles are presented in Chart 2–2.

An accurate and complete baseline muscle test will allow comparison to future findings. This is especially important when the cord injury has occurred very recently because at this stage it is not unusual for neurological return to occur or for the lesion to progress. Progression of the cord lesion may be shown by loss of motor function, and neurological return may manifest itself in return of function to previously paralyzed muscles.

Muscles to Be Tested. A specific manual muscle test is required for accurate assessment of motor function following spinal cord injury. In extremities where any motor function is present, a complete muscle test is indicated.

The exception to this rule is an extremity that is innervated above the level of the lesion. Although a complete muscle test may not be necessary in these extremities, the therapist should never simply assume that all musculature above the diagnosed level of lesion is functioning normally. A therapist

---

[1] Neurological level of injury is explained in Chapter 2.

who makes this assumption will miss any preexisting weakness or previously undetected signs of neurological damage. For this reason, a gross test is indicated in extremities that are innervated above the diagnosed level of lesion. If any areas of weakness are found, a complete muscle test should follow.

When evaluating an extremity that appears to lack any motor function, it can be tempting to check only a muscle or two or even to forgo the muscle test altogether. One reason for this is that performing a muscle-by-muscle test is very time consuming. It can also be discouraging to both the patient and the therapist to run through a long series of unsuccessful attempts at motion in a single extremity. However, testing only one or two muscles can lead to inaccurate results. To avoid this problem, it is usually best to test a representative muscle from each myotome.[2] Doing so will be less time consuming and frustrating than performing a complete muscle test and will avoid the problem of the therapist overlooking motor sparing that is not immediately apparent.

Substitution. When performing a muscle test, the therapist should *watch for substitution!* People with spinal cord injuries quickly learn to use functioning musculature to perform the actions of muscles that are weakened or absent. For example, the anterior deltoid can be used to extend the elbow in the absence of triceps, and the radial wrist extensors can be used to flex the fingers in the absence of any functioning finger flexors (tenodesis grasp). These compensations can be very deceptive, giving the appearance of normal or partial functioning in musculature that is paralyzed.

Substitution is an important skill for improving functional status, but it can wreak havoc on the evaluation results of an unwary therapist. This is especially true when a long time has passed since the injury, as the cord-injured person will have become more adept at muscle substitution. To prevent substitution during a muscle test, the therapist should eliminate motions at other joints. In addition, he should carefully palpate the muscle being tested to verify that it is contracting.

Stabilization. Musculature normally used for stabilization during manual muscle testing may be weak or absent. Failure to accommodate for this impaired ability to stabilize can make muscles appear to be weaker than they are. For example, someone with normal (5/5) deltoids and a weak serratus anterior

may give the appearance of having weak deltoids. He may be able to perform the test motion without resistance, but scapular instability will enable the therapist to "break" the position with less than 5/5 force.

A person's ability to stabilize his entire body must also be taken into account during muscle testing. For example, someone who has recently sustained a cervical or thoracic injury may not have learned how to stabilize his trunk while sitting upright in a wheelchair. During manual muscle testing of his deltoids, he will be unable to maintain the test position against 5/5 force; his inability to stabilize his trunk will make his deltoids appear weak. Thus if a therapist does not provide the needed trunk stabilization during muscle testing, the test results will be inaccurate.

To obtain accurate results, the therapist must stabilize the patient appropriately. Whenever stabilizing musculature is weak or absent, the therapist must provide the needed stability.

Spasticity. Spasticity can also influence muscle test results. Reflexive contraction can occur when a muscle is being tested, making the muscle appear to be stronger than it actually is.

Since spasticity can affect muscle test results, its presence should be noted when muscle strength is documented. In addition, the therapist must attempt to distinguish between voluntary muscle strength and spasticity. To make this distinction, the therapist should ask the patient to contract and relax the muscle on command.

Limiting Conditions. Orthoses and medical restrictions often interfere with standard positioning for manual muscle testing. When this is the case, the therapist should simply adapt the tests by performing them in the best positions possible within the limitations. The adaptations in muscle test procedure should be documented.

Precautions. If vertebral injury is very acute and the spine is not yet stable, the therapist should exercise caution when testing musculature. Strong contraction of muscles that may exert a pull on the affected vertebral area should be avoided. For example, it is prudent to avoid maximal resistance to the hip flexors if the patient has an unstable lumbar fracture.

Trunk Musculature. Testing trunk musculature presents a unique problem. The standard tests for the abdominals and back extensors assume that the musculature is functioning along its entire length.

---

[2] Muscles representative of different myotomes are presented in Chart 2–2.

This is often not the case after a spinal cord injury. A given person may have strong contraction of the rectus abdominis from the ribs to the umbilicus and no contraction below this level. What grade can be assigned to this person's rectus? Instead of trying to assign a grade to the musculature in such instances, it may be more meaningful to focus instead on identifying (through palpation and observation of umbilical motion) the approximate myotome levels in which the musculature functions.

The position of the umbilicus during muscle testing can be used as an indicator of function in the abdominal musculature. If it remains central during testing, this indicates that there is a uniform pull in the abdominals; abdominal musculature functions uniformly above, below, and to either side of the umbilicus. For this condition to exist, the abdominals are either absent or functioning along their entire length; the level of motor paralysis must be either above T5 or below T12. The therapist should palpate to determine which of these is the case. If the umbilicus moves upward (cephalad) during testing, the muscular pull is greater above the umbilicus than below; the lesion lies between T5 and T12. If the umbilicus moves to the side, the musculature is stronger on the side toward which it moves.

When testing the back extensors, the therapist should determine the level of motor function by palpating while the patient attempts back extension.

Sensation

Like motor function, sensation is directly affected by spinal cord injury and is a reflection of neurological status. Sensation should be monitored closely when a person has recently sustained a spinal cord injury.

Sensation also has an impact upon function, though to a smaller degree than strength. Someone who has intact proprioception and touch sensation in an extremity will find it easier to learn to use that extremity. For example, learning to propel a wheelchair will be easier if some touch sensation is present in the hands.

Pain sensation is particularly important because it serves to protect the skin. The normal reaction to pain is to withdraw from the stimulus, thus avoiding or reducing damage to the skin. Without this protection, an area that lacks pain sensitivity is more vulnerable to trauma. People with spinal cord injuries need to know about this vulnerability and must take measures to avoid trauma to insensate areas.[3]

The sensory evaluation should include proprioception in all joints of the affected extremities and pain and light touch in all dermatomes. (See Fig. 2-22 for a dermatomal chart.) Because pain and temperature are carried in the same tract of the spinal cord, they will be affected equally by a spinal cord injury. For this reason, it is not necessary to test both.

When performing sensory tests, it is important for the therapist to prevent substitution from other senses. In his eagerness to "do well" on the test, a patient may "cheat," possibly without even being aware of it. A variety of senses can be used for this sensory substitution. The patient can watch the therapist performing the test. The therapist's voice intonation and choice of words can also provide hints. A patient who lacks proprioception in a joint can often detect movement through other sensory cues. For example, someone who is lying in bed and has his hip flexed passively may feel his body being pushed toward the head of the bed. To increase the accuracy of sensory testing, the therapist should take measures to eliminate these sensory cues.

Muscle Tone

Muscle tone is another area that has a major impact upon functional capabilities. Spasticity generally makes physical activities more difficult and when severe can seriously impair function. Occasionally people can use spasticity to their advantage. For example, some people with incomplete lesions depend upon their spasticity to augment their voluntary quadriceps function when walking.

Muscle tone can also provide information regarding physical status. Following spinal cord injury, an increase in muscle tone can be a sign that something is wrong physically, since a noxious stimulus below the lesion can cause an increase in spasticity. For example, sometimes an increase in spasticity is an early indication of a urinary tract infection.

When testing muscle tone, the therapist should check deep tendon reflexes and resistance to passive stretch. If spasticity is present, the therapist should note its severity and whether it is constant or intermittent. If certain conditions or bodily motions are seen to influence tone, this observation should also be documented. Chart 5-1 presents a rating scale for grading spasticity.

Range of Motion

Range of motion,[4] like strength and muscle tone, can have a profound impact on functional capabil-

---

[3] Skin care is addressed in Chapters 3, 8, and 19.

[4] The phrase "range of motion" in this section is used to refer to both joint range of motion and the flexibility of two-joint musculature such as the hamstrings or the biceps brachii.

Chart 5—1. Modified Ashworth Scale for Grading Spasticity[a]

0	No increase in muscle tone.
1	Slight increase in muscle tone, manifested by a catch and release or by minimal resistance at the end of the range of motion when the affected part(s) is moved in flexion or extension.
1 +	Slight increase in muscle tone, manifested by a catch, followed by minimal resistance throughout the remainder (less than half) of the ROM.
2	More marked increase in muscle tone through most of the ROM, but affected part(s) easily moved.
3	Considerable increase in muscle tone, passive movement difficult.
4	Affected part(s) rigid in flexion or extension.

During testing, the clinician asks the patient to relax and moves the patient's extremities passively through the available range of motion.

Bohannon & Smith (1987).

[a] From *Physical Therapy* with the permission of the American Physical Therapy Association.

ities after spinal cord injury. Even mild restrictions in motion at crucial joints such as the elbows or shoulders can severely limit a person's functional potential.

The therapist should check range of motion of all joints, starting with a gross test and specifically examining any areas where limitations exist. The evaluation should also cover flexibility of the biceps brachii, pectoralis major, long finger flexors and extensors, rectus femoris, hamstrings, and gastrocnemius. Flexibility in these muscles has a significant impact on function.

When testing someone with a very acute spinal injury, the therapist should avoid stress to areas of vertebral instability. For example, if a patient with an unstable lumbar fracture has limited hip range of motion, the hip should not be forced beyond the point at which resistance to motion occurs. Even when range does not appear to be limited, it may be prudent to avoid hip flexion past 90 degrees or straight leg raising past 60 degrees in the presence of an unstable lumbar fracture. Motion past these points may cause undesirable motion in the lumbar area.

Hamstring flexibility should be tested in supine. Having a cord-injured person long-sit and reach for his toes is not an appropriate technique for performing this assessment, as excessive back flexibility can mask hamstring tightness.

Functional Abilities

A functional evaluation investigates what a person is capable of doing, how much assistance he needs, and what equipment he requires to perform various activities. Since the major thrust of the physical therapy component of rehabilitation is to increase functional capability, this part of the evaluation is very important. The functional evaluation provides a starting point for goal setting and program development.

The functional evaluation performed upon completion of the therapeutic program is also critical, as it provides a measure of the program's success. A physical rehabilitation program usually results in improvements in other areas such as strength and range of motion, but these gains are significant only if they contribute to an increase in function. If the patient is no more independent at discharge than he was initially, the functional training program has failed.[5]

Evaluation and documentation of functional skills should be specific enough to provide a complete picture of the patient's abilities. Blanket statements about areas of functioning do not provide adequate information, as these statements can be interpreted differently by various readers. For example, a statement that an individual is "independent in wheelchair propulsion" does not provide enough information. Does this refer to even surfaces only? 100 feet or 10 miles? How long does it take for him to propel a given distance? Can he negotiate stairs with the wheelchair? Are specific wheelchair accessories such as pegged handrims required?

The therapist should also be specific when documenting the assistance required. Merely noting that a person "needs assistance" does not provide adequate information. For example, the statement that a patient "requires assistance in even transfers" could be true with an individual who is totally dependent (unable to contribute to the process), someone who requires only stand-by spotting, or anyone who falls between the two extremes. Chart 5-2 presents terminology appropriate for documentation of assistance required during functional activities.

Finally, documentation of functional abilities must be as accurate as all other areas of the evaluation. It can be tempting to "give the patient the benefit of the doubt" in the functional evaluation,

---

[5] This is not meant to imply that functional gains are the only relevant outcomes of a comprehensive rehabilitation program. Certainly gains made in other areas such as breathing ability, skin integrity, psychosocial adaptation, patient and family education, bowel and bladder regulation, equipment procurement, and home modification are also extremely important.

Chart 5—2. Functional Assessment Terminology[a]

Independent	The patient can safely perform the activity without any form of assistance from another person.
Guarding assist	The patient is capable of performing the activity but is unsafe; another person must be present to provide support when needed.
Verbal assist[b]	The patient requires verbal cues from another person to perform the activity safely.
Minimal assist	The patient requires a small amount of physical assistance to perform the activity but contributes most of the effort required to accomplish the task.
Moderate assist	The patient requires a greater amount of physical assistance to perform the activity but is still able to contribute significantly to the accomplishment of the task.
Maximal assist	The patient contributes minimally to the performance of the task, requiring almost full physical assistance to accomplish the task.
Unable to perform	The patient is unable to perform the task and cannot contribute physically to its accomplishment.

[a] Documenting Quality Care, 1988; Zimmerman, 1988
[b] Verbal assistance may be combined with other forms of assistance. For example, a patient may require both guarding and verbal cueing.

calling him independent in an activity when he actually falls slightly short of the mark. For example, a therapist may report that an individual is independent in level transfers, even though he requires spotting because he occasionally loses his balance and falls. A patient should not be called independent in an activity unless he is capable of performing the task alone, without anyone in the area to set him up or spot him.

To ensure accuracy in the functional evaluation, the therapist must observe the patient performing the activity; he should not take the patient's (or anyone else's) word on his capabilities.[6] An inexperienced person may feel that he is safe in a given activity when in fact he is not. For example, the author once had a patient report that he could negotiate ramps safely. When asked to demonstrate, he careened down the ramp at a breakneck speed,

stopping only when he struck a glass door (fortunately, a sturdy one) about 20 feet beyond the bottom of the ramp. Following this hair-raising display, the patient still maintained that his technique was safe.[7]

The areas commonly covered in a functional evaluation include mat and bed abilities, transfers, wheelchair skills, ambulation, and the ability to instruct others in dependent activities.

Mat and Bed Abilities. The therapist should evaluate the patient's capabilities in rolling, coming to sitting, and gross mobility (moving to the right or left, forward or backward) on an exercise mat. These activities should also be evaluated on a bed because functioning on beds is much more difficult.

Transfers. The evaluation should address even and uneven transfers, also called level and unlevel transfers. Even transfers involve moving between the wheelchair and a surface that is level with the wheelchair seat.[8] An uneven transfer involves moving between the wheelchair and a higher or lower surface such as a bathtub, toilet, couch, truck, car, plinth, or the floor.

An independent transfer involves more than merely moving the body from one surface to another. To be independent in a transfer from a wheelchair, a person must be able to set up for the transfer. This includes positioning the wheelchair, locking the brakes, removing or repositioning an armrest, positioning the legs and footrests, and positioning the sliding board, if one is used. The person must be able to move his entire body onto the surface, including his legs. To be independent in a transfer to the wheelchair, he must be able to prepare to leave the area following the transfer. This involves positioning his body appropriately on the wheelchair seat, removing the sliding board (if used), positioning his footrests and armrests, placing his feet on the footrests, and unlocking the brakes.

To transfer safely, a cord-injured person must move from one surface to another without falling and *without traumatizing his skin.* Someone who scrapes his buttocks across the wheelchair's tire while transferring is *not* performing the transfer safely.

[6] If direct observation of the skill is not indicated, the documentation should make it clear that it is the patient's judgment of independence, not the clinician's, that is being reported.

[7] This example illustrates both the need to observe a patient's performance of functional activities and the need to *guard* him while doing so!

[8] An even transfer is actually between the wheelchair and a surface that is level with the sitting surface. If a wheelchair cushion is used, its top is the sitting surface.

Wheelchair Skills. If a patient will require the use of a wheelchair, wheelchair skills should be included in the functional evaluation. The therapist should check the person's capabilities in propulsion over even surfaces, specify the distance that he is able to travel, and note the time required to propel this distance. Obstacle negotiation is also important to address. Evaluation of obstacle negotiation should cover the ability to maneuver over uneven terrain (grass, dirt, gravel, sidewalk), curbs (the therapist should specify the height that can be managed independently), inclined surfaces, doorways, and stairs. The evaluation report should note any special equipment that is required for propulsion, such as pegs or surgical tubing on the wheelchair handrims.

Pressure reliefs in a wheelchair are critical to a spinal cord-injured person's health. Someone who cannot perform pressure reliefs independently must have assistance throughout the day if he is to avoid decubiti. For this reason this is an extremely important functional skill to assess. The evaluation should determine both whether the person is capable of performing pressure reliefs and whether he assumes the responsibility to get the relief at appropriate intervals.

Ambulation. If a cord-injured person is ambulatory, the therapist should determine how far he can walk, the time required to walk this distance, the gait pattern used, and the level of assistance required. Capabilities in obstacle negotiation (obstacles listed above in wheelchair skills section) should also be assessed. Additional ambulatory skills that should be addressed include donning and doffing the orthoses, walking backward and to the side, safe falling techniques, coming to stand from the floor, coming to stand from sitting, and returning to sitting from a standing position.

Instruction of Others. The therapist should determine whether the patient is able to instruct others in safe techniques to assist him with activities in which he is dependent.

Skin Integrity

Skin breakdown is a complication of spinal cord injury that can lead to severe medical problems, even death. If precautionary measures are not taken, a decubitus ulcer can develop in a matter of hours. Once a decubitus develops, it can take months to heal.

During the evaluation, the therapist should note any decubiti or early signs of skin breakdown. If a problem is found, pressure over the area must be relieved to prevent a worsening of the condition. The therapeutic program must be modified to avoid any further trauma to the area. The therapist should also notify other members of the team if they are not already aware of the breakdown.

Areas of scarring from healed decubiti should also be noted in the evaluation. Because scar tissue is more susceptible than normal skin to breakdown, care must be taken to minimize trauma to scarred areas.

Scarred areas provide a history of past skin problems. The presence of healed decubiti may indicate that the cord-injured person has neglected his skin care in the past and needs to learn better habits in this area. These scars may also be the legacy of poor medical care.

Respiration

Most spinal cord injuries result in at least partial impairment of breathing ability. As a result, respiratory complications are a significant source of mortality among cord-injured people. The respiratory evaluation investigates the patient's ability to breathe and clear secretions from his lungs.[9]

Equipment

Equipment has a significant impact upon function. Someone who lacks needed equipment, or has equipment that is inappropriate or in disrepair, will not be able to function optimally.[10] An equipment check during the initial evaluation helps to focus attention early on this important area. As soon as a patient's equipment needs have been identified, the process of meeting those needs should be started. If arrangements for equipment purchase or repair are initiated early, the results are likely to be more satisfactory than if equipment procurement is attempted in a rush just prior to discharge.

The therapist should record any orthoses, wheelchairs, or other equipment in the patient's possession and note whether it is rented, on loan, or owned by the patient. The fit, function, and condition of the equipment should be evaluated.

Home Environment

One important task of rehabilitation is to prepare the newly disabled person to return home. This involves a combination of acquiring functional skills and adapting the home environment as necessary.

During the initial evaluation, the therapist should find out what environment the patient in-

---

[9] Chapter 3 addresses respiratory evaluation and rehabilitation.
[10] Chapter 19 addresses equipment.

tends to return to upon completion of his rehabilitation. During discharge planning it will be helpful to know, for example, if the patient plans to live alone in an isolated trailer park or with a large family in an apartment building in the city. The therapist should also investigate whether the home has architectural barriers, such as stairs or small bathrooms.

A more detailed assessment of the home should follow. Ideally a health professional should visit the home and get a detailed picture of the environment, including door and hall widths, layout of the bathrooms and kitchen, accessibility of kitchen and bathroom fixtures, accessibility of the entrance to the home, and a variety of other features of the home environment. A family member or the patient can also provide this information if given guidelines for the home evaluation.[11]

Other

The evaluation should cover any other problem areas exhibited by the patient that may require intervention, impact on prognosis, or influence treatment strategies. Possible problem areas include edema or pain.

SUMMARY

Evaluation provides an opportunity for both the therapist and patient to learn about the patient's physical and functional status and to investigate other areas of concern. The information gathered during initial and subsequent evaluations is the basis for goal setting and for the design, evaluation, and revision of the therapeutic program.

REFERENCES

Bohannon, R., & Smith, M. (1987). Interrator reliability of a modified Ashworth scale of muscle spasticity. *Physical Therapy, 67*(2), 206–207.

Documenting Quality Care, Inc. (1988). *Functional Rating Scales for Physical Therapists*. Washington, DC: Documenting Quality Care, Inc. (Available from Documenting Quality Care, Inc., PO Box 33978, Washington, DC, 20033-0978.)

Zimmerman, J. (1988). *Goals and objectives for developing normal movement patterns*. Rockville, MD: Aspen Publishers.

---

[11] Chapter 18 addresses architectural design.

6

Goal Setting

Goals give direction in the development of therapeutic programs. They also provide a measure with which the therapist and patient can judge the program's effectiveness.

Patient Involvement

In rehabilitation, people who have experienced a significant loss of bodily function acquire new skills to live more independently. For this process to be successful, patients must be involved in establishing their own goals. Participation of the patient in goal setting ensures that the program is directed toward mastering skills that he values. It also gives him some control over his problem, promoting independence.

Setting Meaningful Goals. Rehabilitation is an active process, requiring patient participation. Functional gains come only after a cord-injured person has worked long and hard. Setting goals that the patient values may result in better motivation to work in the program, which in turn will enable him to achieve a higher level of independence.

Setting goals that are meaningful to the patient will also increase the likelihood that he will use the newly acquired skills following discharge. A program that focuses on gaining abilities that the patient has no desire to use will only waste time, effort, and money.

The only way to ensure that a program's goals are meaningful to the patient is to involve him in establishing them. The therapist cannot assume that what he wants a patient to achieve will coincide with what that individual wants to learn. A health professional who sets goals without the patient's input runs the risk of establishing goals that he does not value. The therapist may also neglect areas of functioning that the patient wants to address.

Program Control. A health professional who dictates a patient's goals places him in a position of dependence. The messages given to the patient are "We are in control. We know what is best for you. You need us to make these decisions for you. Do as you are told." In contrast, having a patient set his own goals affirms his autonomy, giving him the responsibility of identifying what he wants to achieve. It emphasizes that he is still in control of his life, despite his cord injury.

Placing a patient in control of goal setting can also improve his motivation in therapy. Having responsibility for the goals may encourage a feeling of greater involvement in his rehabilitation. A person is more likely to feel motivated to achieve goals if he has established them, rather than having had them decreed by a health professional.

Setting the Goals

Having the patient set his goals does not mean that the therapist cannot provide some suggestions and guidance in the process. Someone with a disability may not know what he is capable of accomplishing or may be so used to a dependent role that he resists setting his own goals. In these situations the therapist should provide what input or encouragement is needed while still giving the patient responsibility for goal setting.

Immediately Following Injury. Someone who participates in setting his therapeutic goals experiences control in at least one area of his life. This is particularly important for a recently injured person. In the bulk of his experiences since the injury, it is likely that health professionals, family, and even friends have been in charge. By giving the newly injured person some control over his program, the therapist supports his autonomy.

Although it is important to involve patients in setting their goals, a recently injured person cannot be expected to come up with a complete list of rehabilitation goals without any guidance. He is likely to have no idea of his functional potential or of the skills that he will require to function. Yesterday, perhaps a week ago, the recently injured person was probably oriented toward such achievements as paying off a loan, completing college, getting a pro-

77

motion, or finding a date for the senior prom. The idea of therapeutic goals such as independent transfers or wheelchair mobility is likely to be completely foreign.

To prepare someone who has recently been injured to set his rehabilitation goals, the therapist should share the initial evaluation results with him and provide an estimation of his functional potential. The therapist should explain what skills are possible to achieve and then ask the patient whether he is interested in learning to perform these activities. The patient should also be given the opportunity to identify any other goals that he wants to pursue.

When discussing goals with an acutely injured person, it is a challenge for the therapist to be forthright and yet tactful. It is important to remember that the patient has not had time to adjust to his injury or even to comprehend its impact. The therapist also needs to understand that the patient may not be overly thrilled with the list of functional skills that are presented as possible goals. Rehabilitation is not an appealing option when compared to recovery.

> Rehabilitation's job is to take your body *as it is* and to maximize your capabilities within recognized limitations. This is a difficult acknowledgement. Rehabilitation seems only second best, which is exactly what it is. To fully accept rehabilitation, for most of us, is to effectively abandon recovery. Rehabilitation can give you strength, reeducation, skills and real improvement, but no cure. Many people find this an easy bridge to cross, and a few find it so upsetting that they temporarily want out of the game.
>
> Barry Corbet (1980)

Further Down the Road. A person who sustained a spinal cord injury months or years ago is likely to have a good understanding of the impact of his injury and should be able to identify specific goals to pursue when he comes for rehabilitation. In these cases the therapist should start the process of goal setting by asking the patient what he is interested in achieving in therapy.

The therapist may know of additional functional abilities that the individual has the potential to achieve. These skills may well interest the patient, even though they were not in his list of goals; it may not have occurred to him that these activities were possible. For example, few people would spontaneously come up with the idea of negotiating stairs in a wheelchair. To provide the cord-injured

person with the opportunity to maximize his functional potential, the therapist should let him know what additional skills he has the potential to achieve and allow him to decide whether he wishes to develop these skills.

Content of Goals

Emphasis on Function. The first step in goal setting is specifying exactly what functional skills will be pursued in therapy. As was discussed above, this process involves identifying what skills the patient wants to achieve.

After the patient and therapist have established a list of purely functional goals, the therapist should determine what other elements are prerequisites for these goals. Following spinal cord injury, most new functional skills require an increase in strength, and many require an increase in range of motion. This is because the cord-injured person now has a limited number of muscles with which to perform the functions of all of the musculature that is no longer innervated. This compensation for paralysis requires strength in the muscles left working and flexibility to perform the maneuvers used in functional activities.

The final list of therapeutic goals should include all functional goals plus any prerequisite goals such as improving strength or flexibility. It should also address equipment needs, architectural adaptation, and educational goals.

Goal Specificity. Goals provide direction, focus, and structure for therapeutic programs. They should be specific, with identifiable endpoints, since vague goals allow vague therapeutic programs. A program will flounder if the therapist and patient do not have a clear notion of what exactly they are aiming for.

Goals without specific endpoints do not identify exactly what is to be accomplished. ''Improve wheelchair skills'' is an example of such a goal. Technically if the patient improves even slightly in his wheelchair skills, he has reached the goal as stated. If the objective of the program is for the patient to become independent, this should be stated clearly.

One way to improve the above goal would be to change it to ''independence in wheelchair skills.'' The patient will have achieved the goal only when he can perform wheelchair skills independently. However, this wording is still too vague; it does not clarify which wheelchair skills will be addressed in the program. The goal could refer to mastering wheelchair propulsion over even surfaces, learning to negotiate various obstacles, or performing any number of wheelchair-related activities.

A more appropriate wording would be "independence in wheelchair negotiation of 6″ curbs." This wording communicates a specific skill (negotiation of a particular obstacle) and provides an endpoint (independence).

Goals regarding physical prerequisites (strength, range of motion) should also be specific, with identifiable endpoints. This does not mean that the therapist must state exactly what muscle grade or degree of flexibility will be aimed for. It is not always possible to predict exactly what strength or range of motion a particular individual will need to perform a functional activity because these requirements vary with body build and ability. For this reason, specifying an exact muscle grade or degree of flexibility is often not appropriate.

How, then, can the therapist write a specific goal? Wording prerequisite goals in terms of function will accomplish this end. For example, "increase strength to the degree required to achieve the above functional goals" provides a verifiable endpoint. When the functional goals have been accomplished, the goal of improving strength has also been accomplished. This wording helps to keep the program's focus on function, preventing it from drifting away from its real purpose.

Aiming High. It is almost axiomatic that to achieve great things, one must set high goals. (The popular literature is full of books attesting to this idea.) The same principle holds true for rehabilitation: setting higher goals will lead to higher functional outcomes.

The one problem with striving to achieve is that this striving carries with it the risk of failure. To achieve something, we must first attempt it, and in attempting, we run the risk of failing. However, the only way to eliminate this risk is to avoid striving for challenging goals. The result is mediocrity.

Setting high goals in rehabilitation involves an element of trust. The therapist must trust the patient to have the emotional strength to withstand failure in the event that the goal is not reached. Some schools of thought hold that health professionals should set only readily achievable goals to ensure that patients do not experience failure. This practice prevents disabled people from attempting more challenging activities, robbing them of the opportunity to reach their full potentials.

For a disabled person to achieve his highest potential for functioning, the rehabilitation team must not limit him by refusing to set unlikely goals. (Who are we to deny someone the opportunity to experience walking?) On the other hand, we should not give our patients false hopes, telling them that all functional goals are in their reach if they only try hard enough. If an individual wants to learn a skill that he is not likely to achieve, the goal should be set with a realistic mutual understanding of the prognosis for successful completion.

Although everyone should be given the opportunity to attempt unlikely goals, this does not mean that endless hours and effort should be spent on working toward goals that have little possibility of being achieved. The therapist and patient should agree on a time frame at the outset, specifying what progress must be made within a given time limit if the person is to continue working toward this goal. Doing so will prevent endless pursuit of questionable goals at the expense of achievable functional goals.

SUMMARY

Goal setting should be a cooperative effort involving the disabled person and the rehabilitation professional. This approach serves to reinforce the patient's autonomy and to ensure that the goals established are meaningful to him. Goals should be specific, with identifiable endpoints. Goals that challenge limits instead of imposing them are likely to result in higher levels of achievement.

REFERENCE

Corbet, B (1980). *Options: Spinal cord injury and the future*. Denver, CO: A.B. Hirschfeld Press.

SUGGESTED READING

For additional information on goal-setting, the reader is referred to the following book:

Kettenbach, G. (1990). *Writing S.O.A.P. Notes*. Philadelphia: F.A. Davis.

7

Functional Potentials

This chapter contains descriptions of functional potentials of people with complete spinal cord injuries. It is meant to assist in goal setting by providing information about the functional outcomes that have been achieved in the past by people with various levels of injury.

The descriptions of functional outcomes in this chapter are intended to be presentations of possibilities rather than rigid guidelines for goal setting. The information should not be used to set strict upper limits when setting goals. Therapists who impose inflexible ceilings on patients' goals can limit their functional gains. Moreover, the information presented here may become outdated some day. Through the years, people with spinal cord injuries have achieved increasingly higher levels of independence, and presumably this trend will continue. This can only happen if rehabilitation professionals and cord-injured people attempt to accomplish higher goals, stretching past previous limits.

Variation in Functional Outcome

Following spinal cord injury, an individual's potential for physical activity is determined largely by his motor function. People with more innervated musculature have a greater capacity for independence. The level and extent of a cord lesion determine the motor function that remains after the injury: lower lesions and incomplete lesions leave more of the body's musculature innervated.

If all other factors are equal, a person with a low cord lesion can be expected to achieve independence in more advanced activities than are possible for someone with a higher lesion. Even the degree of motor sparing within a level will have an impact. For example, someone with only 3/5 strength in the muscles of his lowest functioning myotome may not achieve the same level of independence as a person with the same neurological level of injury who has greater strength in the same musculature.

Although the level of injury has a major impact upon a person's functional capacity, it is not the sole determinant. The potentials described below are just that: potentials. There is no guarantee that someone with a given level of injury will be able to master the skills that others with similar injuries have achieved. Many factors can limit progress in functional training. These factors include obesity, contractures, advanced age, spasticity, impaired mental functioning, medical complications, disadvantageous body build (short arms, for example), and low motivation. Unfortunately the rehabilitation that is available to a cord-injured person can also be a limiting factor. If inadequate time is allotted to rehabilitation, functional gains will be limited. Functional gains can be as severely constrained if the person undergoes rehabilitation in a setting that is not oriented toward the aggressive persuit of independence.

Functional Gains After Discharge

Many cord-injured people experience significant functional gains after they leave rehabilitation (Welch, Lobley, O'Sullivan, & Freed, 1986). This improvement is at least in part due to the development of skill through practice. In addition, the strength gains that typically occur for an extended period following cord injury (Ditunno, Sipski, Posuniak, Chen, Staas, & Herbison, 1987; Young & Ransohoff, 1989) may lead to functional improvements.

C3 and Above

People with C3 or higher quadriplegia retain voluntary function in their facial, pharyngeal, and laryngeal musculature, since cranial nerves are not affected. Neck extensors above the level of the lesion also remain innervated. The sternocleidomastoid is partially innervated at the C2 level and is fully innervated at C3. People with C3 quadriplegia also retain partial function in the levator scapulae and trapezius.[1]

---

[1] Kendall, & McCreary (1983) is the reference used throughout the chapter for information on innervation.

Innervation to the diaphragm exits the spinal cord from cervical levels 3 through 5. For this reason people with quadriplegia at C3 or above are unable to breathe without the assistance of a respirator or a phrenic nerve stimulator.[2]

Transfers, Mat and Bed Activities, Self-Care. People with C3 or higher quadriplegia are unable to perform any transfers or mat, bed, or self-care activities.

Wheelchair Mobility. Independent wheelchair propulsion is possible using power wheelchairs. A variety of control options are available that use breathing or motions of the head, chin, or mouth to direct the chair. Most people with this level of lesion require a power-reclining electric wheelchair to perform independent pressure reliefs.

C4 Quadriplegia
Diaphragm function is retained with this level of quadriplegia, making it possible to breathe without assistance from a ventilator or phrenic nerve stimulator.

A person with C4 quadriplegia is capable of scapular adduction and elevation. This is due to the retention of full trapezius function and partial functioning in the rhomboids and levator scapulae.

Transfers, Mat and Bed Activities, Self-Care. People with C4 quadriplegia are unable to perform any transfers or mat or bed activities. If some function is retained in shoulder and elbow musculature,[3] adaptive equipment, such as a mobile arm support, may make self-feeding and facial hygiene possible.

Wheelchair Mobility. The presence of scapular adduction and elevation makes it possible to use a hand-controlled power wheelchair (McClay, 1983).

C5 Quadriplegia
With C5 quadriplegia, the degree of motor innervation that is left intact in the C5 myotome has a large impact upon functional potential. If the elbow flexors and deltoids are strong, this musculature may be used to perform transfers, manual wheelchair propulsion, and mat, bed, and self-care activities. If these muscles remain weak,[4] the individual's functional potential may more closely resemble that described above for C4 quadriplegia. However, more (though still limited) self-care activities may be possible than can be performed by someone with C4 quadriplegia, and a hand-control electric wheelchair will be easier to master.

Transfers. Because transfers require strong deltoids, C5 quadriplegia is the highest level at which independent transfers are feasible. Although it is a great challenge, people with C5 quadriplegia who retain or regain strong deltoids have the potential to perform even transfers independently. This task usually requires the use of a sliding board and sometimes requires an overhead frame with hanging loops.

Mat and Bed Activities. Mat and bed skills require strong biceps and deltoids. For people who retain or regain adequate strength in these muscles, all mat and bed skills (rolling, coming to sitting, gross mat mobility, and leg management) are possible. These skills are more easily achieved using bedrails, loops, or a wheelchair to pull on. Some individuals with this level of quadriplegia are able to achieve independence without any such equipment.

Self-Care. Independent self-feeding and facial hygiene are readily achievable by people with C5 quadriplegia. Upper body dressing can also be achieved. Dressing the lower body presents more of a challenge, but some with strong biceps and deltoids are able to learn the required skills. Independence in personal hygiene, including bowel and bladder care, is possible in exceptional cases.

Wheelchair Mobility. Manual wheelchair propulsion is a reasonable goal for people with strong biceps and deltoids. With adequate instruction and practice, most are capable of propulsion without hand-rim projections (pegs). With or without pegged hand-rims, wheelchair propulsion is limited to even surfaces. Independent pressure reliefs are possible for most people with C5 quadriplegia.

C6 Quadriplegia
With C6 quadriplegia, the deltoids, biceps, brachialis, and brachioradialis are fully innervated, and the clavicular portion of the pectoralis major receives significant innervation. The presence of this

---

[2] With training, many people can learn to breathe for at least brief periods using their neck accessory musculature (neck breathing) or using mouth, throat, or pharynx musculature (glossopharyngeal breathing). (Gilgoff, Barras, Jones, & Adkins, 1988; Wetzel, 1985).

[3] By definition, a person with C4 quadriplegia can have some functioning (less than 3/5 strength) in the C5 myotome (American Spinal Injury Association, 1989).

[4] By definition, people with C5 quadriplegia have at least 3/5 strength in the C5 key muscles (biceps, brachialis, and brachioradialis); (ASIA, 1989).

strong musculature makes the individual better able to manipulate objects in his environment and to move his body through space.

Perhaps more significantly, the radial wrist extensors and the serratus anterior are functional with this level of quadriplegia. Wrist extension provides the capacity to grasp using the tenodesis effect.[5] The serratus anterior has adequate innervation to stabilize the scapula on the trunk. The presence of a stable scapula greatly improves a cord-injured person's ability to lift his body during transfers and pressure reliefs and while moving on a mat or bed. The combination of a functional grasp and a stable scapula make it possible for a person with C6 quadriplegia to achieve all of the skills required to live alone.

Transfers. With proper training, people with C6 quadriplegia can achieve independence in level transfers with or without the use of a sliding board. Many are able to perform some slightly uneven transfers, making it possible to transfer independently between the wheelchair and such surfaces as toilet or car seats.

Mat and Bed Activities. With the added strength and scapular stability that comes with C6 innervation, mat and bed activities become easier to achieve.[6] Many can learn to roll over, come to sitting, and move around on a mat or bed without having to use any adaptive equipment.

Self-Care. All basic self-care activities are achievable with this level of quadriplegia. These activities include dressing, bowel program, self-catheterization, or application of external catheters, bathing, other personal hygiene, and cooking. These activities generally require some adaptive equipment. Eating and drinking are readily achievable without any adaptive equipment.

Wheelchair Mobility. Virtually everyone with this level of injury should be able to propel a manual wheelchair with standard handrims over level surfaces. Many negotiate minor obstacles such as standard public inclines (ramps with a 1/12 slope), slightly uneven terrain (sidewalks or grass, for ex-

ample), and 2-inch curbs. Some strong, highly motivated people are able to ascend and descend 4-inch curbs independently.

C7 Quadriplegia
The triceps are partially innervated with this level of quadriplegia, making elbow extension possible without muscle substitution. Because even moderately weak triceps can provide stronger elbow extension than can the anterior deltoids, their presence has an impact on function. People with C7 quadriplegia also have significant innervation of the latissimus dorsi and the sternal portion of the pectoralis major. The added musculature functioning with C7 quadriplegia makes many activities easier to learn and perform. Moreover, more difficult transfers are possible.

Transfers. Functioning triceps make it possible to perform uneven transfers over greater distances. Many people with C7 quadriplegia are able to transfer between the floor and a wheelchair without assistance.

Mat and Bed Activities. All mat and bed activities (rolling, coming to sitting, moving around on the mat or bed) can be performed independently.

Self-Care. All self-care activities can be performed independently.

Wheelchair Mobility. Most people with C7 quadriplegia can learn to negotiate slightly uneven terrain, low curbs, and standard public inclines in a manual wheelchair. It is also possible to negotiate steeper ramps, and some learn to ascend and descend 4-inch curbs.

C8 Quadriplegia
The flexor digitorum superficialis and profundus retain enough function with this level of quadriplegia to make it easier to use the hands. Transfers and mat/bed activities are also easier due to almost full innervation of the triceps. Despite the greater ease of many activities, the functional potential for C8 quadriplegia is essentially the same as for C7.

Paraplegia
At and below T1, a spinal cord injury is classified as paraplegia rather than quadriplegia. This classification is due to the fact that all upper extremity musculature is innervated. Intact motor function in the upper extremities makes it possible to perform more advanced activities, enabling people to function in less accessible environments.

---

[5] A person who lacks innervation in his finger musculature but retains the use of his wrist extensors can manipulate objects using a tenodesis grasp: he can flex his fingers by extending his wrist and release the grasp by allowing his wrist to flex.

[6] This is not meant to imply that these skills are *easy* to achieve. Rather a person with C6 quadriplegia will achieve them more readily than will someone with C5 quadriplegia. These skills still require a protracted period of functional training.

The functional potentials of people with different levels of paraplegia are not as distinct as those with different levels of quadriplegia (Lazar et al., 1989). People with lower injuries have superior trunk and lower extremity strength, making all activities easier to achieve and perform. Ambulation in particular is more practical at lower levels.

Barring limiting factors such as obesity or advanced age, everyone with paraplegia should be able to achieve independence in all self-care and mat and bed activities. They should also be able to perform even and uneven transfers independently without equipment. Uneven transfers include transfers between the wheelchair and lower surfaces such as the floor and between the wheelchair and higher surfaces such as the seat of a pickup truck.

Full innervation of the upper extremities makes it possible to perform more challenging wheelchair skills. Virtually everyone with paraplegia can learn to negotiate steep ramps and rough terrain. Most can learn to ascend and descend stairs with a wheelchair (either remaining in the chair or transferring out of it) and to negotiate doorways that are narrower than the wheelchair. Highly motivated people can learn to traverse curbs that are 8 inches high or taller.

Functional ambulation using orthoses and Lofstrand crutches is possible with any level of paraplegia,[7] but it is much more feasible with lower lesions. Swing-to, swing-through, and four-point gaits are used. Additional ambulation skills that are possible to perform independently include getting onto and off of the floor, walking over uneven terrain, negotiating doorways, and ascending and descending stairs, curbs, and ramps.

T1 through T4. People with these levels of paraplegia retain full power in their upper extremities and their erector spinae function above the level of injury. Abdominal musculature is absent.

Walking requires KAFOs (knee-ankle-foot orthoses) and Lofstrand crutches or a walker. It is extremely difficult due to the absence of any trunk or lower extremity control. Ambulation is likely to be restricted to even surfaces.

T5 through T12. With these levels of paraplegia, varying degrees of innervation remain in the abdominal musculature. The upper fibers of the rectus abdominis are innervated by T5. In lower levels of paraplegia, progressively lower fibers are inner-

vated. At T12, the rectus abdominis has full innervation. The erector spinae function above the level of injury.

KAFOs and Lofstrand crutches are required for ambulation. The improved trunk control afforded by the abdominal musculature assists in ambulation. Negotiation of obstacles is more readily achievable. However, ambulation remains a real challenge, even on level surfaces.

L1 and L2. People with L1 and L2 paraplegia have fully innervated internal and external obliques and retain partial innervation of the iliopsoas. Though innervation of the iliopsoas is minimal with L1 paraplegia, it may be enough to assist in ambulation with a four-point gait.[8] Partial innervation of the quadratus lumborum can also make walking easier.

L3 to L5. L3 is the highest level of paraplegia with significant (3/5 or stronger) functioning in the quadriceps. If adequate strength is present in this muscle, it is possible to walk with ankle-foot orthoses (AFOs).

The tibialis anterior and posterior, extensor digitorum longus and brevis, extensor hallucis longus and brevis, and peroneus longus and brevis are partially innervated at L4. However, the gastrocnemius and soleus receive sacral innervation. Since the plantar flexors are important contributors to static balance and ambulation, AFOs are indicated for people with lumbar paraplegia. The control that a given person's orthosis should provide at the ankle will depend on the strength of his knee and ankle musculature.

S1 and Below. Innervation of the gastrocnemius and soleus makes safe ambulation possible without AFOs. If muscle imbalance exists in the ankle or foot, orthotics may be needed to prevent the development of deformity (New York University, 1986).

SUMMARY

The functional potential of people with spinal cord injuries is largely determined by their level of lesion. Other factors such as motivation, body build, and quality of rehabilitation services also strongly affect functional outcomes. This chapter provides infor-

---

[7] Ambulation in the parallel bars is possible for very highly motivated and coordinated people with C6 or C7 quadriplegia, but it is not functional.

[8] By definition, a person with L1 paraplegia has less than 3/5 strength in his iliopsoas (ASIA, 1989). But even the capacity to flex the hip in a gravity-reduced position may assist in swing through.

mation on the physical skills that are possible for people with different levels of complete spinal cord injury.

REFERENCES

American Spinal Injury Association. (1989). *Standards for neurological classification of spinal injury patients.* (Available from the American Spinal Injury Association, 2020 Peachtree Road NW, Atlanta, GA, 30309.)

Ditunno, J.; Sipski, M.; Posuniak, E.; Chen, Y.; Staas, W.; & Herbison, G. (1987). Wrist extensor recovery in traumatic quadriplegia. *Archives of Physical Medicine and Rehabilitation, 68*(5), 287–290.

Gilgoff, I.; Barras, D.; Sellers, M.; & Adkins, H. (1988). Neck breathing. A form of voluntary respiration for the spine-injured ventilator-dependent quadriplegic child. *Pediatrics, 82*(5), 741–745.

Kendall, F.; McCreary, E. (1983). *Muscles: Testing and Function, 3rd ed.* Baltimore, Maryland: Williams & Wilkins.

Lazar, R.; Yarkony, G.; Ortolano, D.; Heinemann, A.; Perlow, E.; Lovell, L.; & Meyer, P. (1989). Prediction of functional outcome by motor capability after spinal cord injury. *Archives of Physical Medicine and Rehabilitation, 70*(11), 819–822.

McClay, I. (1983). Electric wheelchair propulsion using a hand control in C4 quadriplegia. *Physical Therapy, 63*(2), 221–223.

New York University. (1986). *Lower-limb orthotics.* New York: New York University Post-Graduate Medical School.

Welch, R.; Lobley, S.; O'Sullivan, S.; & Freed, M. (1986). Functional independence in quadriplegia: Critical levels. *Archives of Physical Medicine and Rehabilitation, 67*(4), 235–240.

Wetzel, J. (1985). Respiratory evaluation and treatment. In II. Adkins (Ed.), *Spinal cord injury* (pp. 75–98). New York: Churchill Livingstone.

Young, W., & Ransohoff, J. (1989). Acute spinal cord injuries: Experimental therapy, pathophysiological mechanisms, and recovery of function. In Sherk H., Dunn, F., Eismont, F. (ed.), *The cervical spine* Philadelphia, PA: J. B. Lippencott. (2nd ed., pp. 464–495).

8

Getting Started: The Acute Stage of Rehabilitation

Too often, health professionals postpone any serious rehabilitative efforts until the acute stage after spinal cord injury is over. It is easy to neglect preparations for independence during the period immediately following injury, when attention is directed toward achieving medical and orthopedic stability. (When the patient is in skeletal traction, on a cardiac monitor, with a chest tube, multiple intravenous lines [IVs] and a respirator, maintenance of elbow range of motion may seem to be of low priority.) The result is that newly injured people often undergo unnecessary physical deterioration prior to their rehabilitation.

In addition to causing physical problems, postponing the rehabilitation process can lead to the development of a dependent outlook. After experiencing a prolonged period of total helplessness, a newly injured person may come to believe that he is incapable of functioning independently.

To prevent this physical deterioration and learned helplessness, rehabilitation should start as soon as possible after injury. Even in the intensive care unit, steps can be taken to move the recently injured person toward physical and psychological independence.

PHYSICAL CONSIDERATIONS

During the acute stage of rehabilitation after spinal cord injury, it is important for clinicians to keep in mind the manner in which the individual will ultimately function. (How will he transfer? How will he grasp objects?) Appropriate measures must be taken to ensure that the cord-injured person will be prepared for the specific physical activities that he will eventually use to function independently.

In the early weeks and months after injury, a variety of medical or orthopedic problems or both can preclude unrestricted activity. The physical therapist must stay informed of these problems and adapt all treatments accordingly.

Range of Motion

Maintenance of appropriate range of motion is critical during the acute stage of rehabilitation. At best, the development of contractures will cause a delay in the rehabilitation process. At worst, contractures will seriously limit the person's ultimate functional potential.

Joint range of motion and muscle flexibility should be increased or maintained (as indicated) through positioning and daily exercises at this stage. Passive and active range of motion exercises, proprioceptive neuromuscular facilitation (PNF) techniques, joint mobilization, prolonged static stretching or a combination thereof may be employed (Zachazewski, 1989). Orthoses can help increase or maintain range between sessions (Redford, 1980). When orthoses are used, however, the health care team must be aware of their potential hazards and take measures to avoid them.[1]

As a rule, normal joint range of motion and muscle flexibility will enhance function. After spinal cord injury, however, *greater than normal* motion is required in some areas, and mild *tightness* is desirable in others. Moreover, range and flexibility in some areas will have greater functional significance than in others. (For example, limited elbow extension will have greater impact than will a comparable limitation in ankle plantar flexion.) The following are areas of particular concern for spinal cord-injured people.

Shoulders. Normal range in flexion and abduction will facilitate upper body dressing. In the absence of functioning triceps, greater than normal shoulder extension combined with external rotation and

---

[1] Chapter 19 addresses orthotic use following spinal cord injury.

elbow extension is ideal for coming to sitting. This particular combined motion may be neglected during bedside exercises because it is not as easily achieved as other motions: when a patient is supine in a standard bed, his shoulders cannot be extended beyond neutral. Therefore this range of motion exercise should be performed in the side-lying position.

When the cervical spine is unstable, shoulder range of motion exercises should be performed cautiously. The therapist should perform the exercises gently to avoid stress to the cervical region. It may be advisable to avoid shoulder flexion or abduction past 90 degrees (Nawoczenski, Rinehart, Duncanson, & Brown, 1987).

Elbows. Elbow range of motion may be one of the most important physical therapy concerns during the acute phase of rehabilitation. Full elbow extension is required for most functional activities; even a mild limitation in range can profoundly interfere with functional gains. Full elbow extension is particularly critical for people who lack innervated triceps.

For most people, daily range of motion exercises and positioning the elbow in extension will preserve range of motion. If tightness begins to develop, an orthosis may help to maintain or increase extension range.

Forearms. In the absence of functioning triceps, elbow extension is achieved and sustained during transfers and many functional mat activities through "locking," a combination of muscle substitution and positioning. Forearm supination is required for this "locking." Thus forearm supination range must be preserved.

Wrists. Full wrist extension is required to "lock" the elbows in the absence of functioning triceps. In addition, both extension and flexion of the wrist are used to achieve a tenodesis grasp and release.[2]

During the early stages following injury, care should be taken to prevent overstretching of wrist extensors with less than fair (3/5) strength. Overstretching of weakened musculature can inhibit its functioning, and wrist extensors are particularly important because they are used to achieve a tenodesis grasp. Positioning the wrists in extension with cock-up splints or hand rolls can prevent overstretching of the wrist extensors.

Fingers. Mild tightness should be allowed to develop in the long finger flexors of people with C7 or higher quadriplegia to facilitate tenodesis grasp and release. With the appropriate degree of tightness, the fingers will close upon wrist extension and open fully when the wrist is flexed (Fig. 8–1). If the long finger flexors are overstretched, a functional tenodesis grasp will not be achieved. At the other extreme, excessive shortening will inhibit release.

To ensure the development of appropriate tension in the long finger flexors, range of motion exercises should include finger extension to neutral (0 degrees in all joints) with the wrist fully flexed and full finger flexion with the wrist fully extended. Finger extension must be avoided when the wrist is positioned in extension.

Preservation of mild tightness in the long finger flexors is particularly important because damage to the tenodesis mechanism may be permanent. Once the finger flexors become overstretched, it is difficult to get them to tighten. An overzealous but uninformed therapist can cause lasting problems by overstretching these muscles during the acute stage after injury.

Although people with C5 and higher quadriplegia do not have the wrist extensors needed for a

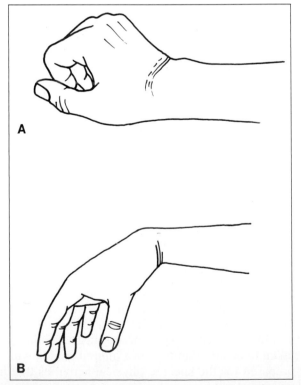

Figure 8–1. Tenodesis grasp used by people with C6 and C7 quadriplegia. Fingers close upon wrist extension (**A**) and open upon wrist flexion. (**B**) (Gravity provides power for wrist flexion.)

---

[2] A person who lacks innervation in his finger musculature but retains the use of his wrist extensors can manipulate objects using a tenodesis grasp: he can flex his fingers by extending his wrist and release the grasp by allowing his wrist to flex.

tenodesis grasp, their long finger flexors should be allowed to tighten. This tightness may make it possible to use the hand as a hook. Moreover, it is common for a spinal cord-injured person's level of motor function to descend one or more levels in the months and years after injury (Young & Ransohoff, 1989). Most people with C5, and a few with C4 quadriplegia, regain function in the C6 myotome during the first eight months after their injuries (Ditunno, Sipski, Posuniak, Chen, Staas, & Herbison, 1987). Thus a person who initially lacks wrist extensor function can regain it and will then require finger flexor tightness for a tenodesis grasp.

Many newly injured people and their families are eager to perform exercises on the paralyzed extremities in the hope that these exercises will bring about a return of function. Often the hands are a focal point of these exercises. For this reason, the cord-injured person and his family should be educated regarding the importance of avoiding overstretching the long finger flexors.

Low Back. Care should be taken to prevent overstretching of the low back. Mild tightness in the low back will allow transmission of head and shoulder motions to the lower body and thus will facilitate transfers and functional mat activities.

Reduced flexibility in the hamstrings can interfere with preservation of low back tightness: when the hamstrings are shortened, sitting with the knees extended (long-sitting) places stress on the low back. For this reason, long-sitting should be avoided when hamstring tightness prevents passive straight-leg raise to 90 degrees. Additionally, hamstring stretching should be performed in supine rather than in long-sitting.

Sitting posture is another important consideration; sitting with lumbar kyphosis can cause overstretching of the low back. When a cord-injured person sits in a wheelchair, his buttocks should be positioned well back on the seat.

Hips. When ambulation is a possible goal, it is important to preserve full extension at the hips. Even when ambulation is not a goal, hip extension to at least neutral will make prone lying and prone mat and bed activities possible.

When the lumbar spine is unstable, hip range of motion exercises should be performed carefully. The therapist should perform the exercises gently and may need to avoid hip flexion past 90 degrees.

Hamstrings. Hamstring flexibility allowing 110 to 120 degrees of straight leg raise will facilitate long-sitting, dressing, mat mobility, and transfers from the floor to a wheelchair. This degree of flexibility is also required for coming to stand from the floor while wearing knee-ankle-foot orthoses (KAFOs).

Hamstring stretching should be performed in supine to preserve tightness in the lower back. When the lumbar spine is unstable, these exercises should be performed carefully. The therapist should perform the exercises gently and may need to avoid straight leg raising past 60 degrees.

Ankle Dorsiflexion. Ankle dorsiflexion to at least 0 degrees (neutral) is important for people who use wheelchairs. If the ankle remains plantar flexed while the foot is on the footrest, excessive pressure will be borne on the metatarsal heads or the toes, and skin breakdown is likely to occur.

Full range in ankle dorsiflexion must be preserved when ambulation is a possible goal. In the absence of hip extensor function, stability in standing is achieved by positioning the hips anterior to the center of gravity (see Fig. 14–1A). Limited ankle dorsiflexion will make it impossible to place the hips in this anterior position.

Proper technique should be used to ensure stretching of the gastrocnemius and soleus rather than of the foot itself. A downward force should be applied to the heel while the ankle is moved into dorsiflexion (Fig. 8–2; Minor & Minor, 1984).

Neck. After a cervical injury, gentle range of motion of the neck should be initiated once the spine has become fully stable. Often, this stability will not be achieved for several months following injury. For this reason it is important to communicate with the physician before initiating neck range of motion exercises.

Strength

Strengthening of all functioning musculature should start as soon as therapy is initiated after injury. Even musculature that exhibits normal (5/5) strength should be strengthened, since abnormal demands will be placed on these muscles during functional activities: muscles that remain innervated must now substitute for all paralyzed musculature. Particular emphasis should be placed on strengthening muscles used in elbow extension, shoulder flexion and horizontal adduction, and scapular protraction and depression, as these muscles are used for most functional activities.

Strengthening exercises should consist of active-assisted, active, or resisted motions, depending on the strength of the functioning musculature. The strengthening program may include any combination of the following: PNF techniques, isometric ex-

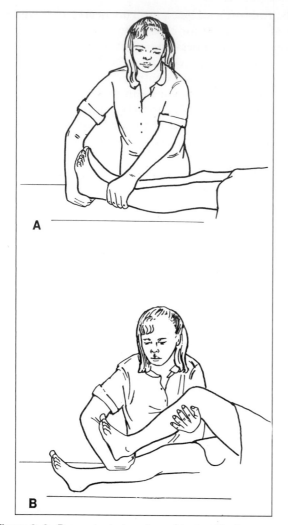

Figure 8–2. Proper technique for ankle dorsiflexion range of motion exercises. A caudally directed force is applied to the heel, and a rostrally directed force is applied to the dorsum of the foot. **A**. Stretching the gastrocnemius: the knee is extended. **B**. Stretching the soleus: the knee is flexed.

ercises, progressive resistive exercises (concentric and eccentric), strengthening through functional activity, isokinetic exercise, and electrical stimulation (Kahn, 1989; Mangine, Heckman, & Eldridge, 1989; Sullivan, Markos, & Minor, 1982). During strengthening exercises, care should be taken to avoid placing stress on unstable vertebral areas.

Whether the cord-injured person has begun out-of-bed activities or remains confined to bed, he should be encouraged to use his functioning musculature as much as possible. While not in therapy, he can maximize his strength by performing isometric exercises, lifting weights, and participating in his care.

Respiration

During the acute stage of rehabilitation after spinal cord injury, respiratory status is an important concern. In the respiratory component of the physical therapy program, the patient works to develop ability in breathing and coughing.[3]

Skin

Pressure ulcers are a serious, common, and preventable complication of spinal cord injury. A lifelong process of skin care beginning at the time of injury is required to prevent decubiti and their sequelae. During the acute phase of rehabilitation, meticulous skin care is particularly important because it sets the stage for future care.

Preventive skin care after spinal cord injury includes a balanced diet, proper management of bowel and bladder incontinence, avoidance of trauma to the skin, and close monitoring of the skin's status.[4] Special attention is given to avoiding prolonged, unrelieved pressure on the skin, particularly over boney prominences.

Pressure Management in Bed. When a cord-injured person lies in bed, his position will determine which areas of his body receive the most pressure and are thus most vulnerable to skin damage. In supine, breakdown is most likely to occur in the skin overlying the occiput, scapulae, sacrum, posterior iliac crests, and heels. In side lying, breakdown is most common over the greater trochanters and both the medial and lateral aspects of the knees and ankles. In prone, the breasts, anterior iliac spines, knees, and toes are vulnerable (Kennedy, Stover, & Fine, 1986; Nawoczenski, 1987; Yob, Wagner, Casson, & Leclerc, 1990).

To prevent the development of decubiti while in a standard bed, a newly injured patient must change positions (turn) at least every two hours. The skin should be inspected each time the patient is turned. As skin tolerance improves,[5] the time spent in each position may be increased gradually. When the time between position changes is increased, the skin over the boney prominences should be monitored especially closely for signs of breakdown.

Eight basic positions are available when lying in bed: supine, prone, and right and left side lying, right and left semiprone, and right and left semi-

---

[3] Respiratory rehabilitation is addressed in Chapter 3.

[4] The skin care program is described in more detail in Chapter 3.

[5] Redness over the boney prominences should disappear within 30 minutes of the position change (Matthews & Carlson, 1987).

supine. In the semisupine position, pressure on the sacrum and greater trochanters is significantly lower than it is in the supine and side-lying positions, respectively (Seiler, Allen, & Stahelin, 1986). The prone and semiprone positions should be used only when the person has a stable spine (Stewart & Wharton, 1976).

Proper bed positioning after spinal cord injury involves more than turning the patient every two hours. The extremities should be placed in positions that preserve range in the key joints discussed above. (For example, the elbows should be placed in extension and the ankles dorsiflexed to neutral.) Pillows or blocks of foam rubber or both can be used for positioning, to relieve pressure on the boney prominences, and to prevent skin surfaces from

contacting each other (Fig. 8–3; Matthews & Carlson, 1987; Stewart & Wharton, 1976).

In the prone position, pillows are used to bridge areas vulnerable to pressure (Fig. 8–3C). One advantage of prone lying is that the hips and knees are extended in this position, preventing the development of flexion contractures. In addition, because the boney prominences are not subjected to pressure, the time spent in this position can be increased to several hours. The person can then sleep uninterrupted through the night (Stewart & Wharton, 1976).

Pressure Management in a Wheelchair. The skin over the ischial tuberosities, sacrum, and coccyx is susceptable to decubiti in sitting (Nawoczenski, 1987).

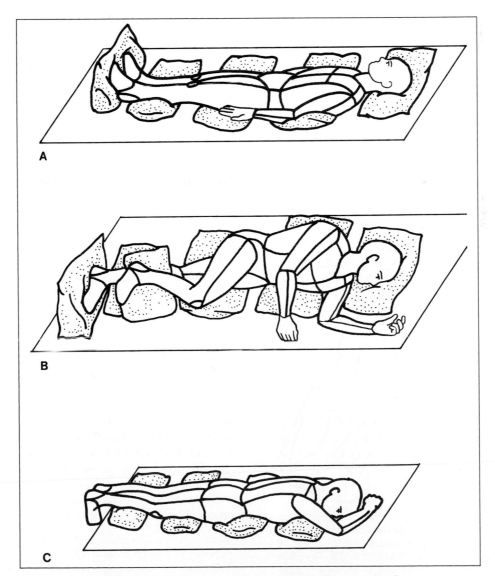

Figure 8–3. Bridging in supine **A**, side lying **B**, and prone **C**.

Proper posture and periodic relief of pressure on the skin will prevent this problem. A good cushion can help reduce the risk of skin breakdown, but it cannot substitute for pressure reliefs.

Appropriate pressure distribution through positioning in the wheelchair will reduce the risk of decubiti. To avoid excessive pressure over the sacrum, the patient's buttocks should be located well back in the chair. Adjusting the footrests so that the knees are at or slightly below the level of the hips will reduce the pressure over the ischial tuberosities by distributing it along the thighs (Brubaker, 1990; Macklebust, 1987; Ragnarsson, 1990). Skin integrity is also protected in sitting through the use of a pressure-distributing wheelchair cushion.[6]

When a cord-injured person sits in a wheelchair, pressure on the ischial tuberosities must be relieved periodically either by lifting the buttocks from the seat (Fig. 8–4) or by shifting weight forward or to the side. Independent pressure relief techniques are presented in Chapter 13.

When sitting is first initiated after spinal cord injury, the pressure over the patient's ischial tuberosities should be relieved every 15 to 20 minutes. The time between pressure reliefs can be increased gradually as the individual's skin tolerance improves. When the time between pressure reliefs is increased, the skin over the ischial tuberosities should be monitored closely for signs of breakdown.

ATTITUDINAL CONSIDERATIONS

A recently injured person may truly be unavoidably dependent. (How could anyone be independent in the intensive care unit?) However, steps can be taken to avoid the feeling of total helplessness and powerlessness that can lead to a lasting attitude of dependency.

From the time of injury onward, the cord-injured person should be educated regarding his condition and his needs and should be encouraged to be his own advocate. For example, he should know his turning schedule and understand the reason for its importance. He should be encouraged to take responsibility for ensuring that he turns on schedule,[7] soliciting assistance when needed.

Starting as soon as possible after injury, a cord-injured person should be asked to do as much as he can for himself. This expectation of active participation will emphasize his remaining abilities and his dynamic involvement in his program. Depending on what musculature is left functioning, a recently injured person may be able to participate in bed positioning, hygiene, and self-feeding. Even if he is unable to perform the above activities, he may be able to assist in his care. For example, someone who cannot feed himself may be able to stabilize the dinner tray when being fed.

To preserve a sense of autonomy, clinicians must include patients in decision making. At this early stage in rehabilitation, goal setting provides an excellent opportunity to involve the recently in-

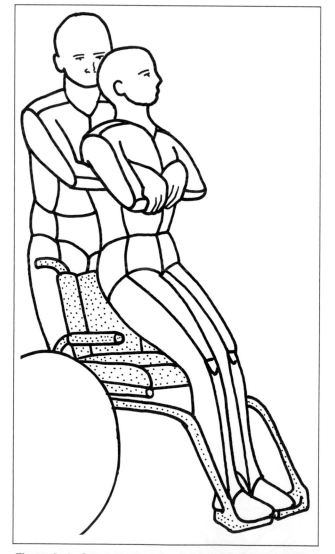

Figure 8–4. One technique for dependent pressure reliefs: while grasping the patient's forearms from behind, the therapist pulls the patient toward himself and lifts. The patient should be encouraged to depress his scapulae and adduct his shoulders ("Squeeze your arms against your body and pull down.") during the pressure relief.

---

[6] Chapter 19 presents cushion options and selection procedures.

[7] This does not relieve health professionals of their responsibilities; at this point the health care team remains ultimately responsible for providing proper care.

jured person in making decisions about his future. The patient's desires regarding functional outcomes and treatment options should be incorporated into the program.

Finally, the manner in which health professionals relate to a recently injured person will influence his self concept. If treated as a pitiable, dependent, and hopeless "victim" for long enough, a patient may begin to adjust to that role. (Who wouldn't?) If all members of the rehabilitation team instead treat the patient as a rational person with a future, they may foster a more positive outlook.[8]

GETTING STARTED

Before a cord-injured person sits upright or begins functional training, his vertebral stability must be established, either with or without a spinal orthosis. As soon as he has been medically cleared to do so, the patient should get out of bed and into a wheelchair. This early mobilization can prevent the physical and psychological ill effects of prolonged bedrest.

Skin Care. When out-of-bed activities are initiated, care must be taken to avoid the development of decubiti while in sitting. A wheelchair cushion, appropriate sitting posture, and frequent pressure reliefs will prevent this complication. The patient should be educated regarding the importance of pressure reliefs and should be encouraged to take responsibility for this aspect of his care. Even if he is physically unable to perform a pressure relief independently, he can keep track of the time and remind nearby clinicians when it is time for one. This early responsibility may facilitate the development of good pressure-relief habits.

Upright Sitting Tolerance. When upright activities are first initiated, people with spinal cord injuries may experience orthostatic hypotension. This is a transient problem that is most prevalent among people with lesions above T6 (Buchanan & Ditunno, 1987; Cole, 1988; Lehman, Lane, Piepmeier & Batsford, 1987; Yashon, 1986). Especially after prolonged bedrest, moving directly to an upright sitting position can cause a drop in blood pressure with resulting dizziness, vomiting, and loss of consciousness. For this reason it is best to allow cord-injured people to accommodate gradually to upright sitting postures.

A reclining wheelchair is useful for developing tolerance to upright sitting. When a recently injured person is first placed in this type of wheelchair, the chair's back can be almost fully reclined and the legrests elevated. As the patient adapts to sitting, the wheelchair's back can be raised in small increments to a progressively more upright position, and the elevating legrests can be lowered.

If a reclining wheelchair is not available, sitting tolerance may be developed in bed. The patient should be able to accommodate to increasingly upright positions by sitting with the head of his bed elevated and his feet dangling over the side of the bed. When his sitting tolerance has increased sufficiently, the patient can use a nonreclining wheelchair.

Thigh-high antiembolic stockings and an abdominal binder[9] can be worn initially to reduce orthostatic hypotension by facilitating venous return. Once the patient has accommodated to sitting, the binder should be discontinued. If abrupt discontinuation of the abdominal binder causes prolonged dizziness, the patient can be weaned more gradually from its use through loosening over a period of days.

Mild dizziness is common and will need to be tolerated by the cord-injured person as he adjusts to sitting. If the patient becomes very nauseated, loses consciousness, or loses vision or hearing, these symptoms can be eliminated by elevating the legs, tipping the wheelchair back into a more reclined position, or both. It is important to remember that the above-described symptoms are not dangerous and to treat them accordingly.[10] A calm attitude on the therapist's part can result in an easier and more rapid adjustment to sitting.

The time allotted to developing sitting tolerance need not be spent with the patient passively watching the clock and waiting for nausea or dizziness (or sudden death from boredom) to strike. While the patient adjusts to sitting, he can perform strengthening exercises and begin working on wheelchair propulsion. He can also practice stabilizing his trunk and leaning from side to side in the wheelchair, controlling the motion by pulling on the armrests. These skills are used in independent maintenance of an upright sitting posture and can be used for relief of pressure.[11]

---

[8] Strategies for enhancing psychosocial adaptation after spinal cord injury are presented in greater depth in Chapter 4.

[9] An abdominal binder is an elasticized band that encompasses the entire abdomen.

[10] Orthostatic hypotension should not be confused with autonomic dysreflexia, which is a dangerous condition. Autonomic dysreflexia is characterized by a *rise* in blood pressure rather than a fall and is brought on by noxious stimulation below the lesion. Its management is addressed in Chapter 3.

[11] Techniques used in these activities are described in Chapter 13.

Functional Training. To many health professionals, the words "functional training" evoke images of vigorous maneuvers performed on a mat in a physical therapy gym. However, important skills can be developed through a variety of less strenuous activities; functional training need not (and should not) be postponed until the patient is ready for upright or physically strenuous activities. While he remains confined to bed, the recently injured person can begin working toward functional goals through a variety of activities. For example, an individual who lacks functioning triceps may make initial progress toward independence by practicing extending his elbows aginst resistance using his anterior deltoids, positioning his elbows in extension while he lies supine, or isolating shoulder flexion from elbow flexion. More extensive functional training should be initiated as soon as the patient is medically ready for the increase in activity level. Early activities in preparation for transfers, mat skills, and wheelchair skills are presented in Chapters 11, 12, and 13.

SUMMARY

Rehabilitation should begin during the acute phase of treatment after spinal cord injury. During early rehabilitation, the therapist and patient can work together to develop range of motion, strength, respiratory ability, and functional skills. The rehabilitation team should also work to preserve or to develop the recently injured person's sense of autonomy. This early rehabilitation can prevent unnecessary physical and psychosocial problems and can prepare the patient for the postacute phase of his rehabilitation.

REFERENCES

Brubaker, C. (1990). Ergonometric considerations. *Journal of Rehabilitation Research and Development, Clinical Supplement #2*, 37–48.

Buchanan, L., & Ditunno, J. (1987). Acute care: Medical/surgical management. In L. Buchanan, & D. Nawoczenski (Eds), *Spinal cord injury: Concepts and management approaches* (pp. 35–60). Baltimore: Williams & Wilkins.

Cole, J. (1988). The pathophysiology of the autonomic nervous system in spinal cord injury. In L. Illis (Ed.), *Spinal cord dysfunction: Assessment* (pp. 201–235). New York: Oxford University Press.

Ditunno, J.; Sipski, M.; Posuniak, E.; Chen, Y.; Staas, W.; & Herbison, G. (1987). Wrist extensor recovery in traumatic quadriplegia. *Archives of Physical Medicine and Rehabilitation, 68*(5), 287–290.

Kahn, J. (1989). Physical agents: Electrical, sonic, and radiant modalities. In R. Scully, & M. Barnes (Eds.), *Physical Therapy* (pp. 876–900). Philadelphia: J.B. Lippincott.

Kennedy, E.; Stover, S.; & Fine, P. (Eds). (1986). *Spinal cord injury: The facts and figures.* Birmingham, AL: The University of Alabama Spinal Cord Injury Statistical Center.

Lehman, K.; Lane, J.; Piepmeier, J.; & Batsfod, W. (1987). Cardiovascular abnormalities accompanying acute spinal cord injury in humans: Incidence, time course and severity. *JACC, 10*(1), 46–52.

Macklebust, J. (1987). Pressure ulcers: Etiology and prevention. *Nursing Clinics of North America, 22*(2), 359–377.

Mangine, R.; Heckmann, T.; & Eldridge, V. (1989). Improving strength, endurance, and power. In R. Scully & M. Barnes (Eds.), *Physical Therapy* (pp. 739–762). Philadelphia: J.B. Lippincott.

Matthews, P., & Carlson, C. (1987). *Spinal cord injury: A guide to rehabilitation nursing.* Rockville, MD: Aspen Publishers.

Minor, M., & Minor, S. (1984). *Patient care skills: Positioning, range of motion, transfers, wheelchairs, and ambulation.* Reston, VA: Reston Publishing.

Nawoczenski, D. (1987). Pressure sores: Prevention and management. In L. Buchanan, & D. Nawoczenski (Eds.), *Spinal cord injury: Concepts and management approaches* (pp. 99–121). Baltimore: Williams & Wilkins.

Nawoczenski, D.; Rinehart, M.; Duncanson, P.; & Brown, B. (1987). Physical management. In L. Buchanan, & D. Nawoczenski (Eds.), *Spinal cord injury: Concepts and management approaches* (pp. 123–184). Baltimore: Williams & Wilkins.

Ragnarsson, K. (1990). Prescription considerations and a comparison of conventional and lightweight wheelchairs. *Journal of Rehabilitation Research and Development, Clinical Supplement #2*, 8–16.

Redford, J. (1980). Principles of orthotic devices. In J. Redford (Ed.), *Orthotics etcetera* (2nd ed., pp. 1–21). Baltimore: Williams & Wilkins.

Seiler, W.; Allen, S.; & Stahelin, H. (1986). Influence of the 30 laterally inclined position and the "super-soft" 3-piece mattress on skin oxygen tension on areas of maximum pressure—implications for pressure sore prevention. *Gerontology, 32*, 158–166.

Stewart, P., & Wharton, G. (1976). Bridging: An effective and practical method of preventive skin care for the immobilized person. *Southern Medical Journal, 69*(11), 1469–1473.

Sullivan, P.; Markos, P.; & Minor, M. (1982). *An integrated approach to therapeutic exercises: Theory and clinical application.* Reston, VA: Reston.

Yashon, D. (1986). *Spinal injury* (2nd ed.). Norwalk, CT: Appleton, Century, Crofts.

Yob, S.; Wagner, D.; Casson, H.; & Leclerc, J. (1990).

Skin management of the SCI patient. In *Dawn of a new decade: spinal cord injury in the 1990's*. Symposium sponsored by National Rehabilitation Hospital, Washington, DC.

Young, W., & Ransohoff, J. (1989). Acute spinal cord injuries: Experimental therapy, pathophysiological mechanisms, and recovery of function. In H. Sherk (Ed)., *The cervical spine* (2nd ed., pp. 464–495). Philadelphia: J.B. Lippincott.

Zachazewski, J. (1989). Improving flexibility. In R. Scully, & M. Barnes (Eds.), *Physical therapy* (pp. 698–738). Philadelphia: J.B. Lippincott.

9

Overview of the Physical Therapy Functional Rehabilitation Program

The key to designing a successful functional rehabilitation program is understanding the nature of the task: the cord-injured person must learn to use his body in a totally different manner after his injury. To move from one place to another, get dressed, open a door, or perform any other physical activity, he must use his remaining musculature in unaccustomed ways. Each activity requires strength in certain muscles and the joint range of motion and muscle flexibility to perform the motions. In addition to these physical prerequisites, each functional task requires an array of skills. Functional independence requires the development of all of these physical and skill prerequisites.

Program Overview
The functional component of the physical therapy rehabilitation program consists of functional training directed toward achieving the patient's functional goals and exercises to acquire the necessary physical prerequisites.[1]

Strengthening. Strengthening is an essential component of any rehabilitation program after spinal cord injury. Functional activities place great demands on the patient's musculature: muscles that remain innervated must compensate for those that have been paralyzed. As a result, they are often required to perform actions for which they are not ideally suited. For example, the anterior deltoids are used for elbow extension when the triceps are paralyzed. During transfers, these muscles, which normally flex the glenohumeral joints, must extend the

elbows and maintain this extension while the person supports his weight on his arms. The stronger the anterior deltoids are, the more stable the arms will be during transfers.

After spinal cord injury, virtually all innervated musculature is used in various functional activities and thus should be strengthened. The strengthening program should place particular emphasis on musculature that is used to extend the elbows, to flex or horizontally adduct the shoulders, and to protract or depress the scapulae. Most functional activities require strength in these muscles.

Muscle Flexibility and Joint Range of Motion. Muscle stretching is another key part of rehabilitation. Many functional activities involve motions that require greater flexibility than most of us have. For example, a floor-to-chair transfer using a side approach requires very flexible hamstrings.

For patients who have normal passive motion in their joints, range of motion exercises are a minor (though important) part of the rehabilitation program. A few minutes of exercise daily is generally adequate to maintain range. Many cord-injured people are able to perform these exercises independently. Once a patient achieves functional independence, even these exercises may become unnecessary; motion of the joints during the day's activities may preserve the needed range of motion.

Range of motion exercises are a more central part of the therapeutic program for patients who have limitations in key joints. Even a few degrees of limitation can have a severe impact upon function. For example, a mild elbow flexion contracture makes it extremely difficult for a person without functioning triceps to maintain elbow extension during transfers.

---

[1] The physical therapy program also addresses respiration, education, equipment procurement, and home modification, addressed in other chapters.

Functional Training. Strengthening and stretching alone will not improve function. The most important component of a functional rehabilitation program is functional training. Through functional training, the cord-injured individual learns the muscle substitutions and acrobatic maneuvers used to move his body, take care of himself, and manipulate his environment.

Functional training should be initiated as early as possible in the program rather than being postponed until strength and range have been maximized. Early functional training can have tremendous psychological benefit, enabling the newly injured person to do things for himself and experience tangible progress toward his goals. As the patient masters and uses more skills, his increased activity level also serves to further develop his strength and flexibility. A balanced program that addresses skill concurrently with strength, muscle flexibility, and joint range of motion will be most efficient in helping the patient progress toward independence.

Time Requirements. In a rehabilitation program following spinal cord injury, the patient strengthens his functioning musculature, increases his flexibility, and learns an entirely new way of moving. Clearly this is a challenging task that requires a great deal of time and effort. Rehabilitation requires several hours of concentrated work in physical therapy daily, often over a period of months. Anything less will yield lower results.

Forms of Therapy

Strengthening, stretching, and functional training can all be accomplished through one-on-one work, group classes, and independent activities. Each of these therapeutic approaches has its advantages and should be included in a functional rehabilitation program.

One-on-One Work. A therapist can give hands-on training while working directly with a single patient. By providing added stability or muscle power, or simply by guarding, the therapist can enable the cord-injured person to go through the motions used to perform a functional activity. This allows the patient to get a feel for the motor sequence involved in the task.

One-on-one work also enables the therapist to watch the patient closely as he attempts and fails a functional task. This close observation makes it possible to analyze the performance and to determine what is preventing successful completion of the task. It may become apparent, for example, that spasticity is interfering with an individual's ability to perform a given maneuver. A particular muscle may not have enough strength or flexibility. The patient may not yet be ready for the task that he is attempting; he may need to develop a more basic skill first. Or perhaps he simply needs more practice. Whatever the underlying problem or problems, the therapist can revise the therapeutic program to address the specific areas of need.

During one-on-one therapy, the therapist can also give direction and immediate feedback. While or after observing the patient as he attempts to perform an activity, the therapist can determine what he is doing correctly and incorrectly and make suggestions for improving the technique. Better yet, the therapist can involve the patient in this problem solving.

Group Classes. Group classes can be an excellent source of motivation as people with similar abilities work together toward common goals. The group can provide mutual support, encouragement, and peer pressure to maximize performance. With this group interaction, people often work harder than they do when working alone.

Strength, flexibility, and skill can be developed in group work. Group classes can involve a variety of activities, including weight lifting, stretching, balance practice, swimming or other recreational activities, and practice working on mat skills, transfers, wheelchair skills, or ambulation. Classes that take the participants out of the gym (an expedition in pursuit of "real-world" obstacles to negotiate in wheelchairs, for example) can be refreshing as well as educational and functionally beneficial.

Independent Work. People undergoing rehabilitation should spend some time every day working independently on problem areas such as particular muscles that need strengthening or skills that need to be improved. This independent work can occur during regularly schedule time in the physical therapy department as well as during "off" times when the patient is not in therapy.

The most important reason to include independent activities in rehabilitation programs is that these activities help to develop a self-reliant attitude. Independent work enables the person to practice problem solving and self-motivated work toward goals. The experience is one of autonomy and personal responsibility. In contrast, constant, direct supervision conveys the message that the patient needs a therapist around for progress to occur.

A second reason for independent work is that functional rehabilitation after spinal cord injury requires more time in therapy than would be feasible with only one-on-one and group classes. In most facilities there simply are not enough therapists to go around.

Strategies for Functional Training

The task of rehabilitation may seem overwhelming when one is faced with a recently injured person who is unable to roll over or even to stay upright in a wheelchair. How on earth will this person achieve the lofty goals that he has identified?

Building a Foundation. Most functional skills are built upon a foundation of fundamental capabilities. For example, many activities require the ability to sit upright while balancing on one arm. The therapeutic program should develop these basic prerequisite skills early and apply them in functional skills once they have been fairly well mastered.

As a part of building a foundation for functional skills, the cord-injured person needs to develop motor control in the various postures involved in functional activities. The four stages of motor control, progressing from most basic to most advanced, are mobility, stability, controlled mobility, and skill (Sullivan, Markos, & Minor, 1982). Before an individual can exhibit a given level of motor control in a particular posture, he must be capable of the more basic levels of control in that posture. For example, walking on the elbows (skill) requires the ability to weight shift (controlled mobility) in prone on elbows, which presupposes the ability to maintain the prone-on-elbows posture (stability), which in turn requires adequate range of motion and ability to initiate motion (mobility). During functional training, the patient develops basic motor abilities and then builds on them as his control improves.

Breaking Down the Activity into its Component Parts. Many functional activities consist of a fairly complex sequence of actions; a "simple" act such as coming to sitting can require a series of five or more separate steps. Each of these steps requires a different set of prerequisite skills. Rather than trying to tackle a complex activity as a whole, it is more productive to break it down and work toward mastery of each component. Once the patient masters the different steps, he can work on putting them together to perform the functional task.

Making the Task Easier. Certain activities are exceedingly difficult initially, even when broken into separate steps. For example, one step in a side-approach transfer from the floor to a wheelchair involves moving the buttocks all the way from the floor to the wheelchair seat. This maneuver requires great flexibility, strength, and finesse. When working on a challenging task such as this one, functional training may involve practicing an easier version of the task. Using this approach, the patient develops his skill by practicing a maneuver that involves the same technique as the activity in question. As his skill improves, the maneuver that he practices should increase in difficulty, becoming more similar to the functional skill being addressed. For example, a patient can develop his technique for floor-to-chair transfers by performing transfers between the floor and successively higher surfaces. He may begin by transferring to and from a surface 1 inch higher than the floor and gradually increase the surface's height until he can transfer as high as the wheelchair seat.

Learning the Skill in Reverse. Many activities are the most challenging at their starting points. These maneuvers are difficult to initiate and become easier

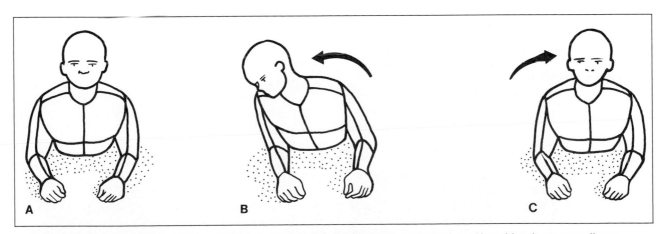

Figure 9–1. Learning a skill in reverse: assuming prone on elbows. **A.** Begin in the end position (prone on elbows in this case.) **B.** Shift a short distance out of the position. **C.** Return to the original position.

as they approach completion. The task of assuming the prone-on-elbows position is an example of such an activity. It takes a good deal of strength for someone with C5 or C6 quadriplegia to lift his trunk off of the mat. The task becomes easier as he rises higher and his arms move into a more vertical position under his trunk.

Working on the skill in reverse is a useful training strategy for this type of activity. Instead of starting at the beginning of the activity where the task is the most difficult, the patient starts at the endpoint and works backward. Emphasis should be placed on the patient controlling his motion as he works on the skill in reverse. For example, the individual learning to assume the prone-on-elbows position can start in that position and practice moving toward side lying or prone. To develop his skill, he should move *slightly* toward side lying or prone *in a controlled fashion* and then actively return to prone on elbows (Fig. 9–1). As his ability improves, he should work on moving progressively further from and returning to the prone-on-elbows position in a controlled fashion.

SUMMARY

Functional rehabilitation after spinal cord injury is a challenging task. The cord-injured individual must increase strength in innervated musculature and preserve or increase joint range and muscle flexibility to be able to perform the maneuvers used to perform functional tasks. He must also develop an array of physical skills, learning to use his muscles and to move his body in new ways. Functional training strategies include building a foundation of prerequisite skills, breaking complex activities into their component parts, making difficult tasks easier,

and practicing certain skills in reverse. The therapeutic program should include a mixture of one-on-one work with the therapist, group classes, and independent work.

REFERENCE

Sullivan, P.; Markos, P.; & Minor, M. (1982). *An integrated approach to therapeutic exercise: Theory and clinical application*. Reston, VA: Reston.

SUGGESTED READING

For additional information relevant to program planning in functional rehabilitation, the reader is referred to the following books:

Basmajian, J. & Wolf, S. (Eds.) (1990). *Therapeutic Exercise* (5th ed.). Baltimore: Williams & Wilkins.

Bauer, D. (1989). *Foundation of Physical Rehabilitation: A Management Approach*. New York: Churchill Livingstone.

Carr, J. & Shepherd, R. (Eds.). (1987). *Movement Science: Foundations for Physical Therapy in Rehabilitation*. Rockville, MD: Aspen.

Morrow, J. (1989). Teaching. In R. Scully & M. Barnes (Eds.), *Physical Therapy* (pp. 1104–1114). New York: J. B. Lippincott.

Sullivan, P., Markos, P., & Minor, M. (1982). *An Integrated Approach to Therapeutic Exercise: Theory and Clinical Application*. Reston, VA: Reston.

Wolf, S. (Ed.). (1985). *Clinical Decision Making in Physical Therapy*. Philadelphia: F.A. Davis.

Umphred, D. (1990). Conceptual Model: A framework for clinical problem solving. In D. Umphred (Ed.), *Neurological Rehabilitation* (2nd ed., pp. 3–26). Baltimore: C. V. Mosby Company.

10

Mechanical Principles Used in Functional Activities

Normal movement involves the coordinated action of an array of skeletal muscles; dozens of muscles function in concert to move the trunk and extremities. Damage to the spinal cord disrupts this normal pattern of motion.

Following spinal cord injury, a person who wishes to regain functional independence faces a difficult task. He must learn to use what muscles remain to perform the tasks of the now absent musculature. With fewer muscles functioning, he must find new ways to move. Three major tools are available to enable a cord-injured person to make the most of what musculature remains functional: muscle substitution, momentum, and the head-hips relationship.

MUSCLE SUBSTITUTION

Muscle substitution can be used when the musculature normally causing a motion is weak or absent. In one method of substitution, agonistic musculature compensates for a strength deficit. For example, the tensor fascia lata can substitute for a weak or absent gluteus medius in hip abduction. This and other substitutions by agonists should be familiar to all physical therapists, who monitor for them whenever performing manual muscle tests.

Agonists are commonly used to substitute after spinal cord injury. Whenever agonists of a weak or nonfunctioning muscle remain functional, they work to compensate for the motor deficit. However, in the paralysis that results from spinal cord injury, agonists often are not available for substitution. In these instances, other methods of substitution are used.

The substitutions used following spinal cord injury may seem mysterious to the uninitiated. (Muscles are used to move joints that they do not even cross!) However, a muscle used to substitute does not do anything out of the ordinary. It simply contracts concentrically, eccentrically, or isometrically, pulling in the same direction that it always did. Unless a muscle is moved surgically, it cannot do otherwise. The key to muscle substitution after spinal cord injury is learning to use a muscle's pull differently.

In addition to substitution by agonists, there are three ways in which a muscle can be used to substitute. Muscle action can be combined with the effects of gravity, tension in passive structures, or fixation of the distal extremity to effect a desired motion.

Substitution Using Gravity

Functioning musculature can be used to reposition a part in such a way that gravity will effect the desired motion. For example, shoulder motion can be used to pronate the forearm. When a person is sitting upright, shoulder abduction and internal rotation can move the forearm to a position in which the palm faces downward slightly. Once the forearm is in this position, the downward pull of gravity will pronate the forearm.

When gravity is used in substitution, the movement's force will be very limited. Any significant resistance will prevent the motion.

Substitution Using Tension in Passive Structures

Tension in nonfunctioning musculature can also be used to effect motion. The tenodesis grasp is an example of this method of substitution. When a tenodesis grasp is used, the extensor carpi radialis longus and brevis are used to extend the wrist. The resulting increase in tension in the long finger flexors causes the fingers to flex (see Fig. 8–1).

This method of substitution can cause a more

forceful motion than is possible in substitutions using gravity; the motion can be performed against some resistance. For this reason, a tenodesis grasp can be used functionally in activities such as eating, dressing, and self-catheterization.

Substitution Using Fixation of the Distal Extremity

This method of muscle substitution involves fixing the distal end of an extremity by stabilizing it on an object and using proximal musculature to cause mo-

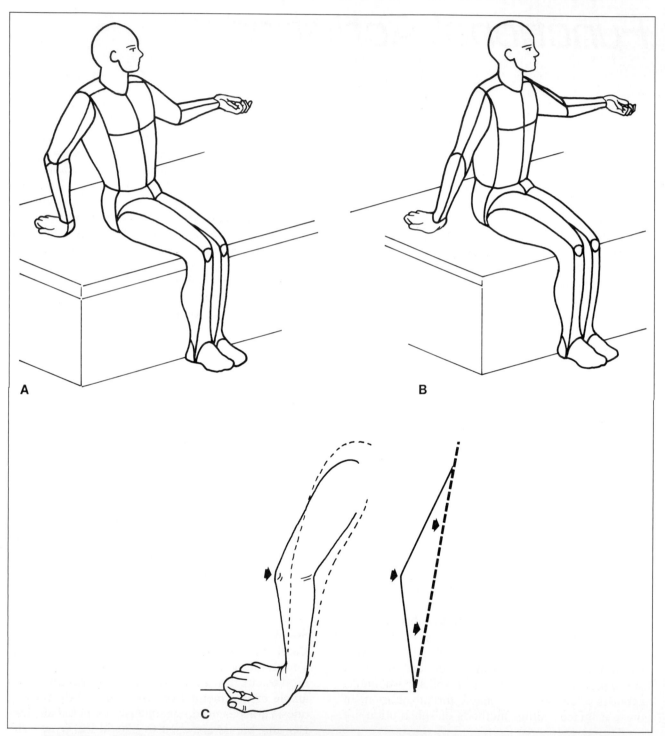

Figure 10–1. Substitution using fixation of the distal extremity. **A** An individual lacking functioning triceps is sitting on a mat, leaning on one arm. The elbow is flexed and the hand is stabilized on the mat. **B** The elbow is extended by adducting the shoudler. **C** When the humerus is adducted, the proximal forearm also moves medially, resulting in elbow extension.

tion at an intermediate joint. The anterior deltoid and pectoralis major can be used to extend the elbow in this manner. When a cord-injured person extends his elbow using proximal musculature, he first stabilizes his hand. He then uses his anterior deltoid and pectoralis major to adduct the humerus. Figure 10–1 illustrates this process. In this example the patient is sitting upright with his hand stabilized beside him on a mat. When the humerus is adducted, the proximal end of the forearm also moves, since it is attached to the humerus. With the hand fixed distally, the forearm moves in an arc (Fig. 10–1C). The result is extension of the elbow.

Using this method of substitution, a fair amount of force can be generated. A patient who has adequate strength proximally will be able to extend his elbows forcefully enough to lift his trunk from a forward lean (Fig. 10–2).

ANGULAR MOMENTUM

Once an object is set in motion, it tends to continue moving in the same direction. This physical property is called momentum. An object that is rotating about an axis has angular momentum, the tendency to continue its rotation.

Angular momentum can be used to augment motion when musculature is weak. A patient who cannot complete an action when he "places" the part, moving it slowly, may be able to complete the same action if he "throws" the part instead. An example would be someone with weak posterior deltoids who is sitting in a wheelchair and wishes to position his arm behind the wheelchair's push handle. He may find that he is unable to "place" his arm behind the push handle but can move his arm into position by throwing it.

In another use of angular momentum, functioning musculature initiates a motion, and the momentum of the moving part(s) causes movement in other areas of the body. This use of angular momentum is exemplified by the technique for rolling used by people who lack functioning trunk musculature. To roll, a cord-injured person throws his head and arms to the side. If the motion is forceful enough, the momentum of the head and arms will carry the trunk from supine.

The angular momentum of a large object (such as a person) is equal to the sum of the angular momenta of all of its parts. Each part's angular momentum is proportional to its velocity, mass, and the moment arm, or distance of the part from its axis of rotation. The effects of these characteristics of angular momentum are important to keep in mind during functional training.

Summation of Momenta

During functional activities, the motions of relatively small body parts are often used to cause larger parts to move. Rolling is an example of this: head and arm motions are used to move the trunk and lower extremities. To move such a large mass in this manner, a person may need all of the momentum that he can muster. If he attempts to roll using only arm motions, he may not be able to move his trunk from supine. The added momentum from head motions may be required.

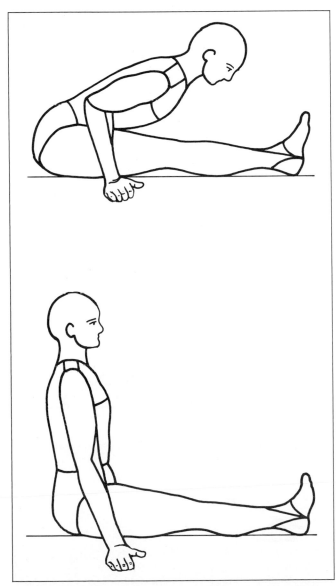

Figure 10–2. Muscle substitution used to extend the elbows and lift the trunk from a forward lean.

Velocity

An extremity that moves slowly will not have as much momentum as one of equal mass that moves with a higher velocity. Thus when a person uses momentum to execute a functional activity, his motions need to be performed with adequate speed. In the case of rolling, someone who moves his arms and head too slowly will not be able to work up enough momentum to move his trunk.

Mass

If all other things are equal, an object with greater mass will have greater angular momentum. Attaching a weight to a patient's arm effectively increases

its mass. This increases the angular momentum that the arm will have at given speed, making rolling easier. Although adding a wrist weight to facilitate rolling is not practical as a permanent measure, it can be used to assist rolling during functional training.

Moment Arm

For a given mass and velocity, an object with a larger moment arm will have greater angular momentum. For this reason, rolling is easier when the elbows are held in extension. Keeping the elbows extended moves the arms' mass further from the body, increasing their moment arms. This enables

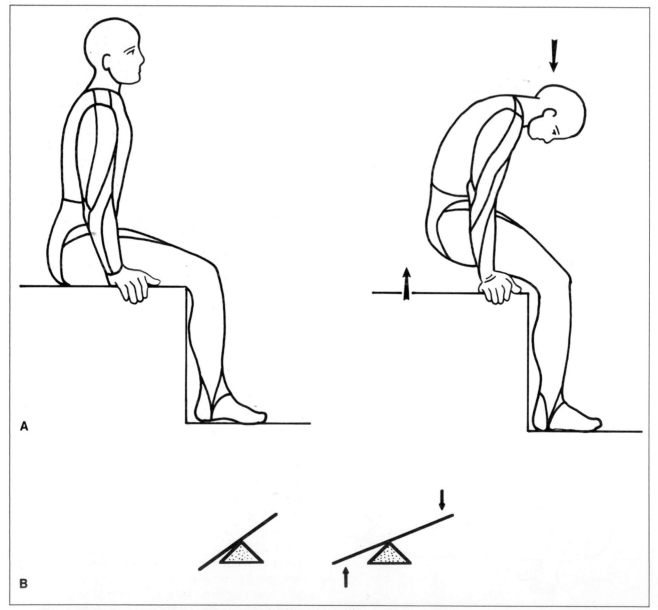

Figure 10–3. The head-hips relationship. **A** The cord-injured person pivots on his arms, moving his head down to lift his buttocks. **B** First-class lever.

the patient to generate more angular momentum when he throws his arms.

HEAD-HIPS RELATIONSHIP

The final tool used in functional activities is the head-hips relationship. When using the head-hips relationship, a person with a spinal cord injury moves his buttocks by moving his head in the opposite direction. To do so, he pivots on his shoulders, which act as a fulcrum in a first class lever (Fig. 10–3).

Transfers provide a good example of the use of the head-hips relationship. Someone who wishes to lift his buttocks up and to the left in a transfer does so by moving his head down and to the right while pivoting on his arms.

SUMMARY

After a complete spinal cord injury, an individual is left with a limited number of innervated muscles with which to function. He must learn new ways to move his body if he wishes to regain functional independence. During functional training, he learns to use muscle substitution, momentum, and the head-hips relationship to regain physical independence.

SUGGESTED READING

For additional information on biomechanics, the reader is referred to the following books:

Lehmkuhl, L. & Smith, L. (1983). *Brunnstrom's Clinical Kinesiology* (4th ed.). Philadelphia, F.A. Davis.

Luttgens, K. & Wells, K. (1982). *Kinesiology: Scientific Basis of Human Motion* (7th ed.). Philadelphia: Saunders College Publishing.

Soderberg, G. (1986). *Kinesiology: Application to Pathological Motion*. Baltimore: Williams & Wilkins.

von Heijne Wiktorin, C. & Nordin, M. (1986). *Introduction to Problem Solving in Biomechanics*. Philadelphia: Lea & Febiger.

11

Transfers

Transfers are crucial for independent mobility; before a person can go anywhere in his wheelchair, he must first get out of bed. Independent transfers can improve the quality of life by opening up options. A person who can transfer independently can get out of bed in the morning without waiting for assistance and can leave his wheelchair to sit on a couch, get into a car, or get onto the ground for a picnic. Transferring can also be an important survival skill, making it possible to get back into the wheelchair after a fall.

This chapter presents a variety of transfer techniques,[1] as well as suggestions on how to teach them. It is important for the reader to keep in mind that the exact motions used to perform any functional task vary among people. This variability is due to differences in body build, skill level, range of motion, muscle tone, and patterns of strength and weakness. Because of these differences, each individual differs slightly in hand placement, starting position, and the degree and force of head and trunk motion used to accomplish the task.

The descriptions of techniques and training presented in this chapter should be used as a guide, not as a set of hard-and-fast rules. The therapist and patient should work together to find the exact technique that best suits that particular individual.

Role of Legs in Transfers

Legs play an important role in transfers, even in the absence of any motor function. If they are positioned correctly, the legs will bear weight during a transfer. This makes the transfer easier by reducing the weight that the cord-injured person must lift on his arms. The legs can also help to stabilize the trunk during the transfer, making it easier to pivot on the arms.

Preservation of Tenodesis Grasp

People with active wrist extension are able to compensate for nonfunctional finger flexors by using a natural tenodesis grasp (described in Chapter 8.) For this grasp to work, the long finger flexors must not be overstretched.

Whenever the wrists and fingers are extended simultaneously, the long finger flexors are stretched and the tenodesis grasp can be damaged. This can occur during transfers when weight is borne on the palms. To avoid stretching the long finger flexors, an individual who uses a tenodesis grasp (or may use this grasp in the future) should keep his interphalangeal joints flexed whenever he bears weight on his palms. This will preserve his tenodesis grasp.

Preservation of Low Back Tightness

Mild tightness in the low back is desirable for people with complete spinal cord injuries, as it facilitates transfers and functional mat activities. To preserve mild tightness in the low back, long-sitting should be avoided when shortening of the hamstrings prevents passive straight leg raise to 90 degrees.

PHYSICAL AND SKILL PREREQUISITES

Each functional activity involves a particular set of skills. Each activity also has strength, joint range of motion, and muscle flexibility requirements. A deficiency in any of these skill or physical prerequisites will impair a person's performance of the activity.

The descriptions of functional techniques presented below are accompanied by charts that summarize the physical and skill prerequisites. Exact values for the physical prerequisites are not given because the requirements vary among individuals.

---

[1] This chapter does not attempt to present all possible transfer techniques. An individual who is unable to master a transfer described in this chapter may fare better with a variation of that transfer or with an altogether different method.

For example, a person who is thin, coordinated, and has relatively long arms will probably require less anterior deltoid strength to perform a particular transfer than someone who is overweight, uncoordinated, and has short arms.

ACCESSORY SKILLS

When most of us think of transfers, we consider only the leap from one surface to another. In fact, a great deal more is involved. To move from a wheelchair to a bed, for example, an individual must be able to position the wheelchair, lock the brakes, reposition or remove an armrest (if armrests are used), and position the footrests. He must also position his legs, buttocks, and torso in preparation for the transfer and pull his legs onto the bed following the transfer. If a sliding board is used, it must be placed before the transfer and removed afterwards.

These accessory skills are an integral part of every transfer. Each technique is used in a variety of transfers. To avoid repetition, the accessory skills will be described separately here.

The physical and skill prerequisites required to perform these accessory skills are summarized in Charts 11–1 and 11–2.

Stabilizing the Trunk in a Wheelchair. While sitting in a wheelchair, someone who lacks functional trunk musculature must use his arms for stability when his trunk is in any position other than resting forward on the legs or resting back on the backrest. He must also stabilize his trunk in any situation in which his trunk is likely to be pulled off balance. An example of such a situation is when he lifts one arm to the side. Even such a minor act can shift a person's center of gravity enough to cause his trunk to fall to the side.

To stabilize his trunk in an upright position, a cord-injured person can simply hook one arm behind a push handle. Someone with adequate triceps strength can push on his thigh or on an armrest to hold himself upright. He can stabilize his trunk in the same manner while leaning forward.

In an alternate method for stabilizing the trunk while leaning forward, one arm is hooked behind a push handle. The arm's position is determined by the angle of the trunk's forward lean. Figure 11–1 shows different arm positions that can be used.

Stabilization can be accomplished in the same manner when leaning to the side: the person can hook his arm behind a push handle. Alternatively, he can hold the far armrest, using his hand, wrist, or forearm.

Chart 11–1 Accessory Skills Physical Prerequisites

		Stabilize trunk in wheelchair	Move trunk in wheelchair	Move buttocks on seat	Position wheelchair	Lock brakes	Position armrests	Manage legs	Position footrests	Manage sliding board
Strength										
	Anterior deltoids	√	√	√	√	√	√	√	√	√
	Middle deltoids	√	√	√	√		√	√	√	√
	Posterior deltoids	√	√	√	√		√	√	√	√
	Biceps, brachialis, and/or brachioradialis	√	√	√	√	√	√	√	√	√
Range of motion										
Shoulder	Extension	√	√	√			√			
	Abduction	√	√	√			√			√
	Flexion			√		√		√	√	
Elbow	Extension	√	√	√	√	√			√	√
	Flexion	√	√	√			√	√		

√: Some strength is needed for this activity, or severe limitations in range will inhibit this activity.

Chart 11–2 Accessory Skills—Skill Prerequisites

	Stabilize trunk in wheelchair	Move trunk in wheelchair	Move buttocks on seat	Position wheelchair	Lock brakes	Position armrests	Manage legs	Position footrests	Manage sliding board
Tolerate upright sitting position			√		√	√	√	√	√
Place arm behind push handle	√	√	√		√	√			
Hold push handle to stabilize trunk	√	√	√		√	√			
Move trunk in wheelchair by pulling with arms		√	√		√	√	√	√	√
Move trunk in wheelchair using momentum		√	√		√		√	√	
Move trunk in wheelchair by pushing with arms		√	√			√	√	√	
Manipulate armrests						√			
Slide buttocks on wheelchair seat			√						
Extend elbows using muscle substitution[a]	√	√	√			√			
Prop forward on extended arms	√								
Lift buttocks by pushing on armrests			√						
Lift on armrests and move buttocks			√						
Propel wheelchair[b]				√					

[a] In the absence of functioning triceps
[b] Skill addressed in Chapter 13.

Moving the Trunk in a Wheelchair. In the absence of functioning trunk musculature, a person with a spinal cord injury uses his arms and head to move his trunk. He can pull on the wheelchair or use momentum from arm and head motions to move the trunk.

One way to lean the trunk forward while sitting in a wheelchair is to pull on an anterior part of the chair such as the front of the armrest or seat. The person can return to upright by pushing on his thighs, the front of the chair, or the armrests.

Momentum can also be used to lean the trunk forward. If the head and arm are thrown forward forcefully enough, the body will fall forward. One arm should remain hooked behind the wheelchair's backrest or push handle to provide stability once the trunk has moved forward. This arm should remain relaxed until the trunk has leaned far enough forward. Holding too tight will inhibit the trunk's forward motion. The cord-injured person can use this arm to pull back into an upright position. The other arm can assist by pushing on a thigh, the front of the chair, or an armrest.

The trunk can also be brought forward by pushing on the wheelchair's tires, behind the seat. The cord-injured person should hook one arm behind a push handle for stability and to return to upright.

Any of the above-three methods can be combined to bring the trunk forward. For example, an individual may push on a tire with one hand while throwing his head and the other arm forward.

To lean to the side, a person lacking trunk musculature can either pull sideways on an armrest or throw his head and an arm to the side and allow their momentum to move his trunk. To return to upright, he can pull on the opposite armrest or push handle.

Moving the Buttocks in the Wheelchair. A cord-injured person uses the head-hips relationship to move his buttocks in the wheelchair: to move his buttocks in one direction, he moves his head and upper torso in the opposite direction.

Someone who has intact upper extremity musculature can move on a wheelchair's seat with relative ease. He can simply lift his buttocks by pushing on the armrests or wheelchair seat and throw his head in the direction opposite to where he wants to move.

In the absence of functioning triceps, the exact

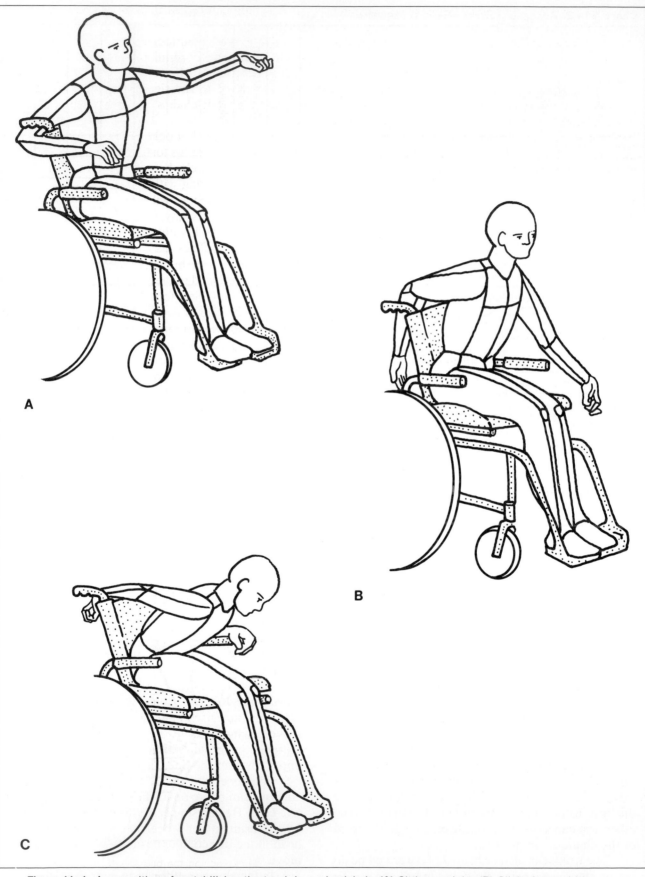

Figure 11–1. Arm positions for stabilizing the trunk in a wheelchair. **(A)** Sitting upright. **(B)** Slight forward lean. **(C)** Pronounced forward lean.

methods used are as varied as the people performing them. What works for one person may not work for the next. The descriptions that follow are some examples.

To move his buttocks forward in the seat, a cord-injured person can throw his head back repeatedly and forcefully. He may be able to improve his performance by pushing on the wheelchair's backrest with his elbows while throwing his head.

Another technique that a person can use to move his buttocks out in the wheelchair seat is to lean his head and upper torso back and to shimmy, twisting his trunk right and left repeatedly. This shimmy is accomplished by throwing the head and arms right and left.

A third method for moving the buttocks out on the wheelchair seat involves larger twisting motions. Using this approach, a person moves his buttocks out and to one side by twisting his head and upper torso in the opposite direction. To twist out and to the left, he hooks his right shoulder behind the wheelchair's right push handle and hooks the left hand on the right armrest. Pulling with his arms, he twists his head and upper trunk to the right and back (Fig. 11–2). This motion will cause the buttocks to slide to the left and forward. The distance that the buttocks will move depends on the magnitude of the head and upper trunk motion. Someone who is unable to move far enough by twisting to one side can repeat the twist in the opposite direction.

To move his buttocks straight to the side for a short distance, a cord-injured person can lean in the opposite direction. For example, someone who desires to move to the right can hook his right arm around the wheelchair's right push handle and lean to the left.

To move his buttocks over larger distances, an individual can lean his torso forward and to the side, pushing his buttocks back and to the other side. If he is already sitting with his buttocks well back in the seat, the buttocks will move laterally only. (The backrest prevents any further motion toward the back.) To move his buttocks back and to the left, the person stabilizes his trunk by holding the right push handle with his right forearm or wrist and twists forward and to the right by pulling on the right armrest with his left forearm (Fig. 11–3).

This method of twisting forward and to the side can also be used to move the buttocks back in the seat. The person should twist first to one side and then to the other while leaning forward. Doing so will ensure that his buttocks are centered instead of being lodged to one side when he has completed the backward motion.

Another method for moving back on the seat involves leaning forward and shimmying. The person leans his body well forward and stabilizes his

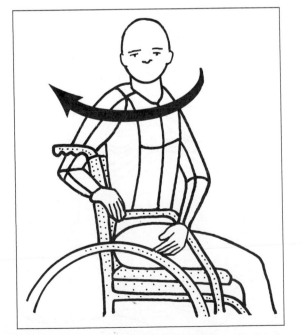

Figure 11–2. Moving the buttocks out in the wheelchair seat. The cord-injured person twists his head and upper torso to the right and back to move his buttocks forward and to the left.

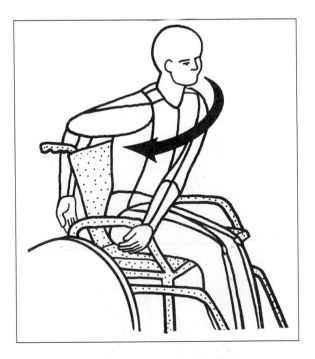

Figure 11–3. Moving the buttocks back and to the left by leaning forward and twisting the head and upper torso to the right.

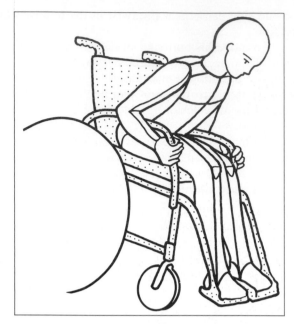

Figure 11–4. Moving the buttocks back in the seat.

be parked at about a 30-degree angle to the object, with the wheel and caster as close as they can get to the other surface. Positioning the wheelchair in this manner will minimize the gap between the surfaces, making the transfer easier and safer.

Someone who has difficulty angling his wheelchair as described above should start by positioning the chair parallel to the object, close enough for the wheel to touch it. He should then lock the brake closest to the object and push forward on the other wheel to angle the chair.

When a person plans to transfer from the floor to his wheelchair after a fall, he may first have to move the chair into an upright position. To do so he should lock the brakes and then pull down on the front of the chair to place the chair upright (Fig. 11–5).

Locking the Brakes. To lock a wheelchair's brakes while sitting in the chair, the person pushes or pulls on the brake lever, depending upon its construction. To reach the brake, he may have to lean forward and to the side.

Positioning the Armrests. Armrest styles vary. Some can be rotated out of the way, either up and back or to the side and back. With these armrest styles, a person can prepare for a transfer by pulling up on the armrest and pushing it out of the way. Other armrests must be removed prior to a transfer. Removing the latter type of armrest involves unlocking it (if locked) and lifting it out of its channels. The

hands against the front of the armrests, as shown in Figure 11–4. He then shimmies his head and shoulders right and left while pushing his hands forward. The result is a backward motion of the buttocks.

Positioning the Wheelchair. During a transfer from a wheelchair to a surface such as a mat, bed, or couch, the wheelchair should be positioned as close to the other surface as possible. The chair should

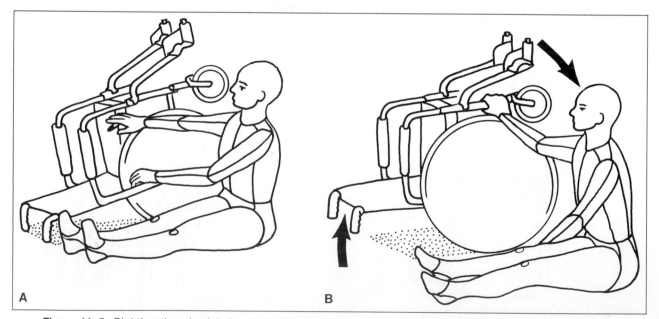

Figure 11–5. Righting the wheelchair prior to transfer. **(A)** Locking the brakes. **(B)** Righting the wheelchair by pulling down on the front of the chair.

lift should be straight upward. Any lateral, forward, or backward pull can jam the armrest in its channels.

It can be tempting to place (or even throw) an armrest on the floor or bed after removing it from the wheelchair. The problems with this practice are twofold: the armrest may be damaged, and it is likely to be in the wrong place when needed. (It gets kicked under the bed, moved to the other side of the bed, etc.) To preserve his equipment and to save himself the trouble of hunting down misplaced armrests, it is a good idea for someone who uses a wheelchair to get into the habit of storing the armrest on the wheelchair, out of the way but still accessible. An armrest can be hung on one of the wheelchair's push handles, but it is likely to fall off from this position. The rear armrest channel will provide more stable storage. Figure 11–6 shows the position of the armrest for storage.

Placing an armrest in this position can be more of a bother than putting it onto the floor or hanging it on a push handle. However, it will be less bothersome than having the armrest repaired or locating it after it has fallen off of the chair.

Managing the Legs. Independent leg management is easily achieved by a person with intact upper extremity function. To get his foot on or off of the wheelchair's footplate, he can move his leg by grasping it with one hand and lifting. The other arm can be used to stabilize the trunk.

In the absence of active hand function, leg management is slightly more involved. To remove his foot from a footrest, a person leans forward, stabilizing his trunk with one arm. The arm opposite the leg being lifted is placed between the legs, and the forearm is used to lift the leg. To add power to the lift, he can stabilize his proximal forearm on the other leg, using this leg as a fulcrum. As the thigh lifts, the foot will slide back off of the footrest. If the shoe gets snagged on the heel loop of the footrest, the person can push the leg back with his hand.

Before performing an even transfer, a cord-injured person should position his feet flat on the floor with the legs vertical. This can be done by pushing or pulling on the legs to move the feet into position.

To place his foot back on the footrest, the person can use the same lifting technique. As his foot gets high enough, he pushes it forward with his forearm and places the foot over the footrest.

To be independent in transfers between a wheelchair and a mat (or bed), a person must be able to get his legs onto and off of the mat. When lifting his legs onto a mat following a transfer, the cord-injured person balances on one arm and lifts with the other arm. He starts by propping on one extended arm, leaning away from the wheelchair. He then places his free arm under the thigh of the leg furthest from the wheelchair (Fig. 11–7A). Balancing on the extended arm, he pulls the thigh onto the mat (Fig. 11–7B). He can add power to the lift by leaning away from the leg. Once his foot is well onto the mat, the person straightens his knee by pushing his foot and leg with his hand (Fig. 11–7C). He then repeats the process to lift the other leg. Getting the feet back onto the floor involves the same process, done in reverse.

Positioning the Footrests. After the feet have been placed on the floor, the chair's front rigging should be positioned out of the way. This involves either folding the footplates or positioning the entire front rigging[2] out of the way.

For many transfers, folding the footplates provides adequate clearance for the transfer. To fold a footplate, a wheelchair user first places his foot on the floor. If he is stabilizing his trunk by holding on to the back of the wheelchair, he needs to shift his hold more distally on his arm so that he can lean forward further. He then can reach down with his free hand and fold the footplate by pulling it up. If he cannot grasp the footplate, he can move it by getting his hand or forearm under the plate, pulling upward and against it.

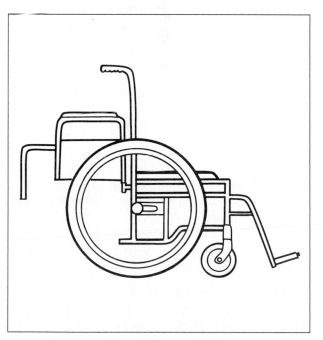

Figure 11–6. Position of armrest for storage.

---

[2] A footplate (footrest) and front rigging (front end) are illustrated in Figure 19–1**B**.

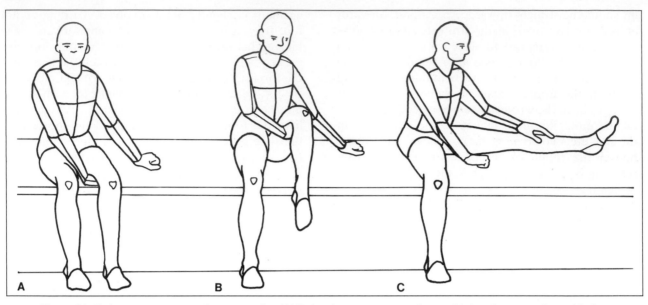

Figure 11–7. Leg management after a transfer. **(A)** Balancing on one arm, the cord-injured person places his free arm under the thigh of the leg furthest from the wheelchair. **(B)** Pulling the leg onto the mat. **(C)** Straightening the leg on the mat.

During some transfers, such as floor transfers, one or both footrests must be swung out of the way rather than merely folded. To reposition a footrest, the person leans forward and operates the footrest release, using the arm on the same side of the chair as the footrest. The other arm is used to stabilize the trunk.

Managing the Sliding Board. To place a sliding board, a cord-injured person grasps the far end of the board and pulls the near end under his proximal thigh and buttocks. Moving the board back and forth laterally while pulling will help to work the board into position. The board should be angled with the far end higher than the near end, so that it will slide under the thigh instead of being pushed into it. Leaning away from the board will make placement easier.

Someone with an impaired grasp can pull on the sliding board using either his forearm or the back of his hand. If neither of these techniques works, the board can be adapted. A loop of webbing or a hole for the hand can make the board easier to maneuver, as will a shorter board.

Someone with good hand function can remove a sliding board by grasping it and pulling it out. In the absence of good hand function, he can use his palm to push outward on the board, pushing on the top surface or on the sides. Leaning away from the board and working it back and forth will make this task easier.

EVEN TRANSFERS

Even transfers, also called level transfers, involve moving between two surfaces of equal height. During even transfers a cord-injured person pivots on his arms, using the head-hips relationship to lift and swing his buttocks.

An even transfer to a mat or bed can be performed with the legs down (feet on the floor) or up (on the mat or bed). In the descriptions below, the legs are down. This is due to the author's preference rather than any particular advantage.

Whenever an even transfer is done with the legs down, the feet should be positioned with the soles flat on the floor and the legs perpendicular to the floor. This positioning will maximize the weight accepted through the legs during the transfer. Charts 11–3 and 11–4 summarize the physical and skill prerequisites for even transfers.

Even Transfers Without Equipment
The presence of well-innervated deltoids makes it possible for people with C5 quadriplegia to perform even transfers without equipment. In C6 and lower quadriplegia, superior functioning of the serratus anterior makes this goal more readily achievable.

In the Absence of Functioning Triceps. In the absence of functioning triceps, a cord-injured person must lock his elbows whenever he bears weight through

Chart 11—3 Even Transfers Physical Prerequisites

	No equipment	Sliding board, upright method	Sliding board, alternate method	Board and loops
Strength				
Anterior deltoids	☑	☑	☑	✓
Middle deltoids	✓	✓		✓
Posterior deltoids			☑	✓
Biceps, brachialis, and/or brachioradialis			☑	✓
Serratus anterior	●	●	●	
Range of motion				
Shoulder Extension				☑
Abduction			✓	☑
Flexion	✓	✓	✓	
External rotation	☑	☑		
Internal rotation				☑
Elbow Extension	☑	☑		
Flexion		✓		
Forearm supination	☑	☑		✓
Wrist extension	☑	☑		✓

✓: Some strength is needed for this activity, or severe limitations in range will inhibit this activity.
☑: A large amount of strength or normal or greater range is needed for this activity.
●: Not required, but helpful.

his arms during transfers. This locking is done through a combination of positioning and muscular contraction.

The following is a description of a technique for transferring from a wheelchair to a mat. The same technique is used to transfer to a bed and is used in reverse to return to the wheelchair.

After moving his buttocks forward in the wheelchair, a cord-injured person sits upright and positions his hands in preparation for the transfer. His hands should be anterior to his hips, far enough forward to enable him to lean on them during the trans-

fer. They should not be so far anterior that he cannot pivot on them when leaning forward.

The hand on the wheelchair should be placed next to the person's thigh. The hand on the mat should be positioned far enough away to leave adequate space on the mat for the buttocks at the end of the transfer.

The arms should be positioned with the shoulders externally rotated fully, the elbows and wrists extended, and the forearms supinated. This position makes it possible to lock the elbows in extension. The Interphalangeal (IP) joints should be flexed to preserve the tenodesis effect. Figure 11–8A shows the starting position of the transfer. The person maintains his elbows in extension during the transfer through strong contraction of his anterior deltoids.

To transfer, the cord-injured person leans for-

Chart 11—4 Even Transfers Skill Prerequisites

	No equipment	Sliding board, upright method	Sliding board, alternate method	Board and loops
Tolerate upright sitting position	✓	✓	✓	✓
Accessory skills	✓	✓	✓	✓
Extend elbows using muscle substitution[a]	✓	✓		
Lock elbows[a]	✓	✓		
Prop forward on extended arms[b]	✓	✓		
Prop forward on one extended arm[b]	✓	✓		
Unweight buttocks by leaning forward on extended arms[h]	✓	✓		
Control pelvis using head and shoulders	✓	✓	✓	✓
Move buttocks laterally while propping on extended arms[b]		✓		
Lift buttocks by pivoting on extended arms[b]	✓			
Lift buttocks and move laterally	✓			

[a] In the absence of functioning triceps.
[b] Arm(s) with elbow(s) positioned in extension.

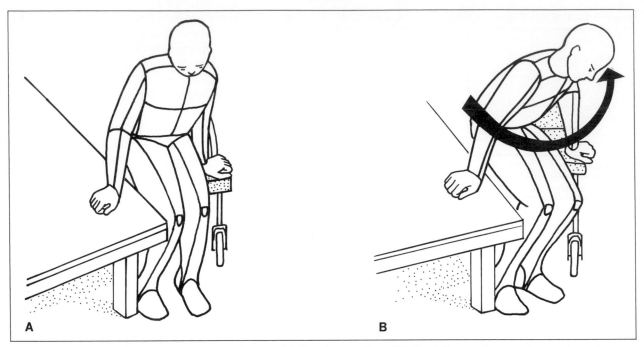

Figure 11–8. Even transfer without equipment. **(A)** Starting position. **(B)** Head thrown down and away from the bed to lift the buttocks up and toward the bed.

ward on his arms, tucks his chin, and rolls his head downward. By pivoting on his arms in this manner, he lifts his buttocks from the wheelchair seat. If any serratus anterior function is present, he should protract his scapulae to increase the height of the lift.

When pivoting on his arms, the person needs to lean forward enough to get adequate clearance of the buttocks. At the same time he must not pivot so far forward that he moves past his balance point. Doing so will result in a forward fall.

While he pivots on his arms, the cord-injured person swings his buttocks toward the mat: keeping his head down, he forcefully swings his head and twists his shoulders away from the mat (Fig. 11–8B). This twisting motion causes the buttocks to swing toward the mat. It is important for the head to remain down during the transfer to maintain the lift.

The sideways motion of the buttocks during the transfer is *not* accomplished by pushing laterally with the arms; it is achieved by swinging the head and twisting the shoulders. Pushing laterally on the wheelchair will cause the chair to slide. If this problem is to be avoided, the arms must push straight downward throughout the transfer.

In the Presence of Functioning Triceps. Innervated triceps make it easier to support the body's weight on the arms during transfers. If the triceps are strong enough to maintain elbow extension while the in-

dividual pivots on his arms, he does not need to lock his elbows with positioning and muscle substitution. The transfer technique described above is used, with the exception that the shoulders do not need to be held in external rotation.

Even Transfers With Equipment
Weakness, contractures, obesity, spasticity, confusion, or low motivation can keep an individual from achieving independence in even transfers without equipment. In these instances, many people can learn to transfer using a sliding board or using a sliding board and loops.

Even Transfers With a Sliding Board
During a transfer, a sliding board bridges the gap between the wheelchair and the other surface, making it possible to transfer without lifting the buttocks.

Like any piece of equipment, a sliding board has its disadvantages. Although a board may appear to make a transfer easier, it adds an extra step to the process. Worse, it *must be there* for the transfer. Someone who depends upon a sliding board will be out of luck if the board is ever misplaced or left behind.

This is not to say that sliding boards are inherently bad or should never be used. Many people who are unable to transfer without equipment can gain independence using a sliding board. If a board makes independent transfers possible for someone who would otherwise be dependent, it is certainly indicated. But if an individual has the potential to transfer without equipment, the extra time and effort required for training will be well worth it.

Upright Method. This method is similar to an even transfer without equipment. The person first positions his buttocks forward in the chair and places the sliding board. During the transfer, his hands should be anterior to his hips, far enough forward to enable him to lean on them. The hand on the wheelchair should be placed next to the thigh, and the hand toward which the individual is transferring should be placed on the sliding board. If the transfer is to be done in one motion, the hand on the sliding board should be far enough away to make room for the buttocks to slide across the board. If the transfer is done in several steps, the hand can be placed relatively close to the thigh and repositioned when necessary.

In the absence of functioning triceps, a cord-injured person uses his anterior deltoids to lock his elbows using the technique described above: his upper extremities are positioned with the shoulders externally rotated fully, the elbows and wrists extended, and the forearms supinated. If the triceps are functioning with adequate strength to maintain the elbows in extension during the transfer, this positioning is not required.

Although the buttocks do not need to be lifted when using a sliding board, the person does need to shift some of his weight off of them to make it possible to slide. To unweight his buttocks, a cord-injured person leans forward onto his arms. While doing so he twists his head and shoulders away from the mat. This twisting motion causes the buttocks to slide toward the bed. If the individual has sufficient strength and skill, the transfer can be executed in one twist.

An individual who lacks adequate strength or skill or both may have to twist repeatedly during a transfer with a sliding board. The twist of the head and upper torso away from the mat should be forceful, causing the buttocks to slide toward the mat. When moving back into position to prepare for another twist, the motion should not be forceful. A forceful motion toward the mat will cause the buttocks to slide back toward the chair.

Alternate Method. Biceps spasticity, poor balance, or contractures can make it impossible to prop and twist on the arms with the elbows in extension. Some people with these limitations who are unable to perform an upright transfer with a sliding board are able to use an alternate method, although finding a method that works for a given individual can be difficult. The therapist and patient will need to be creative in coming up with a solution to the problem.

The following is a description of one alternate method for transferring from a wheelchair to a bed. For clarity, the transfer will be described with the person moving toward the right.

After positioning the sliding board, the person turns away from the bed. To do so, he first hooks his left arm behind the wheelchair's left push handle and hooks his right forearm around the wheelchair's armrest. This position is shown in Figure 11–9A. Some people are more successful performing this maneuver with the left hand stabilized against the chair's left wheel.

The person twists his head and shoulders back and to the left by pulling on the push handle and the armrest. This twist causes the buttocks to slide forward and to the right toward the bed (Fig. 11–9B). Depending on the individual's strength and ability, positioning the buttocks on the right front corner of the seat may take one or several twists.

From the right front corner of the seat, the person pushes his buttocks across the sliding board toward the bed. To do this, he first places his left palm against the inside of the armrest. Keeping his head low, he pushes on the wheelchair's push handle and armrest and shimmies his head and upper trunk back and forth. This shimmy involves rapid lateral flexion to the right and left alternately.

Once the person has moved his buttocks as far as he can with his arms in the initial position, he needs to move his arms to a position in which weight is borne on the elbows on the left side of the wheelchair seat (Fig. 11–9C). Keeping his head low, he moves toward the bed by pushing with his arms and shimmying his head and upper trunk. The push and shimmy are continued until the buttocks and thighs are completely on the bed.

To sit up, the person can push on the wheelchair seat, extending his elbows with his anterior deltoids. In the presence of elbow flexion contractures, he may have to use overhead loops to come to sitting.

Even Transfers With Sliding Board and Loops

If an individual does not have adequate strength or range of motion to perform a transfer with a sliding board, he may be able to achieve independence using a board and loops hanging from an overhead frame. Hanging loops should be used only as a last resort. The loops and frame are bulky, unsightly, and not very portable.

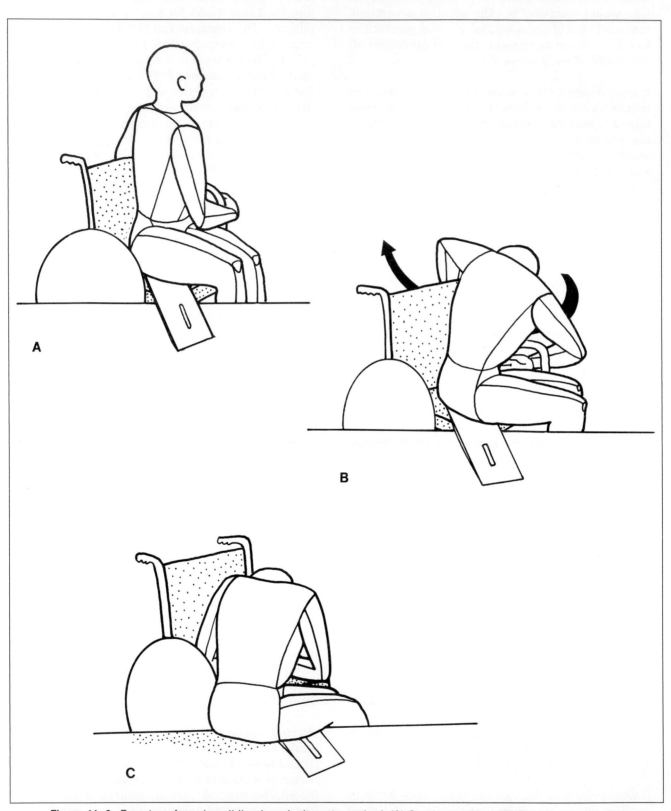

Figure 11–9. Even transfer using sliding board, alternate method. **(A)** Starting position. **(B)** Twisting to slide the buttocks out and toward the bed. **(C)** The transfer is completed with the weight borne on the elbows.

An overhead loop system is shown in Figure 11–10. The exact spacing and length of the different loops will vary between individuals. During transfer training, the therapist and patient should work together to find the best configuration.

The following is a description of a chair-to-bed transfer, moving to the left. A transfer in the reverse direction will simply involve reversing the steps.

The person moves his buttocks forward in the chair and places the sliding board. He then positions his hands for the transfer. The left hand should be placed in the nearest loop, palm facing downward. The right hand should be placed on the wheelchair cushion beside the right thigh, well forward on the seat. An alternate position for this arm is over the wheelchair's backrest, with the weight borne above the elbow.

The next step involves positioning the arms and trunk for the transfer. The transfer will be performed with the trunk leaning well forward to unweight the buttocks. The person assumes this position by leaning forward, supporting his weight on both arms. Both elbows should point upward, with the shoulders internally rotated and the elbows flexed. Figure 11–11 shows the starting position for the transfer.

The buttocks are moved toward the bed using the head-hips relationship. While supporting his weight on his hands, the person forcefully throws his head and upper trunk away from the bed. This motion is repeated multiple times.

Some are able to perform this transfer using one loop. Others need to reposition their hands when they have moved as far as they can from the starting

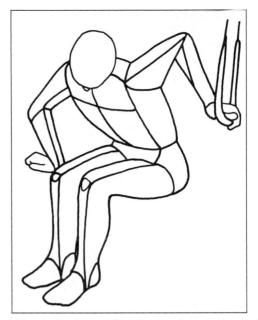

Figure 11–11. Starting position for even transfer from wheelchair to bed using sliding board and overhead loops.

position. An individual repositioning his hands should place his left hand in the next loop and his right hand next to his thigh. He can then resume the twisting motion. The process should continue until the buttocks and thighs are securely on the bed.

UNEVEN TRANSFERS

Uneven transfers include any transfers between surfaces of unequal height. These transfers require greater strength and skill than do even transfers.

Able-bodied people live in a multilevel world. They can stand, sit on surfaces of various heights, and get onto and off of the ground. Someone who uses a wheelchair and is unable to perform uneven transfers has few alternatives. He can choose to be in his wheelchair or on a surface (usually a bed) that is exactly as high as the wheelchair seat. He is "confined" to his wheelchair.

A spinal cord-injured person who can perform uneven transfers has more options open to him. He can leave his wheelchair to sit on a couch or on the floor if he likes and can get back up if he falls. He can get into a car or truck independently, freed from the necessity of a lift. All of these options make for a more flexible lifestyle.

The prerequisite skills required to perform uneven transfers are summarized in Charts 11–5 and 11–6.

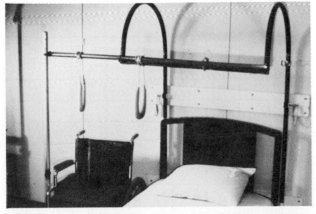

Figure 11–10. Suspended loops for transfers between wheelchair and bed. (Reproduced with permission from Ford, J., & Duckworth, B. [1987]. *Physical management for the quadriplegic patient.* Philadelphia, PA: F.A. Davis. [2nd ed.].

Floor Transfers

Transfers between the floor and a wheelchair enable a person to get onto and off of the floor or ground. This ability can be life enriching, enabling someone to get into the water at the beach, take a picnic on the ground, or get onto the floor to play with children. Independent floor transfers are also an important survival skill. Even if a patient does not foresee using the skill by choice, it is quite likely that he may find it helpful at some time in the future. Many people who use wheelchairs over a period of time eventually fall. At those times it is useful to be able to get up from the floor, the street, or the basketball court.

The first step in transferring from the floor to a wheelchair involves ensuring that the chair is upright with the brakes locked. Once the chair is positioned and locked, the individual can transfer using a side, front, or back approach.

Side Approach. This technique for transfers between the floor and a wheelchair has the advantage of being fast. Speed is important when a cord-injured person finds himself on the street in the middle of an intersection or on the floor in the middle of a basketball game.

Using the side approach method, a person utilizes finesse to move his body from the floor to a wheelchair seat. A great deal of strength is not required. For this reason, people with C-7 quadriplegia can perform the transfer. As can be seen in Figure 11–12, loose hamstrings are necessary.

During the actual lift of the transfer, one hand stays on the floor and one stays on the wheelchair

Chart 11–5 Uneven Transfers—Physical Prerequisites

		Side approach floor to chair	Front approach floor to chair	Back approach floor to chair	Intermediate levels	Wheelchair to higher surfaces	Toilet	Bathtub
Strength								
	Anterior deltoids	☑	☑	☑	☑	☑	☑ᵃ	☑
	Middle deltoids	☑	√	√	√	√	√	√
	Posterior deltoids	√	√	√	√	√	√	√
	Biceps, brachialis, and/or brachioradialis	√						
	Serratus anterior	☑	☑	☑	☑	☑	√	☑
	Triceps	√	☑	☑	√	☑		√
	Pectoralis major		☑	☑		☑		√
	Latissimus dorsi		☑	☑				√
Range of motion								
Shoulder	Extension	☑	√	☑	√	√		√
	Abduction	☑			√	√	√	√
	Flexion	☑	√		√	√	√	√
	Internal rotation			☑		√		√
Elbow	Extension	☑	√	√	√	√	☑ᵃ	√
	Flexion		√	√	√	√		√
Wrist extension		√		√		√	☑ᵃ	√
Combined hip flexion and knee extension		☑						

ᵃ In the absence of functioning triceps.

√: Some strength is needed for this activity or severe limitation in range will inhibit this activity.

☑: A large amount of strength or normal or greater range is needed for this activity.

Chart 11–6 Uneven Transfers—Skill Prerequisites

	Side approach floor to chair	Front approach floor to chair	Back approach floor to chair	Intermediate levels	Wheelchair to higher surfaces	Toilet	Bathtub
Tolerate upright sitting position	✓	✓	✓	✓	✓	✓	✓
Accessory skills	✓	✓	✓	✓	✓	✓	✓
Extend elbows using muscle substituion[a]					✓		
Lock elbows[a]					✓		
Control pelvis using head and shoulders	✓	✓	✓	✓	✓	✓	✓
Lift buttocks by pivoting on extended arms	✓			✓	✓	✓	
Lift buttocks and move laterally	✓			✓	✓	✓	
Lift buttocks to the side from floor to higher surfaces	✓						
Straight lift from floor		✓	✓				✓
Turn body to drop onto wheelchair seat		✓					

[a] In the absence of functioning triceps.

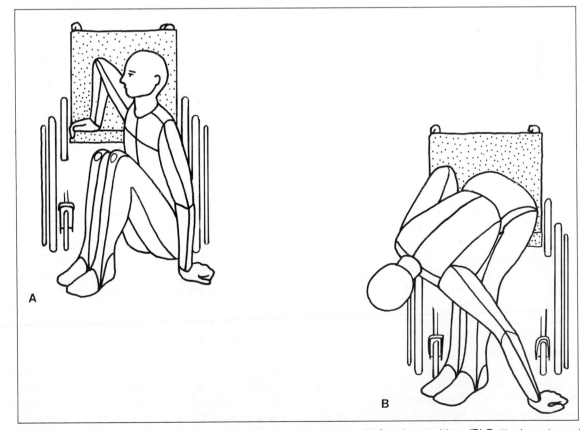

Figure 11–12. Side-approach transfer from the floor to a wheelchair. **(A)** Starting position. **(B)** Buttocks onto seat. (*Continues.*)

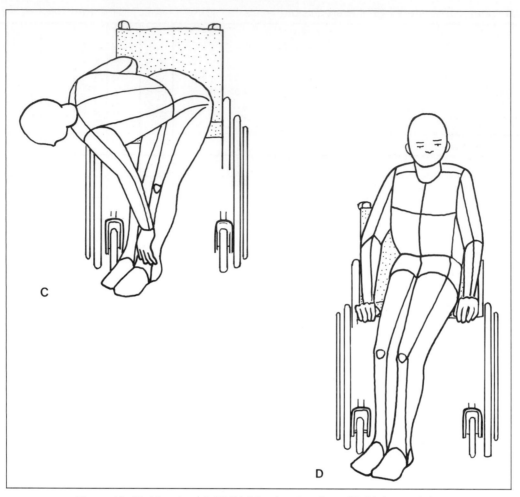

Figure 11–12 (*Continued*) **(C)** Walking hand up legs. **(D)** Sitting upright.

seat. For the purpose of this discussion, the hands will be referred to as the floor hand and the chair hand, respectively.

The starting position for a side-approach floor-to-chair transfer is shown in Figure 11–12A. The person sits in front of the wheelchair with his legs at a 30- to 45-degree angle to the chair. The transfer will be much easier if his knees are bent, pointing upward. The buttocks should be slightly in front of the casters, closer to the one behind the person. The hand closer to the wheelchair is placed on the seat, on the furthest front corner. The palm should face down, and the elbow should point upward. The other hand is placed on the floor, a few inches lateral and anterior to the hip.

To lift his buttocks onto the seat, the person swings his head and upper torso down and away from the wheelchair while pushing downward with his arms. The twist must be forceful and the downward motion of the head must be very pronounced to lift the buttocks high enough. To provide extra

lift, the person should protract the scapula of the floor arm at the end of the transfer. He ends in the position shown in Figure 11–12B.

The next task is to assume an upright sitting position. This involves placing the floor hand on the legs and walking it up the legs (Fig. 11–12C). Once he has placed his hands on his legs, the person unweights the hand by pushing on the leg and throwing his head back. Some people use their other arm to assist in this process, pulling on the armrest or on the push handle of the wheelchair. When the hand on the legs is unweighted, the person quickly moves it and catches his weight on a more proximal handhold. This step is repeated until he achieves an upright sitting position (Fig. 11–12D).

The same procedure (with minor changes) is used in reverse when transferring down to the floor. After moving his buttocks to the front of the wheelchair seat, the person positions his legs at a 30- to 45-degree angle to the chair. The hand facing out from the chair becomes the "floor hand." To position the floor hand, the individual can either walk his hand down his legs or place it directly on the floor while holding onto the wheelchair's push handle with the other hand.

The next step involves moving the buttocks onto the floor. The person slides his buttocks off of the seat by twisting his head and upper torso slightly toward the back of the chair. Once the buttocks have moved from the seat, gravity provides the downward force moving the buttocks. The person's task at this point is to control the motion so that he lands without trauma. To do so, he slows the downward motion by resisting the upward and chairward twist of his head and upper torso. He *should not* swing his head and upper trunk up and toward the chair forcefully during the transfer, as that would increase the speed of his descent and result in trauma to his buttocks.

Front Approach. This transfer technique requires less finesse and hamstring flexibility than does a side-approach transfer, but it requires greater strength. Fully innervated upper extremities are necessary.

The starting position for this transfer is shown in Figure 11–13A. The person is side sitting with his knees flexed. The knees are located in front of the wheelchair's casters, centered between them. One hand is on the wheelchair seat, and one is on the floor.

The person lifts his buttocks off of the floor, using the head-hips relationship to do so. Pushing downward on both hands, he twists his head and upper torso down and away from the chair (Fig. 11–13B).

In the next step the person pushes on the chair and raises his trunk to assume an upright kneeling position in front of the wheelchair (Fig. 11–13C). While doing so he must push downward on the chair, as pulling on it will tip it over.

During the transfer, a forceful downward push on the armrests is used to lift the body (Fig. 11–13D). Again, the person must refrain from pulling on the chair. While pushing on the armrests, he tucks his head, protracts his scapulae, and raises his buttocks high above the level of the seat. He then releases one hand and twists, turning and landing on the wheelchair seat.

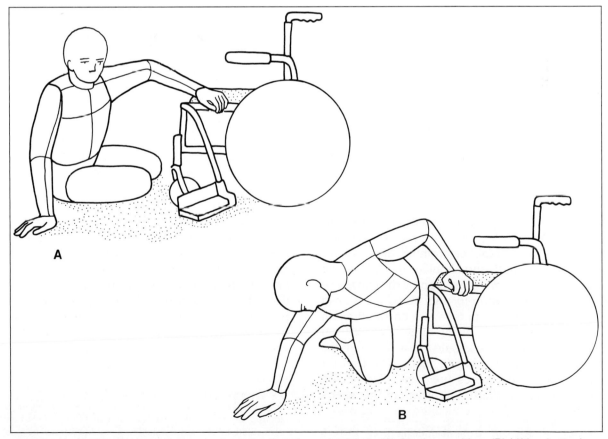

Figure 11–13. Front-approach transfer from the floor to a wheelchair. **(A)** Starting position. **(B)** Lifting buttocks from floor. (*Continues.*)

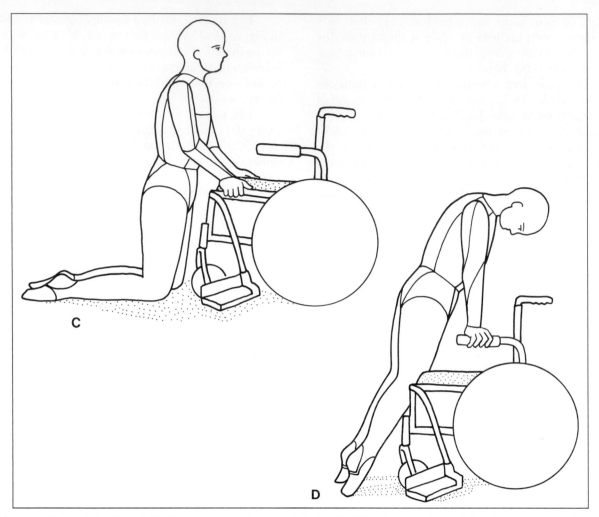

Figure 11-13. (*Continued*) **(C)** Kneeling in front of wheelchair. **(D)** Lifting buttocks by pushing down on armrests.

This transfer is not a particularly good method for returning to the floor. The side-approach technique is much faster and easier to perform.[3]

Back Approach. The third method for floor-to-wheelchair transfers requires fully innervated upper extremities. The person performing this transfer needs greater strength and shoulder flexibility than is required to perform a front-approach transfer.

The starting position for this transfer is shown in Figure 11-14A. The person sits on the floor in front of the wheelchair, facing directly away from the chair. His buttocks should be in front of the casters and centered between them. The transfer will be easier if his knees are bent. The person places his palms on the front corners of the wheelchair seat, with the fingers facing forward. This hand position requires a great deal of flexibility in shoulder internal rotation and extension. Many people are not able to perform this transfer because they are unable to assume the starting position.

The person lifts his buttocks from the floor by pushing down hard on the wheelchair seat. This maneuver requires the muscles to function in a position of extreme stretch, making this step prohibitively difficult for most people.[4] As he pushes down, the person should lean back with his head and upper torso until his buttocks reach the seat level (Fig. 11-14B).

---

[3] In contrast to a side-approach transfer from the floor to a wheelchair, loose hamstrings and a high level of skill are not required when using a side approach to transfer *down* from a wheelchair.

[4] People who cannot achieve independence in a direct transfer from the floor to a wheelchair may be able to transfer using an indirect approach: they transfer first from the floor to an intermediate-height surface such as a stool and from the stool to the wheelchair seat. The techniques used are as described for a direct floor-to-chair transfer.

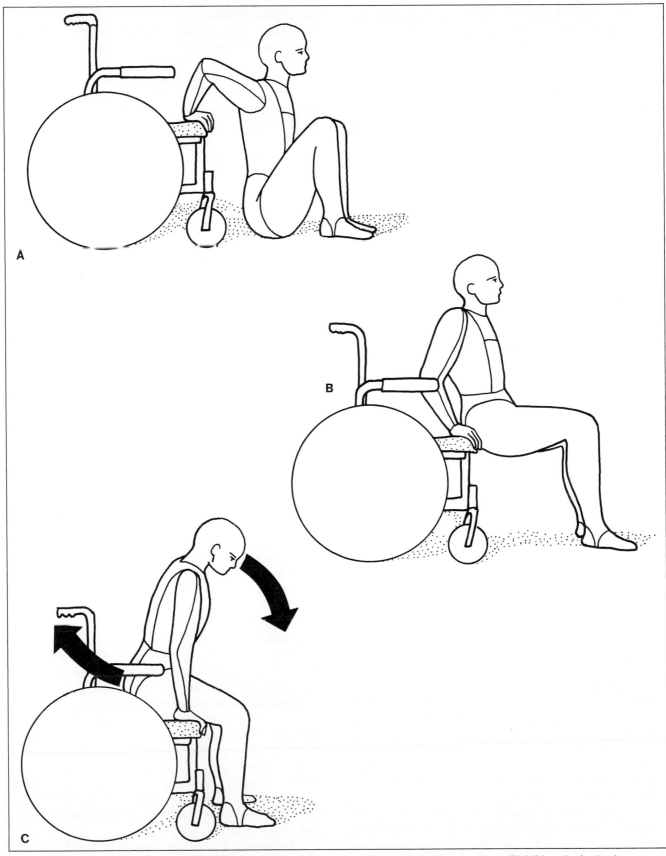

Figure 11–14. Back-approach transfer for the floor to a wheelchair. **(A)** Starting position. **(B)** Lifting the buttocks from the floor. **(C)** Moving the buttocks back on the seat.

Once the wheelchair seat has been cleared, the person uses the head-hips relationship to lift his buttocks higher and to move back further on the seat. He pivots on his arms, leaning forward and curling his head downward (Fig. 11–14C). Additional lift is achieved through strong protraction of the scapulae. Like the front approach, this transfer method can be used to return to the floor but is less convenient than the side approach.

Transfers to Intermediate Levels

To transfer between a wheelchair and a lower surface such as a couch, a cord-injured person uses a method similar to that used for even transfers without equipment. The difference is that the head and upper torso motion used to lift the buttocks must be more forceful and exaggerated to get adequate lift. When transferring down from the wheelchair, gravity supplies the power to move the body. The person's task is to control the motion so that he can land without injury.

Wheelchair to Higher Surfaces

The ability to transfer from the wheelchair to a higher surface is another useful skill. Many beds are significantly higher than wheelchair seats, as are many "accessible" toilets in public restrooms. An uneven transfer is also required to get into trucks, vans (without lifts), or tractors.

The person planning to transfer first locks his brakes with the wheelchair positioned as close as possible to the surface toward which he plans to transfer. If moving toward the right, he places his right hand on the higher surface, several inches in front of the wheelchair seat. The other hand is placed on the wheelchair's seat or armrest, depending on the height of the surface. Placing the hand on the armrest makes a higher transfer possible but increases the risk of the chair sliding to the side during the transfer. Figure 11–15A shows the starting position for the transfer.

While pushing straight down and pivoting on both arms, the person tucks his head and upper torso downward and swings them away from the higher surface. To achieve an adequate lift, the downward motion of the head must be pronounced. To move his buttocks further onto the surface and to gain a more stable position, the person protracts his scapulae strongly.

Once the individual is sitting securely on the higher surface, he leans his torso to a position over the surface (Fig. 11–15B). He can then move his hand from the wheelchair to the higher surface and push himself upright.

Bathroom Transfers

Most bathrooms are very small, with little room for maneuvering a wheelchair. The approach that is used for a toilet or tub transfer may be dictated by the bathroom's layout. During transfer training, the therapist and patient should develop a method of transferring that will be applicable in the patient's home bathroom.

Toilet. If space permits, a cord-injured person can transfer to a toilet using a transfer technique that is essentially the same as the even transfer without equipment described above. The wheelchair is positioned against a front corner of the toilet seat, angled in as with a mat transfer. Using the methods described above, the person removes the armrest closest to the toilet, positions his legs, moves the footplates out of the way, and gets into position for the transfer. One hand is placed on the far side of the toilet seat, and the other hand is placed on the wheelchair seat next to the thigh. The person then pivots forward on his arms, twisting his head and upper torso down and away from the toilet. The transfer is likely to be slightly uneven, so a higher lift will be required. This can be accomplished by throwing the head and upper torso into a lower position when pivoting the arms. To return to the chair, the same steps are performed in reverse.

In an alternate method, the patient straddles the toilet. To use this technique, he approaches the toilet from the front, facing it directly. The footrests are swung out of the way, and the feet are placed on either side of the toilet. The chair is moved into position against the front of the toilet. After the person moves his buttocks forward in the chair, he leans forward and props on his arms (elbows extended) with one hand on either side of the toilet seat. He then pushes down hard with his arms and depresses his shoulder girdle while leaning forward. This maneuver lifts his buttocks onto the toilet seat. To return to the chair, the person first places his hands on the wheelchair seat, one on each side. He then moves his buttocks back by pushing down with his arms and depressing his scapulae.

Bathtub. A cord-injured person with impaired pain and temperature sensation may sustain serious burns if he transfers into a bathtub full of hot water or fills the tub while sitting in it. To prevent burns, an individual with impaired sensation should fill the bathtub and check the water temperature before transferring into the tub.

To prepare for a tub transfer, the cord-injured person approaches the tub directly facing its side. The chair should be positioned toward the end op-

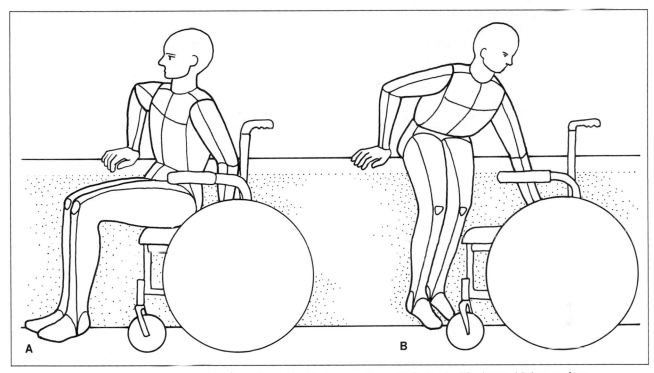

Figure 11–15. Transfer to higher surface. **(A)** Starting position. **(B)** Buttocks lifted onto higher surface.

posite the faucet. The person transferring swings his wheelchair's front rigging out of the way, lifts his legs, and places his feet in the tub. After positioning the chair close to the side of the tub, he locks the brakes. He may find the transfer easier with the chair directly against the tub or slightly back from it.

The actual transfer is performed in two steps: from the wheelchair to the side of the tub and from there into the tub. To transfer to the side of the tub, the person places one hand on the near side of the tub and one on the front of the wheelchair's seat or armrest. He then pushes down to lift his body and lower his buttocks onto the side of the tub.

Stabilizing his trunk by balancing on an arm with the hand placed on the far side of the tub, the person uses his free hand to move his feet toward the faucet. He then lowers himself into the tub, with one hand on each side of the tub. To transfer back to the chair, the same steps are performed in reverse.

Vehicle Transfers

The skills used for the basic even and uneven transfers described above can be applied to transfers between a wheelchair and a car, truck, or van. The cord-injured person angles his wheelchair as close as possible to the vehicle's seat and moves the arm-

rest and footplates out of the way. With one hand on the vehicle's seat and one on the wheelchair seat, he pivots on his arms and transfers. As the therapist and patient work together on the transfer, they can experiment with different hand holds.

After transferring into a car, the cord-injured driver places his feet in the footwells and loads the wheelchair. He can load it either behind or next to himself.[5] If the chair has a folding frame, he turns the chair so that it faces the car (footplates toward the car) and folds the chair. He then lifts the casters through the door and finally pulls the chair into the car. If the chair has a rigid frame, the driver removes the wheels, folds the backrest, and places the chair and wheels in the car.

THERAPEUTIC STRATEGIES

General Strategies

To accomplish a functional goal, the patient must acquire both the physical and skill prerequisites for that activity. For example, when working on a side-approach floor-to-chair transfer, a cord-injured per-

---

[5] If loading chair with a folding frame in the front, the driver must perform the initial transfer into the passenger side of the car and slide across the seat to the driver's side.

son must develop adequate hamstring flexibility and upper extremity strength as well as the ability to pivot on the arms to lift the buttocks.

When developing skill prerequisites for a functional goal, the patient should start with the most basic prerequisite skills and progress toward more challenging activities. (There is no point in working on lifting the buttocks by pivoting on the extended arms if the individual cannot independently maintain an upright sitting position by propping forward on his arms with the elbows extended.)

It is generally best to work on even transfers first and to progress to uneven transfers. As a cord-injured person develops the strength, range of motion, flexibility, and skills to perform an even transfer, he lays the foundation for more advanced transfers.

Before asking a patient to attempt a new skill, the therapist should explain and demonstrate the technique. The demonstration should provide a clear idea of the motions involved and the timing of these motions. The patient should also be shown how the new skill will be used functionally.

During functional training, the therapist should remember that every patient will perform a particular activity differently. Each person has a unique combination of body build, coordination, strength, and flexibility, and these characteristics influence the manner in which he performs functional tasks. As a result of these individual variations, each person is unique in the exact placement of his hands; the timing of his pushes, pivots, and twists; and the degree to which he must dip his head to get an adequate lift of this buttocks. What works for one patient may be a total disaster for the next. The challenge of functional training is finding the timing and maneuvers that best suit the individual involved.

As a therapist and patient work together on a skill, they can learn from failed attempts by analyzing the problem. Is the patient strong enough to perform the maneuver? Is he flexible enough? Did he pivot too far forward on his arms, or did he fail to pivot far enough? Were his hands too far anterior or not anterior enough?

Trial and error can be another useful strategy for functional training. For example, the best way to determine whether the hands were too far forward in a failed attempt may be to try the maneuver with the hands positioned further back. The relative success of the attempt may provide an answer.

It is important for the therapist and patient to keep in mind that functional training can take a long time; a given transfer may take months to achieve. It is a mistake to give up on a functional goal after

only a few trials. (Assuming that the patient has adequate innervation, of course!)

Strategies to address the various prerequisite skills are presented below.

Specific Strategies

Tolerate Upright Sitting Position. Before a cord-injured person can perform any transfers, he must be able to tolerate an upright sitting posture. To develop this capacity, the therapist gradually moves the patient from a horizontal position to upright sitting. This process is described in Chapter 8.

Unsupported Sitting Balance. A spinal cord-injured individual will probably never need to sit with both hands in the air to perform a transfer. However, practicing unsupported sitting balance can be a useful therapeutic activity. Developing the ability to use head and arm motions to maintain upright sitting will make other activities easier.

To sit unsupported, a person must be able to tolerate an upright sitting position. Once he can tolerate an upright sitting posture, a patient's first task in working on unsupported sitting balance is finding his position of balance, the position in which his trunk is balanced over its base of support. In long- or short-sitting, the therapist supports the patient at his shoulders and helps him find his balance point. When the patient's trunk is balanced, the therapist will not feel him pushing forward, backward, or laterally.

The therapist should explain and demonstrate how the patient can maintain an upright position with his hands in the air, using hand and head motions: if his trunk starts to fall, the patient moves his hands and head in the opposite direction.

The patient should practice this skill, getting a feel for how his head and arm motions cause his trunk to move. He will need to experience the loss of balance and learn to regain the balance point using head and arm motions. His reactions may be slow at first, and he may tend to overcorrect. The therapist can help the process by giving verbal feedback.

As the patient becomes more adept at maintaining his balance point, the therapist should reduce the support being provided at his shoulders. The patient can progress from practicing with light support, then with the therapist's hands hovering inches away, and finally practice without spotting.

To develop the patient's unsupported sitting balance further, the therapist can disturb his balance or have him catch and throw objects. The patient can also practice maintaining his balance while he reaches his arms in different directions.

Independent Work: The patient can practice alone while long-sitting on a mat or short-sitting between mats.

Extend Elbows Using Muscle Substitution. This skill should be addressed very early in the patient's program; it can be developed while the patient is still confined to bed. The therapist can start by manually stabilizing one of the patient's hands and asking him to push. When approached in this manner, many patients will make the substitution without having to think about it. For an individual who is not able to do so, the therapist can cue him to use his anterior deltoid, reminding him verbally, or touching the skin over the muscle, or both. Once the patient has learned to extend his elbows using muscle substitution, the process can be repeated in a variety of positions.

From a Forward Lean in Sitting, Push Trunk to Upright. To work on this skill, the patient must be able to tolerate upright sitting. He must also be able to extend his elbows against resistance, using either his triceps or muscle substitution.

Probably the best position for working on this activity is short-sitting between two mats, with the mats positioned as shown in Figure 11–16. With his hands stabilized on the mat in front of him, the patient lowers his trunk slightly by allowing his elbows to flex a few degrees and then pushes himself back

upright. He should lower his trunk only as far as he can, maintain full control of the motion, and should not move past where he can push back to upright. As the patient's ability improves, he should increase the distance of his pushup.

Some time should also be spent practicing this activity while sitting in a wheelchair. The hands can be placed on or beside the distal thighs.

Independent Work: The activities described above are ideal for independent work.

Lock the Elbows. When bearing weight on extended arms, a cord injured person who does not have functioning triceps needs to lock his elbows using positioning and muscle substitution. The position for locking is as follows: shoulders externally rotated, elbows and wrists extended, forearms supinated. Weight is borne on the palms. The elbows are held in extension using the anterior deltoids and shoulder external rotators.

After demonstrating the techniques for elbow locking, the therapist can help the patient position his arms. The patient then holds the "locked" position while the therapist applies resistance, pushing the elbow toward flexion.

Once the patient has a feel for the position and muscle contraction involved, he can practice locking and unlocking his elbows. If necessary, the therapist can help by supporting the trunk as the patient leans on an arm and practices moving it in and out of position.

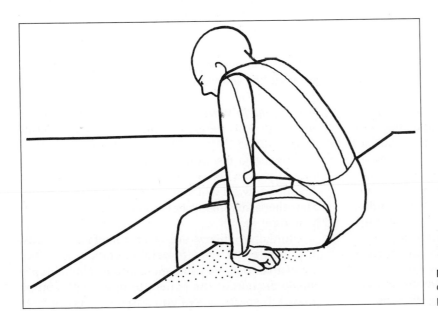

Figure 11–16. Short-sitting on mat with second mat placed in front to allow independent practice of transfer skills.

Independent Work: Sitting in a wheelchair, the patient can stabilize his palms on the wheelchair seat or on a nearby mat and practice locking and unlocking his elbows. This is a good "homework" activity for him to work on when not in therapy.

Place an Arm Behind Wheelchair Push Handle. Before practicing this skill, the patient must be able to tolerate an upright sitting position.

Many people with spinal cord injuries are able to place an arm behind their wheelchair's push handle without any practice. Someone who finds the maneuver more difficult may need to use momentum to get the arm into position. Starting with his arm crossed across his torso, he can throw the arm back and up. The motion should be forceful enough to provide adequate momentum to carry the arm to a position behind the push handle.

The therapist can help at first by assisting with the throw to give the patient a feel for the motion. An individual who continues to have difficulty can practice with a small wrist weight. The weight will add to the arm's momentum, making it easier to throw the arm back.

Practice of this skill should start with the patient sitting upright in a wheelchair. Once the person has become proficient in this position, he should work to develop the skill while leaning forward, to the side, or both. As his ability improves, the patient should practice in increasingly tilted positions.

Independent Work: This skill can be practiced at any time when the patient is in his wheelchair. It is another good "homework" activity to be performed when not in therapy.

Stabilize Trunk by Holding Wheelchair Push Handle. To work on this skill, a person must be able to tolerate an upright sitting position. It is not necessary for him to be able to place his arm behind the push handle independently.

With his arm hooked behind the wheelchair's push handle, the patient practices holding his body stable. Starting in an upright sitting position, he uses one arm to hold his body upright while he moves the other arm to various positions. This activity can be made more challenging by adding weight to the free arm and by throwing this arm more forcefully.

Once an individual has mastered the skill in upright, he should practice with his trunk leaned in various directions. The degree of lean can increase as he becomes more proficient.

In addition to developing the ability to stabilize his trunk as described above, the patient needs to learn how to adjust his hold on the chair's push handle to allow his trunk to lean. When sitting upright, the trunk is stabilized using the upper arm. When moving from upright, the person must relax his arm enough to allow the hold to slide more distally. The therapist can help with initial practice of this skill by lowering the patient's torso while he adjusts his hold on the chair. As his skill improves, the patient can participate in the control of his trunk's descent, lowering himself as he relaxes his hold on the push handle. He should work to the point where he can lower himself independently and can stop the descent at any point.

Independent Work: This skill can be practiced whenever in a wheelchair.

Move Trunk in Wheelchair by Pulling With Arms. To work on pulling upright from a forward or backward lean, a cord-injured person must be able to tolerate upright sitting. Practice leaning the trunk laterally in a wheelchair can begin before this point.

From an upright or partially reclined position, the patient can practice pulling on his armrest to tip his body to the side and pull back upright. He should start with small excursions, leaning only as far as he can maintain control and return to upright. As his skill increases, he should move through longer arcs of motion.

To lean forward or return to upright, a patient can pull on the wheelchair's armrest(s) or a push handle, respectively. A patient who has adequate strength should not have difficulty with these maneuvers. Someone who has difficulty moving can use momentum from head motions to augment the pull. To return to upright, one hand can be used to push while the other pulls.

Independent Work: These skills can be practiced any time the individual is in a wheelchair.

Move Trunk in Wheelchair Using Momentum. To address this skill, the patient must be able to tolerate upright sitting.

To move his trunk using momentum, a cord-injured person throws his head and an arm in the direction toward which he wants his trunk to move. The other arm remains behind the wheelchair's push handle for stability.

Initially patients are often reluctant to throw their heads and arms forcefully. As a result, they are unable to move using momentum. The therapist should encourage the patient to move with abrupt, powerful, and exaggerated motions. It can be helpful for the therapist to give the patient a feel for the motion by moving his arm passively. A wrist weight can also be helpful, adding to the arm's momentum and enabling the person to move his trunk. As his skill improves, he should practice without the weight.

Independent Work: A patient can practice these skills any time he is in a wheelchair.

Manipulate Armrests. To work on managing his armrests, a patient must be able to stabilize his trunk in the wheelchair.

A cord-injured person with intact upper extremities should be able to manipulate his armrests without difficulty, once he has been shown how they work. People who lack active finger flexors have more difficulty with the task. If the armrest can be repositioned by rotating it up or to the side, the person lacking hand function moves the armrest by pulling/pushing on it with his forearm or the back of his hand (wrist extended). A conventional armrest can be pulled out of and replaced in its channels using either of the holds shown in Figure 11–17. The person can balance the armrest in his lap while turning it around.

Learning to remove and replace armrests is simply a matter of practice. With conventional armrests, the patient needs to spend time lifting the armrests, turning them around, and placing them in the rear channels.

Independent Work: Armrest manipulation can be practiced whenever the patient is in a wheelchair.

Slide Buttocks on Wheelchair Seat. To practice sliding his buttocks on a wheelchair seat, a patient needs to be able to move and stabilize his torso in the wheelchair.

The methods used to slide the buttocks are described above. All of these techniques utilize the head-hips relationship. During early practice of this skill, the therapist can help the patient perform the head and upper torso movements while he tries the maneuvers. This can give the patient a feel for the required force and excursion of the motions.

It is difficult at first for people with spinal cord injuries to move on their wheelchair seats. A therapist can aid the process by pulling on the patient's buttocks to enable him to move. The therapist should time the assistance to coincide with the patient's efforts and should apply just enough force to effect some motion. As the patient's skill improves, the therapist can reduce the assistance given.

Independent Work: The patient can practice moving his buttocks on the seat whenever he is in the wheelchair.

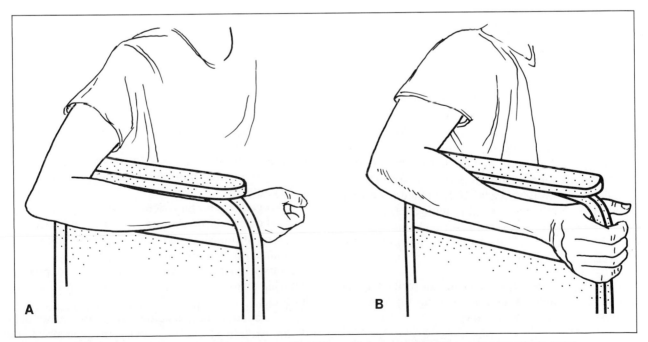

Figure 11–17. Methods for lifting armrest. **(A)** Lifting with forearm. **(B)** Lifting using tenodesis grasp.

Prop Forward on Extended Arms in Sitting. Before someone can learn to prop on extended arms,[6] he must be able to tolerate upright sitting. He must also be able to extend his elbows and hold them in extension against resistance, using either triceps or muscle substitution.

When propping forward on extended arms, a cord-injured person leans forward slightly and supports his trunk on his arms. His palms are lateral to his thighs and anterior to his hips.

After assisting the patient into position, the therapist asks him to help hold his elbows straight. As the patient's ability to support himself improves, the therapist's support is reduced.

The patient should also practice placing his arms in position to support his trunk. As the therapist stabilizes his trunk, he positions his hands and extends his elbows. The patient will soon be able to support his trunk independently by propping forward on extended arms. To prepare for more advanced activities, he can hold the position as the therapist applies resistance, pushing his shoulders in various directions.

Independent Work: Once assisted to a position of propping forward on extended arms in sitting, the patient can practice bending and extending his elbows, lowering and raising his trunk. This can be done long-sitting on a mat or short-sitting between two mats (Fig. 11–16).

Prop Forward on One Extended Arm in Sitting. Before someone can prop forward on one extended arm in sitting, he should be able to prop forward on two extended arms.

After being assisted into the position of propping forward on two extended arms, the patient should be instructed to shift his trunk laterally. At first the therapist can facilitate the weight shift by placing a hand on the lateral surface of one of the patient's shoulders and having him push against it.

The patient should shift *under control* through increasing arcs of motion until he is able to lean far enough to support his trunk on one arm. He can then lift the unweighted arm and balance in that position. He should practice this with each arm. To increase his skill, he should practice balancing with the supporting arm in various positions and reaching the free arm in different directions.

Independent Work: The activities described above can be performed alone, long-sitting on a mat or short-sitting between two mats.

---

[6] "Extended arms" refers to arms with the elbows positioned in extension.

Unweight Buttocks by Leaning Forward on Extended Arms. To develop this skill, a cord-injured person must first be able to prop forward on two extended arms in sitting.

Starting with the patient propped forward on extended arms in sitting, the therapist should instruct him to lean forward and tuck his chin. The therapist can facilitate the lean by placing his hands on the anterior surface of the patient's shoulders and having him push against them.

Independent Work: The patient can practice this skill while long-sitting on a mat or short-sitting between two mats.

Control Pelvis Using Head and Shoulders. To perform any transfer independently, a cord-injured person must use the head-hips relationship. By moving his head and upper torso in one direction, he causes his buttocks to move in the opposite direction.

Many of the activities described below can help develop this ability. However, the therapist and patient may find it helpful to address head-hips control more directly. In doing so, they develop a basic skill that is crucial to all transfers.

Quadruped is an excellent position for working on this skill. This is true whether or not upper extremity motor function is intact. In the absence of functioning triceps, the elbows must be locked using muscle substitution.

When first working in quadruped, the therapist assists the patient to his hands and knees, and the patient attempts to maintain the position. The therapist helps at first, reducing the assistance as the patient's skill improves. The patient can progress to maintaining the position while the therapist applies resistance in various directions.

Once the patient is able to stabilize himself in quadruped, he can progress to moving his buttocks forward and back or side to side using head and shoulder motions. He should move only as far as he can control the motion, increasing the arc as his ability improves.

Someone who has triceps can also practice utilizing the head-hips relationship to assume the quadruped position. Starting in prone, the patient places his palms on the mat next to his shoulders. Simultaneously pushing down and forward (cephalad) with his arms, he pushes his head down to lift his buttocks.

If an individual has elbow flexion contractures or inadequate strength to work in quadruped, he may be able to work on head-hips control while positioned on elbows and knees.

Move Buttocks Laterally While Propping on Extended Arms. To perform this activity, the patient must be able to unweight his buttocks by leaning forward on his extended arms.

During a transfer, a cord-injured person twists his head and upper trunk away from where he wants his buttocks to go. The motion should be forceful and abrupt to provide enough force to move the buttocks.

The patient starts in sitting, propped forward on extended arms. He then attempts the motion as described above. Initial attempts are often done without adequate force, and as a result the buttocks do not move. Verbal encouragement to increase the force and excursion of the twist may not work. In these cases the therapist can help the patient to feel the required motion by assisting him during the attempt, applying force at the patient's shoulders.

Once an individual gets a feel for the head and upper torso motions required, the therapist can help with the lateral slide. Timing the assistance to coincide with the patient's efforts, the therapist applies just enough lateral force to the buttocks to cause motion. As the patient's skill improves, the therapist should reduce the assistance given.

A transfer often requires more than one twist. To make a series of twists possible, the patient moves his head and upper torso back in the other direction between twists. This return motion should not be done forcefully, or the buttocks will slide in the wrong direction.

Occasionally an inexperienced patient twists in both directions with equal force. As a result, the buttocks move back and forth over the same spot. The therapist should give verbal and tactile cues to help him correct this problem.

Independent Work: A patient can practice moving his buttocks to the side while long-sitting on a mat or short-sitting between mats.

In Sitting, Lift Buttocks by Pushing Down on Armrests. To perform this activity, an individual must be able to tolerate upright sitting. Functioning triceps are also required. A patient who has adequate strength should not have difficulty lifting his buttocks by pushing down on his armrests.

Independent Work: A patient can practice lifting his buttocks whenever he is in his wheelchair. To develop some balance skills while practicing this skill, he can short-sit between two mats and do pushups on blocks.

In Sitting, Lift on Armrests and Move Buttocks. Before practicing this skill, the patient must be able to lift his buttocks by pushing down on the wheelchair's armrests.

To perform this maneuver, a cord-injured person throws his head and upper torso forward, back, to the side, or in a rotary direction while lifting his buttocks off of the wheelchair's seat. A patient who moves too timidly while practicing should be encouraged by the therapist to move more forcefully.

Independent Work: This skill can be practiced independently while sitting in a wheelchair.

Lift Buttocks by Pivoting on Extended Arms. To lift his buttocks, a person must first be able to prop forward on extended arms in sitting and hold this position against resistance.

The patient should be shown how to lean forward over his extended arms while tucking his head and protracting his scapulae. It is often helpful for the therapist to assist him into position. This can give the patient a feel for the motion and a sense of just how far he needs to pivot forward to lift his buttocks. The patient should accept full weight on his upper extremities while the therapist helps him to lift his buttocks from the mat by leaning forward over his arms, rolling his head down, and protracting his scapulae. Once in position, the patient can attempt to maintain the lift. As the individual gets a feel for the maneuver, he should progress to practicing with spotting and verbal cueing and then to practicing independently.

One of the challenges of learning to lift the buttocks is finding the balance point. A cord-injured person must move his body fairly far forward over his arms to lift high enough for a transfer. If he tips too far forward, however, he will fall. When an individual is at his balance point, he has moved as far forward as he can (and thus has lifted as high as he can) without falling. The patient should learn to lift to his balance point and hold there briefly.

Moving past the balance point is not the only cause of falls while performing this maneuver; people lacking triceps can also fall forward due to an inability to stabilize their elbows in extension. To correct this problem, a patient may need further strengthening, practice in locking his elbows, or both.

Often a patient will develop the ability to pivot and raise his buttocks, but the lift will still be inadequate for a transfer without equipment. This problem can occur when the patient does not protract his scapulae enough during the lift. The therapist should check for scapular protraction as he attempts the lift.

An individual who does not protract his scapulae adequately when he attempts to lift his buttocks may have serratus anterior weakness. The problem may also be caused by improper technique. If the latter is the case, the therapist can call the person's attention to the problem and provide further instruction. One useful strategy involves placing a hand between the patient's scapulae as he pivots forward on his arms. While pivoting, the patient is asked to push against the therapist's hand by lifting his trunk between his scapulae. If the individual is still unable to perform the motion, the therapist can assist with the scapular protraction during the lift. As the patient pivots forward on his arms, the therapist lifts his thorax between his scapulae (Fig. 11–18). The patient should attempt to hold the position. Once he gets a feel for the scapular protraction, he can attempt the motion on his own.

Independent Work: This skill takes much practice to develop. Once a patient is able to initiate some lift, he can practice on his own while short-sitting between two mats. He should emphasize lifting his buttocks as high as he can, controlling the motion. He should also work on finding his balance point, getting a feel for the limit of his forward pivot.

Lift Buttocks and Move Laterally. Before working on this skill, a person must be able to lift his buttocks by pivoting forward on extended arms.

The therapist should explain and demonstrate how the buttocks can be moved laterally by throwing the head and upper torso to the side while lifting. The motion should be quick and forceful. While first learning the skill, the patient can lift his buttocks first, then twist to move laterally. He should progress to a single combined lift and twist motion.

A common problem that occurs while a patient learns this maneuver is that the buttocks drop as the patient attempts the lateral motion. This is due to a tendency to raise the head when throwing it to the side. The therapist should direct the patient's attention to this problem and encourage him to keep his head low.

Patients also tend to fall forward as they learn the skill. In some cases this is due to the difficulty of keeping the elbows locked in extension during the maneuver. A forward fall also happens when a patient pivots past his balance point. People who fall forward may require more practice in this activity, strengthening of the anterior deltoids, or practice in the prerequisite skill of raising the buttocks by pivoting on extended arms.

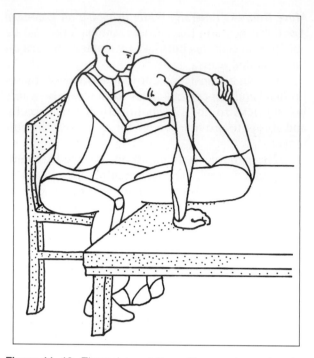

Figure 11–18. Therapist assisting with scapular protraction by lifting patient's thorax between his scapulae while he pivots forward on his arm.

Independent Work: The patient can practice this skill while short-sitting between two mats. He should start by hopping his buttocks over small distances and gradually increase the distance.

Lift Buttocks from Floor to Higher Surface (Side Approach). Before working on this skill, a patient should be able to lift his buttocks and move laterally while pivoting on extended arms. He must also be able to assume the transfer's starting position. The skills required to get into this position are covered in Chapter 12.

At the start of the transfer, the person sits in front of the higher surface, facing at a 30- to 45-degree angle from the higher surface. His knees should be flexed, pointing upward. One hand is on the higher surface and one is on the floor, slightly lateral and anterior to the hip. From this position the person lifts his buttocks by pushing on his arms and throwing his head down and away from the higher surface.

To lift his buttocks high enough for a floor-to-wheelchair transfer, the person must execute his head and upper torso motions in a forceful and exaggerated manner. As can be seen in Figure 11–12, the head must angle toward the floor for the buttocks to lift high enough. During functional training, the therapist should emphasize the magnitude of the head motion required.

Initially patients are often reluctant to throw their heads down far enough and with enough force. A therapist can help a patient to get a feel for the maneuver by moving him passively through the motion as he pivots on his arms.

When first working on this skill, it is best to start by transferring between the floor and a very low surface. The patient should transfer up and down, moving under control in both directions. As his ability improves, he can gradually increase the height of the surface.

Folding mats are useful for this process: the patient can transfer from a floor mat to progressively higher stacks of folded mats. Starting with minimal height, he can gradually build up to the full distance from the floor to a wheelchair seat. Mats should be added to increase the height of the transfer only when the individual has mastered the technique at a given height, performing the transfer consistently and with good control.

An individual who runs into difficulty with higher transfers may need to throw his head further down to get a better lift. Another possibility is that he needs to protract his scapulae more forcefully as his buttocks approach the level of the higher surface.

The patient should remember that when he transfers from a higher to a lower surface, gravity provides the downward force. The head should not be thrown forcefully up to move the buttocks downward. Instead, the patient should resist the downward motion to control the descent.

During functional training, it can be useful to approach the transfer from both directions: in addition to practicing transfers between the floor and higher surfaces, a patient can practice moving between the wheelchair and progressively lower surfaces. During these transfers, his feet should rest on the floor rather than on the piled mats. This position closely replicates the body's orientation at the end of a floor-to-chair transfer.

Once a patient is consistently able to move between the floor and mats stacked to the height of a wheelchair seat, he is ready for practice with a wheelchair. Since a seat cushion adds height to the transfer, the patient should first practice without it. A cushion can be added when the patient masters the transfer without it.

During practice of floor-to-wheelchair transfers, it is common for a patient to catch his buttocks under the wheelchair's seat. This occurs when the

individual transfers from a position too close to the chair.

Independent Work: A patient can work independently on transfers from a floor mat to higher surfaces or from a wheelchair to lower surfaces. Tumbles that occur while an individual transfers between the floor and higher surfaces are usually not a great problem. Early on, before he has become very skillful, a patient practices transfers to and from fairly low surfaces and does not have far to fall. By the time he works on higher transfers, he has developed some degree of control.

Transfer practice between a wheelchair and lower surfaces presents more of a problem. Early in the training, when potential falls would occur from the full height of the wheelchair seat, the patient will not yet have developed enough control to break his fall. This problem can be dealt with by placing a pile of pillows or a chair with a pillow in the seat in front of the patient.

Straight Lift From Floor (Front or Back Approach). Before working on these maneuvers, a patient should be able to lift his buttocks by pivoting forward on extended arms. He should also be able to lift his body by pushing down with his arms, starting with his hands positioned close to his shoulders. This ability can be practiced while sitting between parallel bars or while sitting on a mat between two chairs.

This skill is used both in the front- and back-approach transfer from the floor to a wheelchair. Using the front approach, a person starts from a kneeling position facing the wheelchair, with his hands on the armrests. In the back-approach transfer, the transfer's starting position is sitting on the floor facing outward, with the hands on the front of the wheelchair seat. Using either approach, the cord-injured person lifts his body from the starting position by leaning toward the wheelchair and pushing straight downward. Once his buttocks have passed the seat and he has lifted as high as he can in this manner, he tucks his head and protracts his scapulae to lift his buttocks further.

The patient should practice this skill while being spotted. If he has adequate strength, it should not take many attempts to master. If the patient does not lift his buttocks high enough, the therapist may need to give him verbal and tactile cues to encourage him to tuck his head lower and protract his scapulae more forcefully.

Independent Work: If an individual has some degree of control, this skill can be practiced independently over a floor mat. Someone who has difficulty with the lift facing away from the chair can start by practicing transferring from a raised surface to the chair and can work from progressively lower surfaces as his skill improves.

Turn Body to Drop onto Wheelchair Seat. Before practicing this maneuver, the patient should be able to lift his body above his wheelchair seat from a kneeling position. Once he has lifted high enough, he lets go of an armrest and throws his arm and head away from the armrest. This causes his body to turn and drop onto the wheelchair seat.

A patient who lands on a hip rather than on his buttocks may not have lifted his body high enough initially. If this is the case, he needs to tuck his head lower, protract his scapulae more prior to releasing the armrest, or both. The problem may also occur when the lift was adequate but the patient did not turn far enough before landing. In these instances the patient should be instructed to throw his arm and head more forcefully.

Independent Work: Once a person has developed some degree of control over this maneuver, he can practice alone. The wheelchair should be placed on or in front of a floor mat.

PROGRAM DESIGN

When using this text as a resource to assist in working toward a functional goal, the therapist should first read the text's description of the functional activity. Based on that description, on the corresponding charts, both, the therapist can determine what physical and skill prerequisites are required to perform the skill. Taking into consideration the patient's evaluation results, the therapist can determine where he has deficits relevant to the functional goal. The program should then be designed to address these deficits, developing the needed physical and skill prerequisites.

Many strategies are available for increasing strength and range of motion; the field of physical therapy has a variety of approaches for accomplishing these ends. The program may include any combination of the following: proprioceptive neuromuscular facilitation, progressive resistive exercises (concentric and eccentric), strengthening through functional tasks, isokinetic exercise, prolonged stretching, and electrical stimulation. Strengthening and stretching will also occur with increased activity. The patient can exercise independently, in groups, and one-on-one with the therapist.

This chapter presents functional training strategies for each prerequisite skill. The therapist can use these suggestions, coupled with his own imagination, clinical expertise, and problem solving, to design a functional training program. The program should aim first at developing the most basic prerequisite skills and build to more advanced skills as the patient's abilities develop.

In most cases a patient will have many functional goals. The therapeutic program must progress him toward all of these goals. Fortunately there is much overlap of prerequisites between skills. Thus a person working on propping forward on two extended arms is potentially progressing toward independence in a variety of transfers. Furthermore, work aimed at developing one ability can benefit other, seemingly unrelated, activities. For example, the strengthening and motor learning that results from practicing transfers may benefit an individual's mat or ambulation skills.

Example: Move Buttocks on the Wheelchair Seat. To move his buttocks on a wheelchair seat, a cord-injured person who lacks functioning triceps needs adequate strength in his deltoids and elbow flexors and needs adequate range in elbow flexion and extension and shoulder extension and abduction. He must be able to tolerate an upright sitting position, extend his elbows using muscle substitution, place his arm behind a push handle, hold the push handle to stabilize his trunk, move his trunk in the wheelchair, and slide his buttocks on the seat.

An individual's program design will depend on his unique needs. If he has any deficits in prerequisite strength or range, the program should include exercises to address these deficits. Most patients benefit from strengthening of all innervated upper extremity musculature, with emphasis on muscles used in elbow extension, shoulder flexion and horizontal adduction, and scapular protraction and depression.

If the patient has none of the needed skill prerequisites, functional training should start with the most basic skills: ability to extend the elbow using muscle substitution (if the triceps are not innervated), to tolerate an upright sitting position, to stabilize the trunk in a wheelchair, and to move the trunk in the wheelchair by pulling up the arms. When he has developed these abilities, he can work on sliding his buttocks on the wheelchair seat and moving his trunk in the wheelchair using momentum and by pushing with his arms. By building his skill in this manner, the patient progresses to independence in positioning his buttocks on a wheelchair seat.

SUGGESTED READING

For additional information on transfer techniques used by people with spinal cord injuries, the reader is referred to the following books:

Ford, J., & Duckworth, B. (1987). *Physical Management for the Quadriplegic Patient* (2nd ed.). Philadelphia: F.A. Davis.

Nixon, V. (1985). *Spinal Cord Injury: A Guide to Functional Outcomes in Physical Therapy Management*. Rockville, MD: Aspen.

12
Functional Mat Techniques

Functional mat skills include rolling, coming to sitting, gross mat mobility (moving around on a mat), maintenance of an unsupported sitting posture,[1] and leg management. These skills are required for independent mobility; before someone can get out of bed in the morning, he must first be able to sit up and move to the edge of the bed. Mat skills are also required for independent dressing.

This chapter presents a variety of functional mat techniques,[2] as well as suggestions on how to teach them. It is important for the reader to keep in mind that the motions used to perform any functional task vary between people. This variability is due to differences in body build, skill level, range of motion, muscle tone, and patterns of strength and weakness.

The descriptions of techniques and training presented in this chapter should be used as a guide, not as a set of hard and fast rules. During functional training, the therapist and patient should work together to find the exact techniques that best suit that particular individual.

PRACTICE ON MAT AND BED

An exercise mat is a good surface on which to learn mat skills. It is firmer than most beds, making it an easier surface on which to practice. At the same time, a mat is soft enough to allow the inevitable tumbles without injury.

Although the skills presented in this chapter are first practiced on a mat, the ultimate goal should be for the patient to function on a bed. This is the surface on which he will most often find himself when he needs to roll over, come to sitting, or get dressed. Since a bed is a more difficult surface on which to

function, ability developed on a mat will not automatically transfer to bed function. Thus after an individual has mastered these skills on a mat, he should practice them on a bed. This will increase the likelihood that the skills learned in therapy will be utilized outside of therapy.

PRESERVATION OF TENODESIS GRASP

People with active wrist extension are able to compensate for nonfunctional finger flexors by using a natural tenodesis grasp.[3] For this grasp to work, the long finger flexors must not be overstretched.

Whenever the wrists and fingers are extended simultaneously, the long finger flexors are stretched and the tenodesis grasp can be damaged. This can occur when weight is borne on the palms during activities such as coming to sitting. To avoid stretching the long finger flexors, someone who uses a tenodesis grasp (or may use this grasp in the future) should keep his interphalangeal joints flexed whenever he bears weight on his palms. This will preserve his tenodesis grasp.

PRESERVATION OF LOW-BACK TIGHTNESS

Mild tightness in the low back is desirable for people with complete spinal cord injuries, as it facilitates transfers and functional mat activities. To preserve mild tightness in the low back, long-sitting should be avoided when shortening of the hamstrings prevents passive straight-leg raise to 90 degrees.

PHYSICAL AND SKILL PREREQUISITES

Each method of performing a functional activity involves a particular set of skills. Each activity also

---

[1] Unsupported sitting balance is addressed in Chapter 11.

[2] This chapter does not attempt to present all possible functional mat techniques. An individual who is unable to master a skill described in this chapter may fare better with a variation of that technique or with an altogether different method.

[3] Tenodesis grasp and release are described in Chapter 8.

has strength, joint range of motion, and muscle flexibility requirements. A deficiency in any of these skill or physical prerequisites will impair a person's performance of the activity.

The descriptions of functional techniques presented below are accompanied by charts that summarize their skill and physical prerequisites. Exact values for the physical prerequisites are not given because the requirements vary among individuals. For example, when coming to sitting using a given method, someone who is strong and coordinated may require less range in shoulder hyperextension than another person who is weaker or less coordinated.

FUNCTIONAL MAT TECHNIQUES

Rolling

Rolling is one of the more basic mat skills.[4] It is used to turn in bed and is a prerequisite for several methods of coming to sitting. Rolling is also used for self-care activities such as dressing.

The physical prerequisites for rolling using the three techniques described below are summarized in Chart 12–1. Chart 12–2 summarizes the prerequisite skills for rolling.

Supine to Prone Without Equipment. To roll from supine to prone without equipment, a person with a spinal cord injury turns his body using momentum from head and arm motions.

Some cord-injured people who are very coordinated, strong, or have low lesions (or any combination thereof) are able to roll in a single maneuver. An individual with this capability simply throws his head and arms forcefully in the direction toward which he wants to roll.

For most people with complete injuries, rolling requires more effort. Momentum for the roll is built by rocking back and forth. To roll in this manner, the person swings his head and arms forcefully to one side and then the other. His trunk rocks from supine with each swing, rolling partially in the direction of the throw. As his trunk falls back toward supine, he adds momentum to the motion by throwing his head and arms. By repeatedly throwing his head and arms left and right in coordination with the trunk's rocking motion, the person can build enough momentum to roll (Fig. 12–1).

The number of throws that an individual must use to roll will depend upon several factors. Someone with greater strength and skill will be able to roll with fewer throws. Body build will also have an

---

[4] "Basic" is not meant to imply that rolling is easy. In fact, learning to roll from supine can be very difficult for people with cervical lesions.

Chart 12–1 Rolling—Physical Prerequisites

		Supine to prone without equipment	Supine to prone with equipment	Prone to supine
Strength				
	Anterior deltoids	☑	☑	√
	Middle deltoids	√	√	√
	Posterior deltoids	☑	√	√
	Biceps, brachialis, and/or brachioradialis		☑	
Range of Motion				
Shoulder	Flexion		√	√
	External rotation	☑		
	Horizontal adduction	√	√	
	Horizontal abduction	√		
Elbow	Extension	☑		√
	Flexion		√	
	Forearm Supination	√		√

√: Some strength is needed for this activity, or severe limitations in range will inhibit this activity.
☑: A large amount of strength or normal or greater range is needed for this activity.

impact; obesity or wide hips will make rolling more difficult.

A good deal of momentum is required to move the large mass of the trunk and lower extremities. When using the relatively small mass of the head and upper extremities to roll, their momentum must be maximized. Several things can be done to increase momentum. The elbows should be held in extension to maximize the moment arm. Protracting the scapula at the end of the swing will also increase the moment arm. Arm-and-head swings should be performed forcefully, with maximal velocity.

People with innervated triceps can throw their arms in an arc that is perpendicular to the mat. This is not true for people who lack functioning triceps. In these cases the elbows will flex when thrown in this manner. This elbow flexion interferes with transmission of momentum to the trunk. In addition,

Chart 12—2 Rolling—Skill Prerequisites

	Supine to prone without equipment	Supine to prone with equipment	Prone to supine
Supine Skills			
Position elbows in extension	√	√	
Maintain elbow extension while flexing shoulders	√	√	
Throw arm(s) across body, elbow(s) extended	√	√	
Combined arm throw and head swing	√	√	
Roll toward prone using momentum	√		
Position arm to assist in rolling with equipment		√	
Roll body toward prone by pulling on equipment		√	
Prone Skill			
Roll from prone by pushing with arm			√

elbow flexion can result in the person hitting himself in the face. To avoid these problems, someone who lacks functioning triceps should swing his arms in an arc that is approximately 45 degrees above the plane of his body. (The shoulders are flexed to about 45 degrees.) This position, combined with shoulder external rotation, and forearm supination helps maintain the elbows in extension.

Supine to Prone With Equipment. Weakness, contractures, obesity, spasticity, confusion, or low motivation can keep someone from achieving independence in rolling without equipment. In these instances many people can learn to roll by pulling on a bedrail or a wheelchair parked next to the mat or bed. The use of a wheelchair is preferable to a bedrail, as it does not require any special equipment.

To prepare to roll using equipment, a cord-injured person lacking hand function first positions the arm toward which he plans to roll, stabilizing his arm under a bedrail or under his wheelchair's armrest or wheel rim. The arm should be positioned with the shoulder abducted to about 90 degrees and the antecubital fossa facing the ceiling (Fig. 12–2). The forearm should be supinated.

Pulling with his biceps and anterior deltoid, the person rolls his trunk toward his stabilized arm. At the same time, he swings his head and free arm in the direction of the roll, adding momentum. In the absence of innervated triceps, the free arm should be swung in an arc that is about 45 degrees above the plane of the body.

The roll can be completed in one of two ways. At the end of the free arm's swing, this arm can be used to pull on the equipment. Alternatively, the person can reach or punch with his free arm at the end of the swing, protracting his scapula to add momentum to the roll.

Prone to Supine. Rolling from prone to supine is far easier than rolling in the opposite direction. The cord-injured person simply pushes on the supporting surface, using the arm away from which he wants to roll. Once he reaches a side lying position,

Chart 12—3 Assuming Prone on elbows—Physical Prerequisites

		From prone, shoulders abducted	From prone, shoulders adducted	From side lying	At the end of a role from supine
Strength					
	Anterior deltoids	☑	☑	√	☑
	Middle deltoids			√	√
	Posterior deltoids			☑	☑
	Biceps, brachialis, and/or brachioradialis			√	
Range of Motion					
Shoulder	Flexion	√	√	√	√
	Abduction	√	√	√	
	External rotation	√		√	☑
	Horizontal adduction	√	√	√	√
Elbow	Flexion	√	√	√	√

√: Some strength is needed for this activity, or severe limitations in range will inhibit this activity.

☑: A large amount of strength or normal or greater range is needed for this activity.

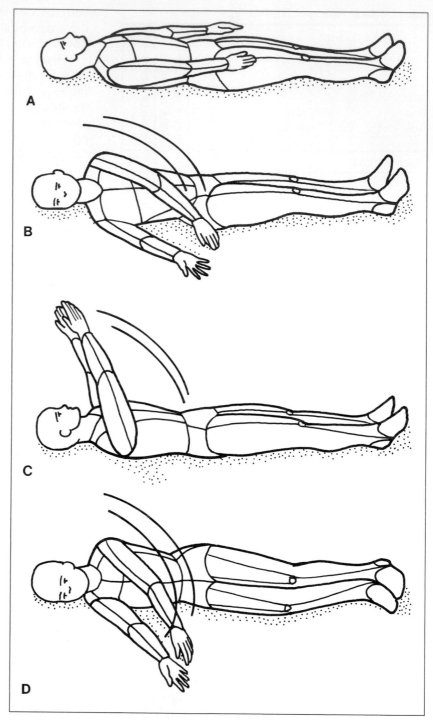

Figure 12–1. Rolling supine to prone without equipment.

he can throw his head and arm in the direction of the roll.

Assuming Prone On Elbows

Assuming prone on elbows is another important basic capability. The prone on elbows position can be used to move in bed, and it is a key position in some methods of coming to sitting.

There are a variety of methods that a cord-injured person can use to get prone on elbows. Four methods are presented below. The physical and skill prerequisites for these techniques are summarized in Charts 12–3 and 12–4, respectively.

From Prone, Shoulders Abducted. When using this method to get onto his elbows, a cord-injured person

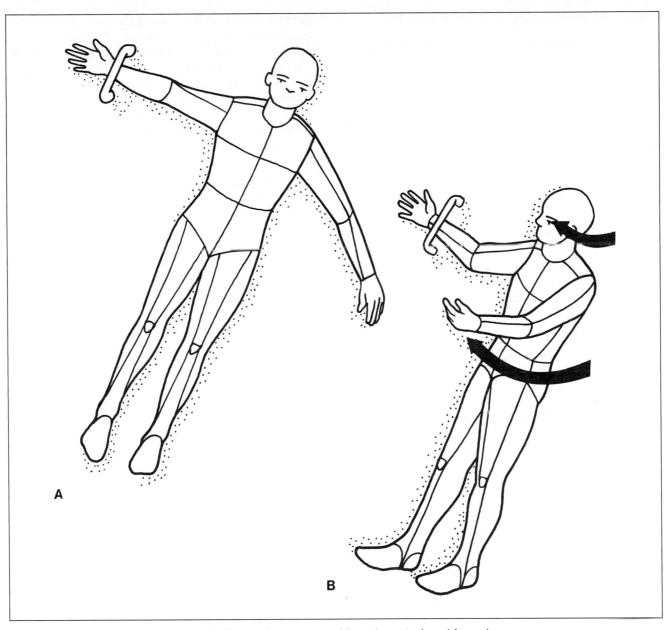

Figure 12–2. Rolling supine to prone with equipment, viewed from above.

starts in prone with his arms resting on the mat in the position shown in Figure 12–3A. His shoulders are externally rotated and abducted to 90 degrees, and his elbows are flexed to approximately 90 degrees.

From the starting position, the person shifts his weight to one side and horizontally adducts and shrugs the opposite shoulder. He then shifts in the other direction and pulls in his other arm in the same manner. Each time he performs this maneuver, the elbow is moved a short distance medially. By repeatedly weight shifting and repositioning his elbows medially, he gradually "walks" his elbows in-

ward until they are positioned vertically under his shoulders.

From Prone, Shoulders Adducted. An alternate method for getting onto the elbows from prone involves shoulder flexion instead of horizontal adduction. The cord-injured person starts with his elbows flexed and his shoulders adducted against his sides (Fig. 12–4A).

From the starting position, the trunk is lifted slightly, using forceful flexion of the shoulders. Shifting his weight to one side, the person flexes the unweighted shoulder. This maneuver brings the

Chart 12–4 Assuming Prone on elbows—Skill Prerequisites

	From prone, shoulders abducted	From prone, shoulders adducted	From side lying	At the end of a roll from supine
Supine Skills				
Position elbows in extension				✓
Maintain elbow extension while flexing shoulders				✓
Throw arm(s) across body, elbow(s) extended				✓
Roll supine to prone without equipment				✓
Prone Skill				
Weight shift in prone on elbows	✓	✓	✓	
Walk elbows in from abducted position	✓			
Walk elbows forward from adducted position		✓		
Side-lying Skill				
Move from side lying to prone on elbows			✓	✓

elbow forward slightly, moving it toward a position under the shoulder. The person then shifts to the other side and pulls the opposite shoulder forward. By repeatedly weight shifting to alternate sides and flexing his unweighted shoulders, he "walks" his elbows into position under his shoulders.

From Side Lying. When using this method to assume a prone on elbows position, the cord-injured person starts in a side lying position with the shoulder and elbow of his lower arm (the arm on which he is lying) flexed. If he does not have fully innervated shoulder musculature, he may need to stabilize his hand against his head. Stabilizing his hand in this manner enables him to use this arm more effectively as a lever. Figure 12–5 illustrates the starting position with the hand stabilized against the forehead. The hand can be stabilized in other positions, such as against either the chin or the side of the head.

Moving to prone on elbows from this position involves simultaneous use of leverage by the lower arm and momentum from the upper arm.

From the starting position, the person pushes the elbow of his lower arm down into the mat, lifting his trunk up and forward over his elbow. Once the lift has been initiated, he can tuck his chin to assist in the motion.

While pushing into the mat with his lower arm, the person forcefully swings his free arm forward, adding momentum to help move the trunk. Upon completion of the arm's swing, he can do one of two things with this arm to help pull his trunk up and over his supporting elbow. He can use momentum by reaching or punching the arm at the end of its swing, protracting the scapula. Alternatively, at the

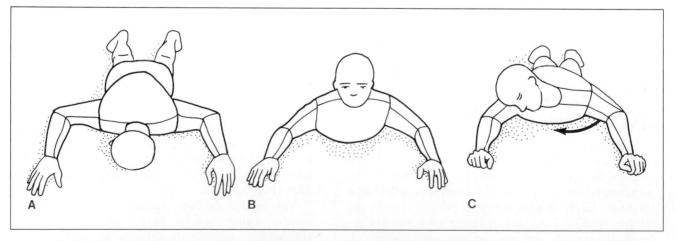

Figure 12–3. Assuming prone on elbows from prone, shoulders abducted. **A.** Starting position, viewed from above. **B.** Part way up, viewed from the front. **C.** Weight shifting and moving unweighted arm medially.

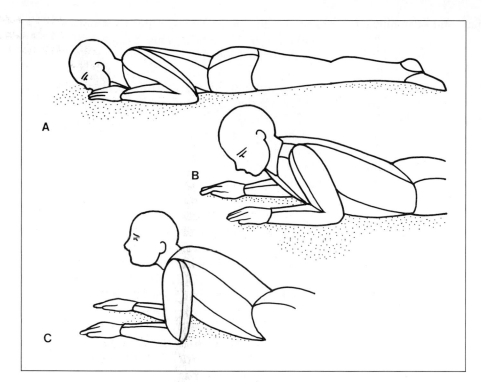

Figure 12–4. Assuming prone on elbows from prone, shoulders adducted, viewed from the side. **A.** Starting position. **B.** Part way up. **C.** Prone on elbows.

end of the arm's swing, he can stabilize his hand against his supporting elbow. With the hand stabilized in this manner, he can use this arm to pull the trunk, helping to move it to a position over his supporting elbow.

At the End of a Roll From Supine. This method for getting prone on elbows is possible for someone with C6 or lower quadriplegia who is both strong in his innervated musculature and skillful in rolling without equipment. Using this technique, a cord-injured person takes advantage of his body's momentum at the end of a roll, using it to get onto his elbows.

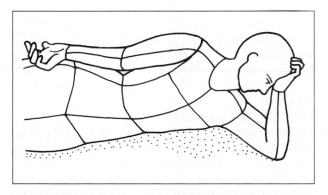

Figure 12–5. Starting position for assuming prone on elbows from side lying.

The person starts the process by rolling forcefully. As he rolls past side lying, he pushes the elbow of his lower arm into the mat. He can use his free arm to assist in the process in either of the two ways described above: he can reach or punch at the end of the arm's swing, or he can stabilize the free hand against his supporting elbow and pull. Whichever method is used, these actions must be performed without interrupting the roll from supine. An uninterrupted roll makes it possible for the trunk's momentum to help carry the trunk over the supporting elbow.

Coming to Sitting Without Equipment
To dress or transfer out of bed independently, a cord-injured person needs to be able to get himself into a sitting position. If he can do so without equipment, he will be spared the stigma, expense, and restrictions of special equipment.

With Functioning Triceps. An individual with intact upper extremity musculature may be able to come to sitting directly from supine by pushing down on the mat with his hands. If he needs, he can rock his trunk side to side slightly as he pushes.

Even without fully intact upper extremities, the presence of functioning triceps makes a large difference in the ability to assume a sitting position. A person with functioning triceps can roll past side lying, plant his hands on the mat, and push himself into a sitting position.

Assuming a sitting posture is a more involved process when functioning triceps are lacking. The three methods presented below do not require triceps. Chart 12–5 provides a summary of the physical prerequisites for these techniques. Chart 12–6 summarizes the skill prerequisites.

Rolling and Throwing Arms. This methods of assuming a sitting position requires very good flexibility.

Chart 12–5 Coming to Sitting Without Equipment—Physical Prerequisites

		Roll and throw	Straight from supine, hands stabilized	Walking on elbows
Strength				
	Anterior deltoids	☑	☑	√
	Middle deltoids	√	√	√
	Posterior deltoids	☑	√	√
	Biceps, brachialis, and/or brachioradialis		☑	√
	Internal rotators			√
Range of Motion				
Shoulder	Extension[a]	☑	☑	
	Flexion	√		√
	Abduction	√	√	√
	External rotation[a]	☑	☑	
	Internal rotation			☑
	Horizontal abduction[a]	☑	☑	√
Elbow	Extension[a]	☑	☑	
	Flexion	√	√	√
Forearm	Supination	√	√	
Wrist	Extension	√	√	

√: Some strength is needed for this activity, or severe limitations in range will inhibit this activity.

☑: A large amount of strength or normal or greater range is needed for this activity.

[a] These motions (shoulder extension, external rotation, horizontal abduction, and elbow extension) must be present in combination.

The shoulder must have greater than normal range in extension. The elbows must extend fully with the shoulders positioned in hyperextension and external rotation.

To come to sitting using this method, the person first gets prone on elbows using any of the methods described above (Fig. 12–6A). He then shifts his weight onto one elbow. With his unweighted arm, he pushes his trunk up and over the supporting elbow, ending in the forearm-supported side-lying position (Fig. 12–6B).

From forearm-supported side lying, the person throws his free arm back in an arc, landing on his palm (Fig. 12–6C). To make the next step possible, the hand must land with the shoulder positioned in external rotation and extreme horizontal abduction and hyperextension. The elbow must be fully extended and the forearm supinated. From this position, the person shifts his weight onto his extended arm and lifts the other arm (Fig. 12–6D).

Balancing on his supporting arm, the person throws his free arm back. When the palm lands on the mat, the elbow of this arm should be extended, the forearm supinated, and the shoulder horizontally abducted, hyperextended, and externally rotated (Fig. 12–6E).

From this position, an upright sitting posture is achieved by walking the hands forward. To walk his hands forward, the person shifts first to one side and then to the other, moving the unweighted hand forward by elevating and protracting the scapula.

Straight from Supine, Hands Stabilized. To assume a sitting position using this method, a cord-injured person must have very strong biceps. Range of motion requirements are the same as those for the method described above.

In the supine position, the hands are stabilized by placing them in the pockets or inside the pants. The person then lifts his upper trunk by flexing his elbows forcefully (Fig. 12–7B).

Once the person has lifted his upper trunk as high as he can, he moves his elbows posteriorly. Shifting his weight from side to side, he walks his unweighted elbows back until he is in a stable position, supine on elbows (Fig. 12–7C).

From supine on elbows, the individual shifts his weight to one elbow and lifts the unweighted arm (Fig. 12–7D). While lifting, he forcefully contracts the anterior deltoid of his supporting arm, turning his upper trunk so that his shoulders are aligned vertically over the supporting elbow.

From this position, the person comes to sitting in the manner described above. He throws back first one arm and then the other (Fig. 12–7E through G)

Chart 12—6 Coming to Sitting Without Equipment—Skill Prerequisites

	Roll and throw	Straight from supine, hands stabilized	Walking on elbows
Supine Skills			
Weight shift in supine, supported on one elbow and one hand	√	√	
From supine, supported on one elbow and one hand, lift elbow	√	√	
Position elbows in extension	√	√	
Maintain elbow extension while flexing shoulders	√	√	
Stabilize hands in pants		√	
With hands stabilized in pants, lift trunk using elbow flexion		√	
Weight shift in supine on elbows		√	
In supine on elbows, walk elbows back		√	
Dynamic shoulder control in single forearm-supported supine	√	√	
From supine on elbows, lift one elbow	√	√	
From single forearm-supported supine, throw one arm back	√	√	
Prone Skills			
Assume prone on elbows position	√		√
Weight shift in prone on elbows	√		√
Move from prone on elbows to forearm-supported side lying	√		√
In prone on elbows, walk elbows to the side			√
Side-lying Skills			
Dynamic shoulder control in forearm-supported side lying	√		
From forearm-supported side lying, throw free arm back	√		
In 90-degree forearm-supported side lying, walk supporting elbow toward legs			√
From forearm-supported side lying, push-pull into sitting position			√
Sitting Skills			
Extend elbows against resistance[a]			√
Tolerate upright sitting position[b]			√
Dynamic shoulder control in sitting, propped back on one hand	√	√	
From sitting propped back on one hand, throw free arm back	√	√	
Weight shift while sitting, propped back on two hands	√	√	
From sitting, propped back on two hands, walk hands forward	√	√	
Push with arms to lift trunk from forward lean[a]			√

[a] Refer to Chapter 11 for a description of this skill and therapeutic strategies.
[b] Refer to Chapter 8 for a description of this skill and therapeutic strategies.

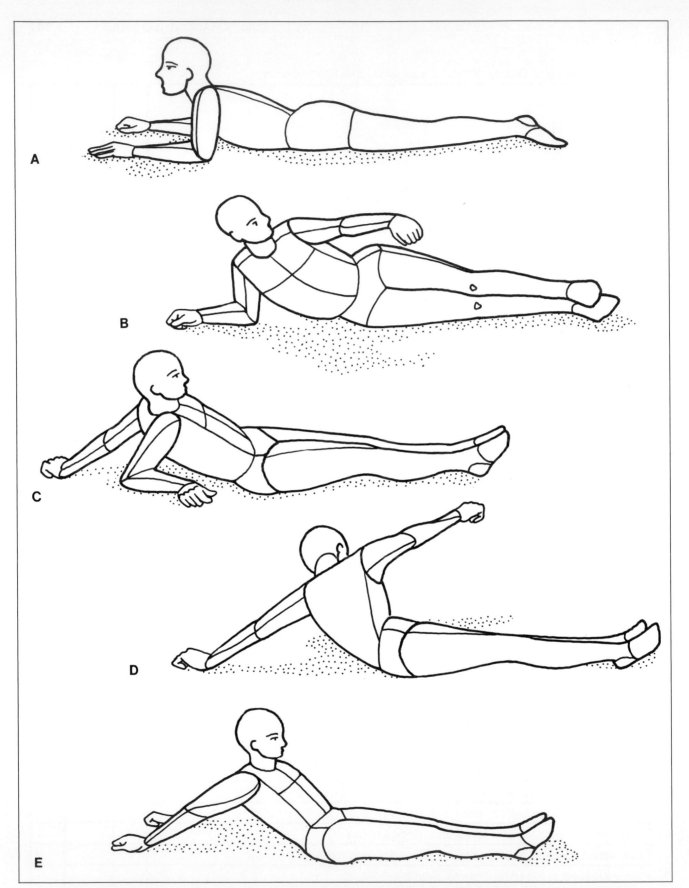

Figure 12–6. Coming to sitting by rolling and throwing the arms. **A.** Prone on elbows. **B.** Forearm-supported side lying. **C.** Supine supported on one elbow and one hand. **D.** Supporting elbow lifted. **E.** Sitting propped back on two hands.

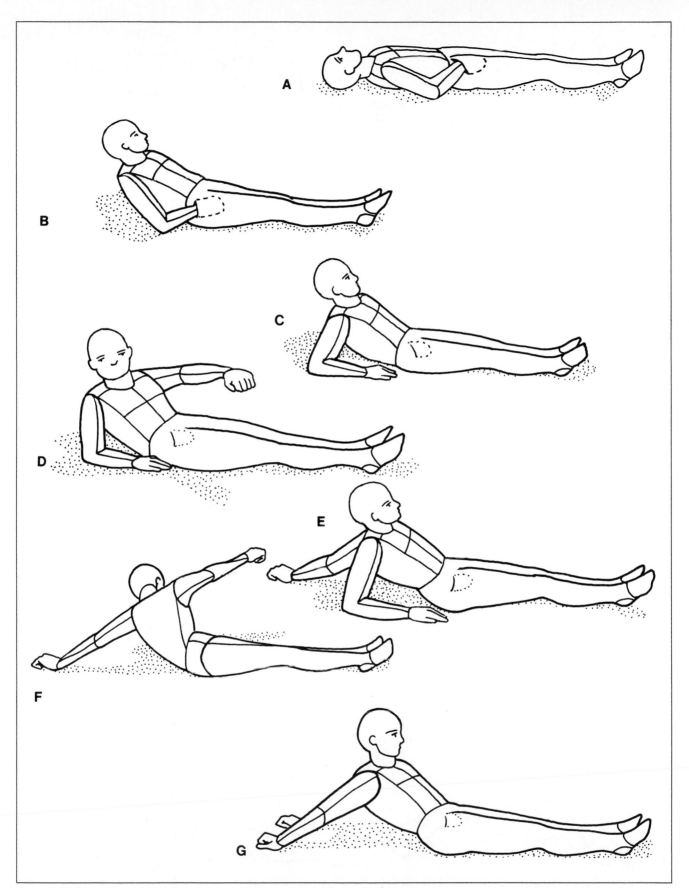

Figure 12–7. Coming to sitting straight from supine, hands stabilized in pants. **A.** Starting position: supine with hands stabilized in pants. **B.** Upper trunk lifted using elbow flexion. **C.** Elbows walked back to a stable position. **D.** One arm lifted. **E.** Free arm thrown back. **F.** Second arm lifted. **G.** Second arm thrown back.

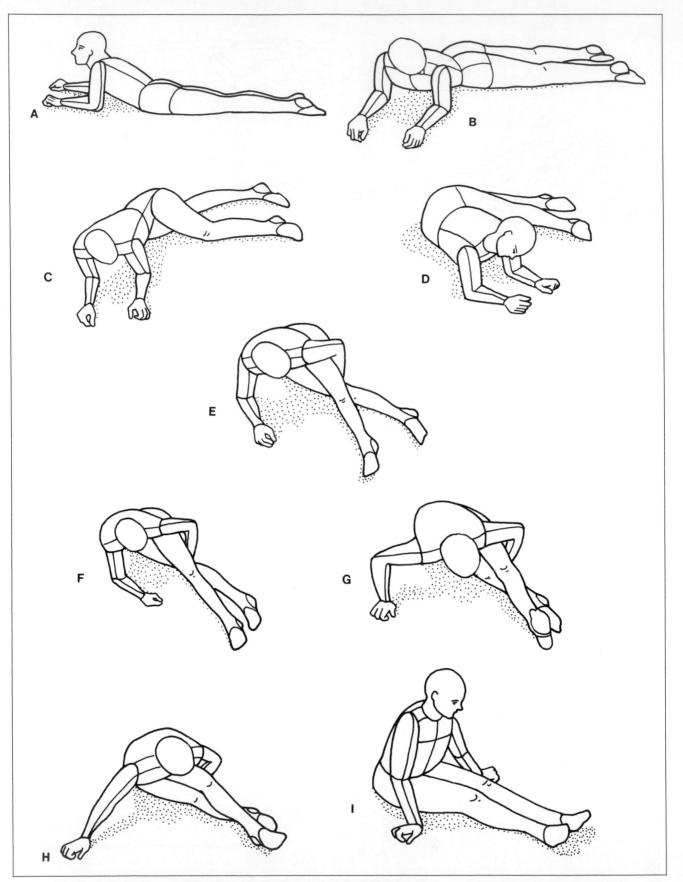

Figure 12–8. Coming to sitting by walking on elbows. **A.** Starting position: prone on elbows. **B.** The elbows are walked to the side until the trunk will not laterally flex any further. **C.** The pelvis is rolled from prone toward side lying. **D.** The elbows are walked toward the legs. **E.** An arm is hooked around the thighs. **F.** The supporting elbow is walked toward the legs. **G.** The palm is planted on the mat. **H.** The body is rocked into position over the legs. **I.** The torso is pushed to upright.

and walks his hands forward until he reaches an upright sitting posture.

This method of coming to sitting has the advantage of being relatively fast. However, since pants are required, it obviously will not be useful when the person is undressed or in the process of dressing. Other methods will be required under these circumstances.

Walking on Elbows. This method of assuming the sitting position does not require the range of motion that is needed to perform the methods described above. Neither shoulder hyperextension nor full elbow extension is needed.

To come to sitting in this manner, the person first gets prone on elbows using any of the methods described above. He then walks his elbows to one side. To do so, he shifts his weight first to one side and then to the other, moving the unweighted elbow.

The person continues walking his elbows to the side until he reaches a point where his trunk will not laterally flex any further (Fig. 12–8B). In the next step he rotates his pelvis from prone toward side lying. This involves pushing with the elbows (using shoulder flexion with the elbows stabilized on the mat) to roll his pelvis from prone (Fig. 12–8C).

With his pelvis tilted from prone, the person can continue walking on his elbows until he is close enough to reach his legs. This position will vary, but it is generally such that the trunk is at a 90-degree or smaller angle to the legs (Fig. 12–8D).

Shifting his weight onto the arm that is furthest from his legs, the person lifts his unweighted arm and hooks the forearm around his thighs (Fig 12–8E). He can then walk the other elbow toward his legs, shifting his weight by pulling with the arm that is stabilized on his legs.[5] In this manner he walks his elbow until it is close enough to his legs for him to perform the next step (Fig. 12–8F). The target position for the elbow will vary, depending on his strength and skill.

Shifting his weight off of his supporting elbow, the person internally rotates this shoulder and plants his palm on the mat (Fig. 12–8G). Pushing with this arm and pulling with the one stabilized on his legs, he then rocks his body into position over his legs (Fig. 12–8H). Once his body is positioned over his legs, he can place both palms on the mat and push his torso to upright (Fig. 12–8I).

---

[5] This step may be omitted if strength and skill allow.

Coming to Sitting Using Equipment

Weakness, obesity, spasticity, and inadequate time for full rehabilitation are among the factors that can prevent someone from learning to assume a sitting posture without equipment. In these cases many can learn to assume a sitting position independently using equipment.

There are various methods that can be used to come to sitting using a loop ladder attached to the foot of the bed or using loops suspended from a bar over the bed. One method for each will be presented below. Charts 12–7 and 12–8 summarize the physical and skill prerequisites for these methods.

Loop Ladder. A cord-injured person who is unable to roll or get into prone on elbows without equip-

Chart 12–7 Coming to Sitting With Equipment—Physical Prerequisites

	Using loop ladder	Using suspended loops
Strength		
Anterior deltoids	☑	☑
Middle deltoids	√	√
Posterior deltoids	√	√
Biceps, brachialis, and/or brachioradialis	☑	☑
Range of Motion		
Shoulder Extension		√
Flexion	√	√
Abduction	√	√
External rotation		√
Horizontal abduction		√
Elbow Extension		☑
Flexion	√	√
Forearm Supination		√
Wrist Extension		√
Combined hip flexion and knee extension	☑	☑

√: Some strength is needed for this activity, or severe limitations in range will inhibit this activity.

☑: A large amount of strength or normal or greater range is needed for this activity.

Chart 12–8 Coming to Sitting With Equipment—Skill Prerequisites

	Using loop ladder	Using suspended loops
Supine Skills		
Position elbows in extension	√	√
Maintain elbow extension while flexing shoulders	√	√
Place arm through loop	√	√
Pulling on loop ladder, move from supine to single forearm supported supine	√	
In single forearm-supported supine, pull on loop ladder and walk supporting elbow toward feet	√	
Lift trunk by pulling on suspended loop		√
Dynamic shoulder control in single forearm-supported supine		√
Sitting Skills		
Tolerate upright sitting position	√	√
With one arm through overhead loop, throw free arm back		√
Dynamic shoulder control in sitting, propped back on one hand		√
In sitting, propped back on one hand, pull on suspended loop and walk supporting hand forward		√
Extend elbows against resistance	√	
Push with arms to lift trunk from forward lean	√	

[a] Refer to Chapter 8 for a description of this skill and therapeutic strategies.
[b] Refer to Chapter 11 for a description of this skill and therapeutic strategies.

ment may be able to come to sitting using a loop ladder.[6] The ladder is attached to the foot of the bed and lies on the mattress (Fig. 12–9**A**).

The starting position is supine, with the loop ladder lying beside the person. The ladder will be used to pull onto the elbow that is closest to the loops. After placing one or both forearms through the nearest loop, the person drives his elbow into the mat while pulling on the loop, lifting his upper trunk onto the elbow (Fig. 12–9**B**).

Balancing on one elbow, he removes his arm(s) from the loop and places the forearm of his free arm through the next loop. Pulling on the loop, he unweights his supporting elbow and inches it toward the foot of the bed (Fig. 12–9**C**). When he has moved as far as he can using that loop, the person moves his free arm to the next one and repeats the process. In this manner he walks his supporting elbow around, bending at the hips. This process can be continued until his torso is positioned over his legs.

Someone who routinely uses a loop ladder to come to sitting needs to plan ahead. When he gets into bed at night, he should place the loops where he will be able to reach them the following morning.

Suspended Loops. Figure 12–10**A** shows an overhead frame with loops.[7] This arrangement is far bulkier, less esthetic, and more difficult to transport than a loop ladder.

Starting in supine, the cord-injured person places a[8] distal forearm through a suspended loop (Fig. 12–10**B**). Pulling on the loop, he raises his shoulders off of the bed (Fig. 12–10**C**). He then places his free elbow on the bed, positioned well under his upper trunk so that he can balance on it (Fig. 12–10**D**).

Balancing on his elbow, the person removes his arm from the first loop and places it through the next one (Fig. 12–10**E**). He then pulls to lift his trunk higher. In doing so, he lifts his supporting elbow off the bed. While suspended from the loop, he throws his free arm back, ending in the position shown in Figure 12–10**F**. The shoulder of the supporting arm must be extended, horizontally abducted, and externally rotated. The elbow is extended fully and the forearm is supinated.

While balancing on his supporting arm, the person moves his other arm to the next loop (Fig. 12–10**G**). Pulling on the loop and throwing his head forward, he unweights his supporting arm and inches the hand forward. When he has moved his hand as far as he can, he balances on his supporting arm and moves his free arm to the next loop. These steps

---

[6] A loop ladder is a series of loops made of webbing material, sewn end to end. The size and number of loops will vary among individuals.

[7] The ideal number, length, and spacing of the loops will vary among individuals.

[8] Two arms may be used for this step.

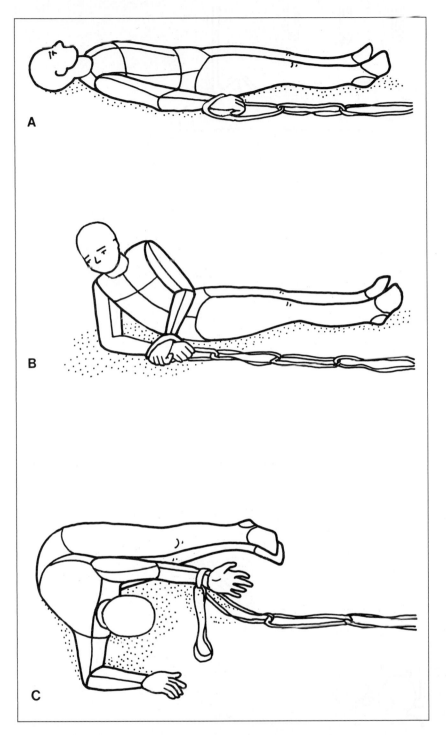

Figure 12–9. Coming to sitting using a loop ladder. **A.** Starting position. **B.** The upper trunk is lifted by pulling on the loop and driving the supporting elbow into the mat. **C.** The supporting elbow is inched toward the foot of the bed. The other arm assists by pulling on the loop ladder.

are repeated until an upright sitting posture is achieved (Fig. 12–10**H**).

Gross Mobility in Sitting
To get in and out of bed without assistance, a cord-injured person must be able to move his buttocks on the bed while in a sitting posture. This skill can also be used for limited mobility without a wheelchair. This mobility can be useful when the person finds himself on the ground, either by choice or after a fall.

Gross mobility in sitting involves pivoting on

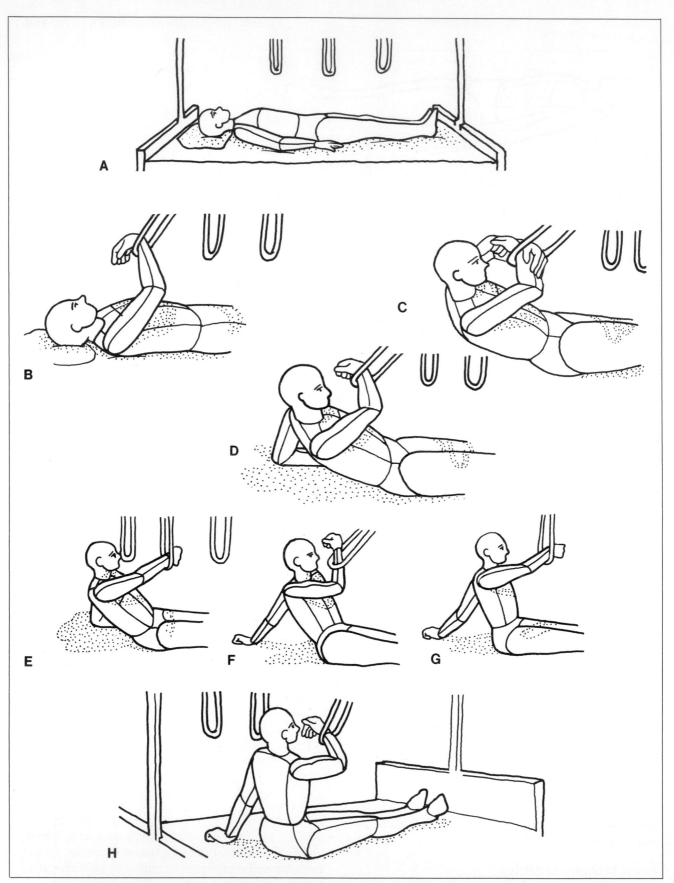

Figure 12–10. Coming to sitting using suspended loops. **A.** Starting position. **B.** One elbow placed through loop. **C.** Upper trunk lifted from bed. **D.** Elbow placed on bed. **E.** Arm placed through second loop. **F.** Trunk lifted and free arm thrown back **G.** Arm placed through third loop. **H.** Supporting hand walked forward.

Chart 12–9 Gross Mobility in Sitting, and Leg Management—Physical Prerequisites

	Gross mobility in sitting	Leg management
Strength		
Anterior deltoids	☑	√
Middle deltoids	√	√
Posterior deltoids	√	√
Biceps, brachialis, and/or brachioradialis	√	☑
Range of Motion		
Shoulder Abduction		√
External rotation	☑	
Elbow Extension	☑	√
Flexion		√
Forearm Supination	☑	√
Wrist Extension	☑	√
Combined hip flexion and knee extension	☑	☑

√: Some strength is needed for this activity, or severe limitations in range will inhibit this activity.
☑: A large amount of strength or normal or greater range is needed for this activity.

the arms. The technique is essentially the same as that used for even transfers without equipment. The cord-injured person lifts or unweights his buttocks[9] by leaning onto his arms and tucking his head. If he lacks functioning triceps, he must lock his elbows in extension.[10] If his serratus anterior is functioning, he can increase the lift of his buttocks by protracting his scapulae. While lifting, he swings his head and upper trunk away from the direction in which he wants his buttocks to move.

The physical and skill prerequisites for gross mobility in sitting are summarized in Charts 12–9 and 12–10.

---

[9] An actual lift is preferable, but unweighting will suffice if the individual is unable to lift his buttocks off the mat.

[10] Even transfers and elbow locking are addressed in Chapter 11.

Leg Management

An individual who lacks lower extremity function must position his legs passively. This skill is relatively easy; anyone who can come to sitting and move on a mat independently should be able to learn to position his legs.

Figure 12–11 illustrates the technique for positioning the legs passively. A cord-injured person maintains his sitting position by propping on one arm. He uses his other arm to move one leg at a time, pulling toward the supporting arm. By forcefully moving his head and torso away from the leg, he can add power to his pull.

Charts 12–9 and 12–10 summarize the physical and skill prerequisites for leg management on a mat or bed.

Chart 12–10 Gross Mobility in Sitting and Leg Management—Skill Prerequisites

	Gross mobility in sitting	Leg management
Sitting Skills		
Tolerate upright sitting position[a]	√	√
In long-sitting, prop forward on extended arms[b]	√	
In long-sitting, lift or unweight buttocks by leaning forward on extended arms[b]	√	
Control pelvis using head-hips relationship[b]	√	
In long-sitting, lift or unweight buttocks and move laterally[b]	√	
In long-sitting, move buttocks forward and back	√	
In long-sitting, prop to one side on one extended arm		√
Dynamic stability in long-sitting, propped to the side on one extended arm		√
Sitting propped to the side on one extended arm, use free arm to move lower extremity		√

[a] Refer to Chapter 8 for a description of this skill and therapeutic strategies.
[b] Refer to Chapter 11 for a description of this skill and therapeutic strategies.

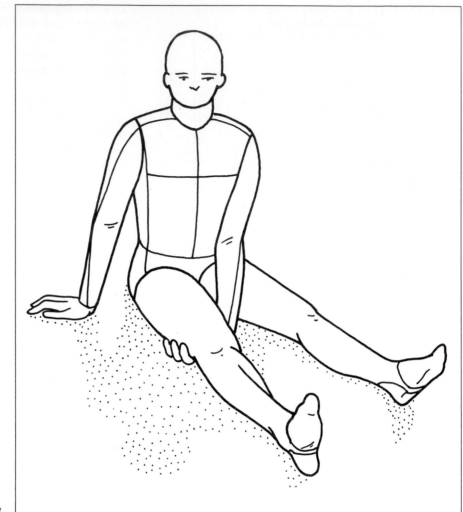

Figure 12–11. Leg management.

THERAPEUTIC STRATEGIES

General Strategies

To perform a functional mat activity, a cord-injured person must first acquire the activity's physical and skill prerequisites. The therapeutic program must work toward developing all of the necessary range, strength, and skills.

Rolling, gross mat mobility, and leg management are relatively simple activities, with few skill prerequisites. As a result, planning a functional training program to develop one of these abilities is fairly straightforward. The patient should start by developing the most basic prerequisite skills and build on these skills until he is able to perform the activity.

In contrast, each method of coming to sitting involves a fair number of steps. Many of the steps are unrelated; the skills required to perform one step are not needed to perform any other steps. As a result, decisions in functional training are less clear-cut. When working toward coming to sitting using the method that involves rolling and throwing the arms, is it best to work first on assuming prone on elbows or on balancing on one extended arm? The two steps involve different skills, and neither step is required to practice the other.

In instances in which an individual has a number of unrelated skills to master, it may be best to work on several skills concurrently. Doing so will add variety to the program. This variety may help to keep the patient's interest in the program. It also will make it possible for him to change activities when a group of muscles becomes fatigued, enabling him to work in therapy for longer periods of time by distributing the demands on his musculature.

Before asking a patient to attempt a new skill,

the therapist should explain and demonstrate the technique. The demonstration should provide a clear idea of the motions involved, as well as the timing of these motions. The therapist should also demonstrate or explain how the new skill will be used functionally.

During functional training, the therapist should remember that every cord-injured person will perform a particular activity differently. Each has a unique combination of body build, coordination, strength, and flexibility, and these characteristics influence the manner in which he performs functional tasks. What works for one patient may be a total disaster for the next. The challenge of functional training is finding the timing and maneuvers that best suit the individual involved.

Strategies for addressing the various prerequisite skills are presented below. The descriptions of skills are grouped according to the patient's position when performing the skills. In instances in which a skill involves moving from one position to another, the skill is defined by its starting position.

Supine Skills

Position Elbows In Extension. People with complete C5 or C6 quadriplegia have active elbow flexion but lack active extension. As a result, a problem that they often experience when lying supine is that they cannot straighten their elbows once they become flexed. Since these people lack functioning triceps, they need to learn an alternate method for extending their elbows. In supine, momentum is used to accomplish this task.[10]

Commonly an elbow is positioned in flexion with the shoulder internally rotated so that the forearm rests on the trunk. To extend his elbow when his arm is in this position, a patient can flex his shoulder and then slam his elbow into the mat by extending and externally rotating the shoulder abruptly. If this maneuver is done with enough force, the forearm's momentum will carry it caudally and the elbow will extend.

The elbow can also be positioned in flexion with the shoulder externally rotated. When this occurs, the elbow can be extended by internally rotating the shoulder while slamming the elbow into the mat. Alternatively, the patient can internally rotate the shoulder to position his forearm across his body and proceed from there as described above.

Many cord-injured people discover these ma-

neuvers on their own. Others require instruction and practice. Those who have difficulty learning to extend their elbows can practice the techniques starting with their elbows only slightly flexed. (Extending the elbows will be easiest from this position.) As they develop skill, they can practice from increasingly flexed positions.

Maintain Elbow Extension While Flexing Shoulders. In the absence of functioning triceps, a cord-injured person must use gravity to hold his elbows in extension when he flexes his shoulders. For gravity to hold the elbows in extension, appropriate positioning is required; the shoulders must be held in external rotation. Internal rotation of the shoulders will result in elbow flexion.

Maintaining elbow extension during shoulder flexion involves more than simply positioning the arms so that gravity extends the elbows. People who lack functioning triceps must also keep their elbow flexors relaxed while they flex their shoulders. After sustaining cervical spinal cord injuries, people often tend to combine these motions. (This may be a result of recruitment in response to a partial loss of deltoid innervation.) To use their arms functionally, these individuals must learn to isolate these motions.

Some patients learn without instruction how to maintain their elbows in extension while flexing their shoulders. However, many require instruction and practice. A therapist may assist by giving verbal and tactile cues as the patient learns to contract his anterior deltoid (and upper fibers of the pectoralis major) while keeping his biceps (and other elbow flexors) relaxed. The patient should first practice flexing his shoulders through only a few degrees of motion and progress through larger arcs as his skill increases.

Throw Arm(s) Across Body, Elbow(s) Extended. The position of the arms during this maneuver will depend upon whether or not the individual's triceps are innervated. People who lack functioning triceps must use positioning to keep their elbows from flexing while they throw their arms across their bodies in supine. The shoulders are held in external rotation and flexed only to about 45 degrees. In this position, the downward force of gravity holds the elbows in extension.

A cord-injured person who wishes to use arm motions to roll must move his arms forcefully. The therapist can help the patient get a feel for the position and force of the arm swings by assisting him through the motions. Once the patient gets a feel for the motion, he can practice on his own.

Some patients are able to throw their arms

---

[10] Muscle substitution using the anterior deltoid is not generally feasible in supine, since it requires the presence of an object on which to stabilize the hand.

across their bodies without prior instruction and do not need to practice this skill separately. These patients may proceed directly to practicing combined head and arm motions.

Combined Arm Throw and Head Swing. To practice this skill, a patient should be able to maintain his elbows in extension while throwing his arms across his body.

The patient should practice turning his head while throwing his arms across his body, turning his head in the direction of the arm throw. To build enough momentum to roll, he must perform the arm and head motions forcefully and simultaneously. The therapist can give the patient a feel for the force of the arm motions by moving him passively.

Roll Toward Prone Using Momentum. This skill can be practiced from side lying without the development of any prior skills. For practice rolling from supine, however, the patient must be able to throw his arms across his body while keeping his elbows extended, simultaneously throwing his head in the same direction.

It can be very difficult to learn to roll from supine to prone without equipment. To facilitate the acquisition of this skill, the therapist should make the task easier. One way to do so is to cross the patient's legs. During practice rolling to the left, the right leg should be crossed over the left.

Rolling is most difficult from supine and gets progressively easier as the individual approaches side lying. For this reason practice should start in side lying. The therapist should position the patient in side lying with legs crossed and instruct him to punch or reach his free arm forward. This motion will move his center of gravity forward, causing him to roll toward prone. Once the patient learns how to rotate his body in this manner, the therapist should move him to a slightly more supine position and have him practice rolling from there. As the patient's skill increases, he should practice rolling from more supine positions. Throughout the practice, forceful head and arm motions should be encouraged.

During initial practice, some cord-injured people benefit from having wrist weights placed on their arms. The added mass of the wrist weight adds to their arms' momentum, making it easier to roll. As a patient's skill increases, the weight should be removed.

The training strategies described above should be used judiciously. The patient should always start from a position as close to supine as possible and use as little weight as he can. Once he is able to roll

from supine, he should practice with his legs uncrossed.

Independent work: To practice this skill independently, the patient should be able to roll back from prone. The therapist can set up the patient for rolling practice by crossing his legs, attaching a wrist weight if needed, and placing him in an appropriate position between supine and side lying. A foam wedge or pillow(s) placed behind the patient's pelvis and lower back will keep him from rolling to a more supine position. The supports should be placed so that they do not restrict arm motions.

Position Arm to Assist In Rolling With Equipment. Before practicing this skill, a patient should be able to extend an elbow, using either triceps or momentum. If he can extend his elbow, positioning the arm to assist in rolling should take little practice.

The therapist should begin by showing the patient the appropriate arm position for rolling with equipment: the shoulder is abducted and in neutral rotation so that the antecubital fossa faces the ceiling. The forearm is supinated and stabilized under either the bedrail or the armrest of a wheelchair (Fig. 12–2).

Once shown the position, the patient should require little practice to learn this skill. An individual who lacks functioning triceps should first position his elbow in extension, then abduct his shoulder to place the arm.

Roll Toward Prone by Pulling on Equipment. Practice of this skill does not require the ability to position the arm.

The patient starts with one arm stabilized against a bedrail or wheelchair, positioned as described above. Using elbow flexion and shoulder horizontal adduction of the stabilized arm, he rolls his body toward the equipment. If he is able, he should add momentum to the roll by swinging his head and free arm toward the equipment. Toward the end of the roll he can use his free arm to assist by reaching or punching in the direction of the roll, by pulling on the equipment, or both.

As was noted in the description of rolling toward prone using momentum, rolling can be a difficult skill to master. The therapeutic strategies used to teach rolling with momentum can be used for rolling with equipment. To make the task easier, the therapist should have the patient practice initially from a side-lying position, with the legs crossed. A weight on the free arm may also be helpful during early practice. (A more complete description is supplied above.)

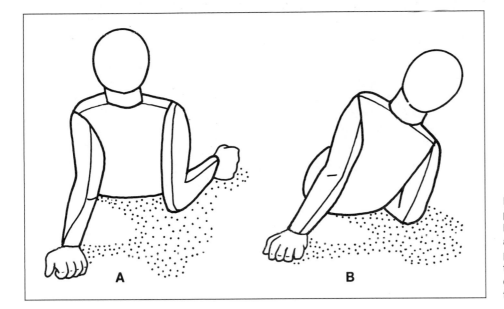

Figure 12–12. Supine, supported on one elbow and one hand. **A.** Shoulder of extended arm positioned in extreme hyperextension. **B.** Shoulder of extended arm positioned in inadequate hyperextension. Note the height of this shoulder.

Weight Shift in Supine, Supported on One Elbow and One Hand. For weight shifting in this position to be possible for someone with a complete cervical lesion, the shoulder of the extended arm[11] must be positioned in extreme hyperextension (Fig. 12–12A). If this shoulder is not in enough extension, it will be higher than the other shoulder (Fig. 12–12**B**). This disparity in shoulder height will make it impossible for the patient to shift his weight onto the higher shoulder. The amount of shoulder extension required will vary among people; an individual with greater strength and skill will not require as much range.

This is a difficult position for weight shifts, and thus it is probably best to develop skill in easier positions first. The patient should first learn to shift his weight while sitting upright, propped back on two hands. As his skill improves, he can progress to shifting weight in supine on elbows. When he is adept at shifting his weight in these positions, he will be ready to practice while propped back on one elbow and one hand.

The therapist should place the patient in position and ask him to shift his weight toward the extended arm. If he has difficulty shifting his weight, the therapist can place a hand against his shoulder and ask him to push. The patient should shift his weight only as far as he can control the motion and return to his original position. He should increase the arc as his skill develops, gradually working up to the point where he can unweight his elbow completely.

From Supine, Supported On One Elbow And One Hand, Lift Elbow. In this maneuver the cord-injured person shifts his weight and lifts the unweighted elbow. As he does so, he pivots his trunk over the shoulder of the supporting arm (Fig. 12–13).

Before practicing this skill, the patient must be able to shift his weight while sitting propped back on one elbow and one hand. The weight shift must be large enough to unweight the elbow completely. The patient also should have dynamic shoulder control in sitting, propped back on one hand.

Lifting an arm while in this position is similar to doing so while propped back on two hands or two elbows. The patient should first practice lifting an arm from the easiest position, sitting propped back on two hands. He can then develop skill in supine, supported on two elbows. Once he has learned to lift an arm from these positions, he will be ready to practice from supine, propped on one elbow and one hand. The strategies for acquiring these skills will be the same in each position.

Once an individual has developed the necessary prerequisite skills (weight shifts and dynamic shoulder control) in a given position, he can work on lifting an arm. The therapist may start by moving the patient passively to give him a feel for the motion. The patient can then practice shifting his weight and lifting his arm.

A patient who is unable to lift his arm can work on developing the skill in reverse, starting in the end position with his arm lifted. From this position he can work on lowering his free arm toward the mat and lifting it again. As he does so, he pivots his trunk on the supporting shoulder. He should move in

---

[11] The arm with the elbow in extension.

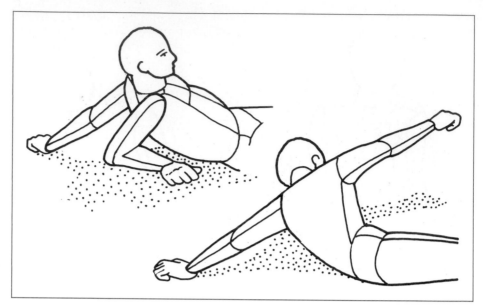

Figure 12–13. From supine on one elbow and one hand, lift elbow. Trunk pivots on supporting shoulder.

small arcs, at first, gradually building to the point where he can lower his elbow or hand to the mat under control and lift it from that position.

Independent Work: Once the patient has developed some skill in this maneuver, he can practice on his own.

Stabilize Hands In Pants. Learning to stabilize the hands in the pants is a relatively easy task. The patient simply needs to practice working his hands into the pants' front pockets or under the waist band. The pants should be made of a nonstretchy material; sweat pants will not adequately stabilize the hands. The pants must be loose enough for the patient to work his hands in without difficulty. This requirement should not present a problem; if the pants are loose enough to allow independent dressing, they should be suitable for this activity also.

With Hands Stabilized in Pants, Lift Trunk Using Elbow Flexion. During the initial practice of this skill, the therapist can stabilize the patient's distal forearms and have him lift his trunk using elbow flexion. Practice can start with the shoulders flexed, since this positioning will make the task easier. As the patient gets stronger and more skillful, the therapist can stabilize his arms in progressively lower positions. Once the patient is able to lift his trunk with his arms stabilized at his sides, he is ready to practice with his hands stabilized in his pants.

Weight Shift in Supine On Elbows. This skill involves leaning to the side while propped on two elbows in supine. The patient's elbows should be positioned medial to or even with (not lateral to) his shoulders.

During initial practice, the therapist can give the patient a feel for the motion by having him push against resistance. To do so the therapist should place a hand against one of the patient's shoulders and ask him to push against it. Once the patient has shifted slightly, he can return to upright by pushing against a hand placed on the opposite shoulder.

The patient should practice leaning to one side, then the other. He should start with small motions, shifting only as far as he is able to control the motion and return to the starting position. As his skill increases, he can increase the arcs of motion.

Supine on elbows is most stable when the cord-injured person's elbows are located directly beneath or cephalad to his shoulders. Early practice of weight shifts should be done with the elbows positioned in this manner. As the patient's skill increases, he should practice in less stable positions, with his elbows located caudal to his shoulders. If he plans to learn to come to sitting using the method in which he stabilizes his hands in his pants, he should build up to the point where he can shift his weight with his hands stabilized in his pants.

Independent Work: After being placed in supine on elbows, the patient can shift his weight to one side and then the other. He should be encouraged to shift as far as he can while maintaining control over the motion; he should shift far enough to make the activity challenging but not so far that he cannot return to upright independently.

In Supine On Elbows, Walk Elbows Back. In supine on elbows, the patient walks his elbows cephalad, moving his shoulders into greater extension. Practice of this skill requires the ability to weight shift in supine on elbows.

The patient starts in supine on elbows with his elbows medial to or even with his shoulders. From this position he weight shifts laterally to unweight one elbow. He extends his unweighted shoulder slightly, moving the elbow a short distance cephalad. He then shifts his weight onto the newly moved elbow and repeats the process with the other arm. In this manner he walks his elbows cephalad.

Walking the elbows back in supine on elbows is most difficult when the elbows are located caudally. The task becomes easier as the elbows move rostrally into more stable positions. Practice of the skill should start in a relatively easy position, with the elbows only slightly caudal to the shoulders. As a patient's skill increases, he can walk his elbows back from progressively caudal positions.

Independent Work: If placed in supine on elbows, a patient can work on his own. Frequent assistance will be needed as the patient either falls or succeeds in walking his elbows and needs to start again.

Dynamic Shoulder Control In Single Forearm-Supported Supine. Dynamic shoulder control in this position is similar to control in sitting, propped back on one hand (described in the sitting skills section below). Dynamic shoulder control is easier in the latter position, so it should be developed there first. The training strategies for the two positions are the same.

From Supine On Elbows, Lift One Elbow. In this maneuver the cord-injured person shifts his weight in supine on elbows and lifts the unweighted elbow. As he does so, he pivots his trunk over the shoulder of the supporting arm (Fig. 12–7**D**).

Before practicing this skill, a patient should have dynamic shoulder control in single forearm-supported supine. In supine on elbows, he must be able to weight shift enough to unweight one elbow completely.

Lifting an elbow from this position involves the same techniques as lifting an elbow from supine,

supported on one elbow and one hand. The training strategies for developing these skills are presented above.

From Single Forearm-Supported Supine, Throw One Arm Back. Before practicing this skill, a patient must have dynamic shoulder control in single forearm-supported supine.

Starting in single forearm-supported supine, the patient throws his free arm back to assume the position of supine supported on one elbow and one hand (Fig. 12–7**D** and **E**). The free arm must land on the palm with the elbow extended, the shoulder externally rotated and hyperextended, and the scapula adducted. For this to occur the throw must be forceful and initiated with the shoulder of the swinging arm positioned as high as possible.

Throwing an arm from this position is similar to doing so from forearm-supported side lying. The reader is referred to the discussion of the latter skill (in the side-lying skills section below) for a more detailed explanation of throwing an arm and for functional training suggestions.

Place Arm Through Loop. Before working on this skill, an individual should be able to position his elbow in extension. To practice with a hanging loop, he must be able to maintain his elbow in extension while he flexes his shoulder.

It can be difficult to place an arm through a loop that is suspended from above. During early training, the task can be made easier by placing the loop on the mat. With the loop in this position, the patient can practice grabbing it and slipping his hand through.

Once a patient has become adept at placing his arm through a loop that is lying on a mat, he can begin working with a hanging loop.[12] To place his hand through a hanging loop, the patient must first bring his hand to the loop, flexing his shoulder while maintaining his elbow in extension. He then slips his hand through the loop. Once the hand is through and the loop is around his forearm, he can internally rotate his shoulder and flex his elbow to "grasp" the loop.

Practice with a hanging loop should begin with a loop that hangs within easy reach. Once the patient becomes adept at placing his arm through the loop, he can practice with loops hung higher.

---

[12] Of course, this is only necessary if the patient plans to use hanging loops.

Independent Work: This skill is ideal for independent work. The patient can practice in therapy or in his room in the evenings.

Pulling On Loop Ladder, Move From Supine To Single Forearm-Supported Supine. In this maneuver the cord-injured person uses a loop ladder to lift his trunk and get onto an elbow (Fig. 12–9A and **B**). With one or both forearms stabilized in the nearest loop, he flexes his elbow(s) forcefully. At the same time he extends the shoulder of the arm closest to the loop, driving the elbow into the mat. With these combined motions, the patient lifts his upper trunk up and over the supporting elbow.

Lifting the trunk is most difficult at the beginning of the lift, when the patient is supine on the mat. The task becomes easier as the supporting shoulder approaches a position vertically over the supporting elbow. Practice of the skill should begin in the easier position: starting in forearm-supported supine with one or both forearms placed through a loop, the patient can practice lowering himself slightly and pulling back up. He should be encouraged to lower himself as far as he can while retaining control of the motion and the ability to return to the staring position. As his skill increases, he can move through larger arcs of motion.

Independent Work: Once a patient has developed the ability to lower and to raise his trunk slightly when positioned in single forearm-supported supine, he will be able to practice on his own.

In Single Forearm-Supported Supine, Pull On Loop Ladder and Walk Supporting Elbow Toward Feet. This skill is performed in forearm-supported supine, with the forearm of the free arm placed through a loop ladder. The upper trunk should be rotated toward the supporting arm, so that the free shoulder is higher than the supporting shoulder (Fig. 12–9**B**).

To unweight his supporting elbow, the person pulls on the loop and throws his head away from the supporting shoulder. The combined pull and head swing should be forceful and abrupt. As he pulls, the person drags his supporting elbow toward the foot of the bed. This maneuver is repeated until he has walked his elbow as far as he can with that loop.

During initial practice, the therapist can assist the patient in the motions to give him a feel for the maneuver. The therapist should emphasize that the motions need to be abrupt and forceful.

Independent Work: Once the patient is able to walk his supporting elbow toward the foot of the bed with

at least minimal success, he can practice the skill independently.

Lift Trunk By Pulling On Suspended Loop. This skill is illustrated in Figure 12–10C. If a patient has adequate strength, he should be able to master this skill with minimal practice. With his forearm(s) stabilized in a hanging loop, he simply pulls to lift his trunk. If he is unable to position an arm through the loop, the therapist can place the arm for him.

Prone Skills

Roll From Prone By Pushing With Arm. To practice this skill, a patient must be able to extend his elbow. He can do so using either triceps or muscle substitution with the anterior deltoid.[13]

Rolling from prone to supine is accomplished by pushing with one arm. To roll toward the left, a patient plants his right hand on the mat and pushes with this arm to roll.

Since rolling toward supine is most difficult from prone, practice can start in side lying. From this position a small push will rotate the body slightly toward supine. Once the patient has moved out of side lying, gravity will take over the roll.

Once a patient is able to roll to supine from side lying, he should practice rolling from a position closer to prone. The therapist can assist him to a position tilted slightly toward prone from side lying and have him roll back by pushing on the mat. As his skill improves, the patient can practice rolling from positions that are progressively closer to prone.

Independent Work: Patients can practice rolling toward side lying from semiprone positions. (A person practicing independently should not roll past side lying unless he is capable of returning from supine.) The therapist should place a pillow or bolster in front of the patient's trunk, positioned so that it supports him in semiprone without blocking his arm.

Weight Shift In Prone On Elbows. This skill involves leaning to the side while in prone on elbows. To do this a person must first be able to stabilize himself in this posture. The therapist can help him develop this ability by placing him in prone on elbows and asking him to hold the position. Applying resistance to the patient's shoulders in various directions while

---

[13] The prerequisite skill of extending the elbow using muscle substitution is covered in Chapter 11.

he holds his posture can help him develop his stability.

Once he has developed the ability to stabilize in prone on elbows, the patient will be ready to practice shifting his weight in this posture. During early weight-shifting practice, the therapist can give him a feel for the motion by having him push against resistance. To do so the therapist should place a hand against one of the patient's shoulders and ask him to push against it. Once the patient has shifted slightly, he can return to upright by pushing against a hand placed on the opposite shoulder.

The patient should practice leaning to one side, then the other. He should start with small motions, shifting only as far as he is able to control the motion and return to the starting position. As his skill increases, he can increase the arcs of motion.

During early practice of this skill, the elbows should be located directly beneath the shoulders. Weight shifts are easiest to control in this position. As a patient's skill increases, he should practice in less stable positions, with his elbows located rostral or caudal to his shoulders.

Independent Work: After being placed in prone on elbows, a patient can shift his weight to one side and then the other. He should be encouraged to shift as far as he can while maintaining control over the motion; he should shift far enough to make the activity challenging but not so far that he cannot return to upright independently.

Walk Elbows In From Abducted Position. This skill is illustrated in Figure 12–3. To practice, a patient must be able to weight shift in prone on elbows.

Walking the elbows in from an abducted position is most difficult at the beginning of the task, when the cord injured person is prone on the mat. The task becomes easier as the arms become more vertical, approaching the stable prone on elbows position. Practice of this skill should start from this easier position.

To practice this skill, the patient starts in prone on elbows with his elbows directly under his shoulders. From this position, he weight shifts laterally to unweight one elbow. He moves the unweighted elbow a short distance laterally and shifts his weight back onto it. He should then shift the weight off again and move the elbow back in, returning to the starting position. Moving the elbow back in involves a combined motion of shoulder shrug and horizontal adduction. The therapist can help the patient learn this motion with verbal cueing and by providing resistance at the shoulder and arm.

When the patient has developed the capacity to move an elbow out and back in, he can progress to moving one elbow a short distance laterally, shifting onto it, and moving the other elbow out. He then reverses the steps, walking the elbows back in.

Walking the elbows out from prone on elbows is relatively easy; bringing them back in is the difficult task. While practicing, it can be tempting for the patient to walk his elbows out too far, reaching a position from which he is unable to return without assistance. The therapist should encourage the patient to walk his elbows out only as far as he can control the motion and return without assistance.

As his skill develops, the patient should walk his elbows out and back over increasing distances. In this manner he can build up to the point where he can walk his elbows all the way out laterally and back in. At this point he will be able to assume prone on elbows from prone.

Independent Work: Once an individual has developed the ability to walk his elbows short distances from and return to prone on elbows, he can work on the skill independently.

Walk Elbows Forward From Adducted Position. This skill is illustrated in Figure 12–4. Before practicing, a patient must be able to weight shift in prone on elbows.

This skill can be developed in the same manner as the skill of walking the elbows in from an abducted position: from a starting position of prone on elbows with the elbows directly under his shoulders, the patient practices walking his elbows back toward his pelvis and returning to the starting position.[14] As his skill develops, he walks his elbows through increasing distances. In this manner he gradually builds to the point where he is able to walk his elbows back until he is prone on the mat and from that position can walk them forward to return to prone on elbows.

Move From Prone On Elbows To Forearm-Supported Side Lying. This maneuver is illustrated in Figure 12–14. To practice, the patient must be able to weight shift in prone on elbows and should have some dynamic shoulder control in side lying with forearm support. In the absence of functioning triceps, he must also be able to extend one elbow using his anterior deltoid.

---

[14] Refer to the section on assuming prone on elbows from an abducted position for more explicit functional training suggestions.

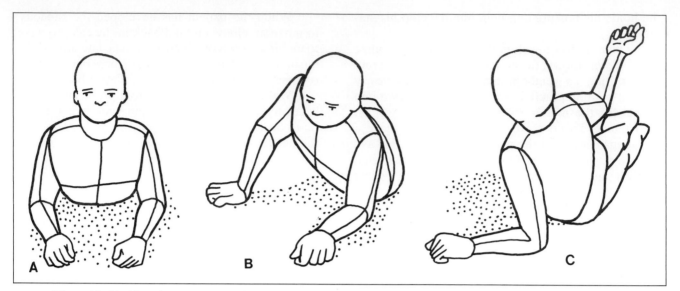

Figure 12–14. Move from prone on elbows to forearm-supported side lying (*Viewed from cephalad*). **A.** Prone on elbows. **B.** Weight shifted and hand planted. Trunk rotates over shoulder of supporting arm. **C.** Supporting shoulder has moved from horizontal adduction to horizontal abduction.

In prone on elbows, the person shifts his weight to one side and plants the hand of his unweighted arm on the mat (Fig. 12–14**B**). He then pushes to rotate his body up and over the supporting arm, ending in the position of side lying with forearm support.

The motions of the supporting shoulder are critical to this maneuver. As the patient pushes his torso up and over his arm, the supporting shoulder moves from a position of horizontal adduction to horizontal abduction (Fig. 12–14**A**–**C**).

Until the patient has developed some skill in this maneuver, he will need assistance to work on it. The therapist can start by demonstrating and passively moving the patient through the maneuver to give him an idea of the motions involved. The therapist can then assist him into a position of side lying with forearm support, with the "free" hand stabilized against the mat. From this position the patient can practice rotating his trunk toward prone and back up (Fig. 12–15). The power for this motion will come primarily from the "free" arm pushing on the mat. The patient's motions should be small enough that they remain under his control, yet large enough to be a challenge. As his skill increases, he can increase his arcs of motion.

This skill is easiest when the trunk and lower extremities are in a line, with the hips in approximately neutral extension. The hips remain in this position while a cord-injured person comes to sitting by rolling and throwing his arms (Fig. 12–6). The maneuver is more difficult when the trunk and lower

extremities are angled, as when coming to sitting by walking on the elbows (Fig. 12–8). Initial practice should be done in the easier position, with the trunk and lower extremities in a line.

Independent Work: Once a patient has developed some skill in this maneuver, he can practice on his own.

In Prone On Elbows, Walk Elbows to the Side. Before practicing this skill, the patient must be able to weight shift well in prone on elbows.

From prone on elbows, the person unweights one elbow by leaning laterally. He moves his unweighted elbow medially a short distance and shifts onto it to unweight the other elbow. He can then move the newly-unweighted elbow laterally. By performing this sequence repeatedly, he walks his elbows to the side.

While practicing walking on his elbows in prone, the patient must make sure that he does not move his elbows too far apart.[15] If he positions his elbows too far apart, he will be unable to shift his weight enough to unweight either elbow. As a result, he will not be able to progress from this position without assistance.

To ensure that his elbows remain close enough together, the patient can make a habit of moving

---

[15] The distance that is "too far" will depend upon the individual's strength and skill.

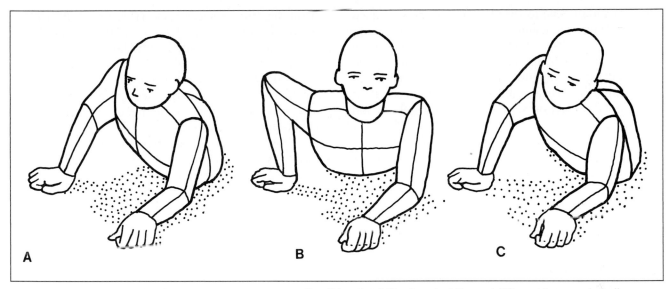

Figure 12–15. In side lying with forearm support, "free" hand stabilized against the mat (*Viewed from cephalad*). **A.** Starting position. **B.** Trunk rotates toward prone. **C.** Return to starting position.

one elbow medially before moving the other one laterally. He should also take small enough "steps" with the laterally-moving elbow.

Side-Lying Skills

Move From Side Lying to Prone On Elbows. This skill is illustrated in Figure 12–16. Before practicing, a patient must be able to weight shift in prone on elbows.

When performing this skill, a patient starts in side lying, lying on a shoulder that is flexed to approximately 90 degrees. He stabilizes the hand of this arm on his chin, forehead, or the side of his head. Pivoting on the strut that is thus formed, he uses forceful shoulder horizontal abduction to push his trunk up and over the supporting arm. Toward the end of the maneuver, he can use neck flexion to augment the lift.

This skill is most difficult at the beginning, when the patient lifts his trunk from the mat. It becomes easier as the trunk is lifted higher and the supporting arm becomes more vertical. Practice should start where the task is easiest: in prone on elbows, with one hand stabilized on the chin, forehead, or side of the head. From this position the

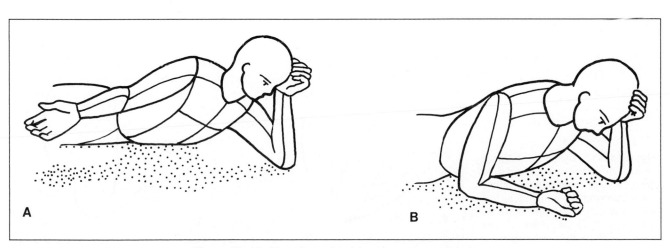

Figure 12–16. Move from side lying to prone on elbows.

patient should lean toward the side of the stabilized (supporting) arm, leaning as far as he can under control. He then lifts his body back over the supporting arm. To do this he uses horizontal abduction of the shoulder of the supporting arm. Since the elbow of the supporting arm is stabilized on the mat, shoulder horizontal abduction serves to lift the trunk up and over the arm.

As the patient's skill increases, he can move through larger arcs of motion. As he leans further from vertical, it will become more difficult to return to upright. He may need to use momentum to augment the supporting arm's push. To utilize momentum, he should swing his free arm forward as he pushes his supporting arm into the mat (Fig. 12–16A).

The patient should practice leaning and lifting through larger arcs of motion. In this manner he can gradually progress to the point where he can lean far enough to touch a shoulder to the mat and return to prone on elbows.

Independent Work: Once a patient has developed the ability to lean slightly from and return to prone on elbows, he can work on the skill independently.

Dynamic Shoulder Control in Forearm-Supported Side Lying. In forearm-supported side lying, the patient maintains his balance while moving the supporting shoulder forward and back. To keep the trunk balanced over the supporting elbow, the patient rotates his trunk in the direction opposite the supporting shoulder's movements; as the shoulder moves for-

ward, his trunk rotates back. (Fig. 12–17 illustrates the motions involved.) Motions of the free arm and head can be used to augment balance.

During initial practice, the therapist can assist the patient into forearm-supported side lying and ask him to maintain the position. At first the patient may just use motions of his head and free arm to maintain his balance.

Once the patient has developed some skill in balancing in forearm-supported side lying, he can practice moving his supporting shoulder forward and back through small arcs of motion. The therapist may first move the patient passively to give him a feel for the motion involved. The patient should then perform the motions with assistance and spotting.

As the patient's skill develops, he can increase the motions of his shoulder until he is able to move through large arcs. He should always practice moving through an arc that is large enough to be a challenge but small enough to be controlled.

The patient should also practice abducting the scapula of his supporting shoulder when this shoulder is positioned directly over the elbow. This scapular motion raises the trunk, increasing the distance between the free shoulder and the mat. This skill is important in coming to sitting using the method that involves rolling and throwing the arms.

Independent Work: Once the patient is able to balance in forearm-supported side lying while moving his supporting shoulder through small arcs, he should be able to practice independently.

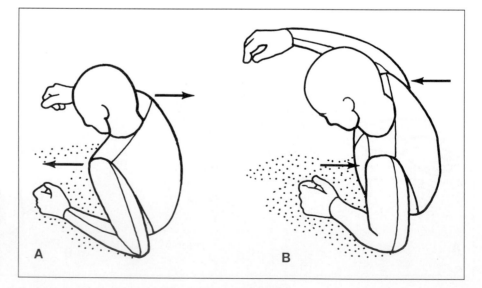

Figure 12–17. Dynamic shoulder control in forearm-supported side lying (*Viewed from behind*). **A.** As the supporting shoulder moves forward, the trunk rotates back. **B.** As the supporting shoulder moves back, the trunk rotates forward.

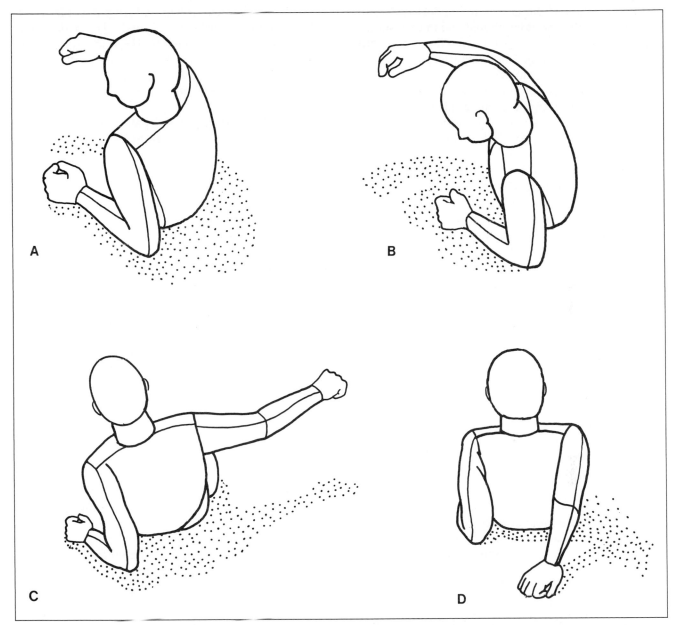

Figure 12–18. From forearm-supported side lying, throw free arm back (*Viewed from behind*). **A.** Forearm-supported side lying. **B.** Ready position to throw: shoulders perpendicular to mat, scapula of supporting arm abducted. **C.** Half-way through throw. Trunk is pivoting on supporting shoulder. **D.** End position.

From Forearm-Supported Side Lying, Throw Free Arm Back. This maneuver is illustrated in Figure 12–18. Dynamic shoulder control in forearm-supported side lying is required for practicing this skill.

Starting in forearm-supported side lying, the cord-injured person throws his free arm back to assume the position of supine supported on one elbow and one hand. As he throws his arm, his center of gravity moves from over his base of support, and he falls in the direction of the swinging arm. The palm must land with the arm positioned so that it can accept weight and catch the falling trunk. The final position of the swinging shoulder is key. When the hand hits the mat, the shoulder must be positioned in extreme horizontal abduction; the hand must land medial to the shoulder. If it lands in a position that is too lateral, the arm will not support the trunk. The elbow will flex, causing the person to fall to the mat.

The thrown arm must land with the hand medial

to the shoulder if the arm is to support the trunk. In addition, the shoulder should end in extreme extension. This hyperextension is required for a cord-injured person lacking functional triceps to come to sitting from this position.

Three factors combine to make it possible for the arm to land with the shoulder positioned appropriately: starting position of the shoulders, velocity of the swinging arm, and direction of the arm's motion.

When the arm throw is initiated, the shoulder of the thrown arm should be as high as possible. Specifically, the shoulders should be aligned perpendicular to the mat (Fig. 12–18**B**), and the scapula of the supporting arm should be abducted. Then as the patient's center of gravity shifts and the trunk falls, the shoulder will fall from as high a position as possible. The further it has to fall, the longer the fall will take. A longer fall will allow the free arm to swing further, so the shoulder can end in extreme horizontal abduction.

The swinging arm will also be able to move further if it is thrown forcefully. An arm that travels at a high velocity will travel further as the trunk falls and as a result will land in a better position.

The patient should throw his arm in the direction of shoulder horizontal abduction rather than extension. If the arm is thrown forcefully in the direction of horizontal abduction, momentum will carry it toward the body's midline at the end of the throw.

The motion of the supporting shoulder is also key to the successful performance of this maneuver. As the patient swings his arm into position, he must pivot his trunk on the supporting shoulder (Fig. 12–18**C**). This pivot will make it possible for the shoulders to end in a stable position when the swing is completed (Fig. 12–18**D**).

It can be quite difficult for a patient to learn to throw an arm back while balancing on the other elbow. For this reason it is advisable to practice first in an easier position. Throwing an arm back while sitting, propped back on one extended arm, is similar to throwing it from forearm-supported side lying. Similar initial positioning and motions are involved, but the more upright posture makes the arm throw easier in sitting. By developing this skill in sitting, a patient can prepare himself for practice in forearm-supported side lying.

Once the patient has some skill throwing an arm in sitting, he can practice from forearm-supported side lying. During early practice the therapist can place the patient in position, with his free shoulder high. By moving the patient's trunk and free arm passively, the therapist can demonstrate how the

supporting shoulder collapses forward as the trunk falls and the free arm swings back. The patient can then practice the technique. He is likely to have many failed attempts as he learns the skill. Verbal feedback from the therapist at this point can help him perfect his technique.

Independent Work: Once a patient has developed some ability in this maneuver, he can practice alone. He is likely to need frequent assistance at first, as he will fall periodically.

In 90-Degree Forearm-Supported Side Lying, Walk Supporting Elbow Toward Legs. Before practicing this skill, a patient must be able to weight shift in prone on elbows. He should also be able to walk his elbows to the side in prone on elbows.

From a position of forearm-supported side lying with the hips flexed to approximately 90 degrees, the patient lifts his unweighted arm and hooks it behind his legs, placing his forearm behind the knees or thighs (Fig. 12–8**E**). Once his arm is stabilized in this manner, the patient is ready to pull his torso toward his legs. To do so, he repeatedly pulls on his legs while throwing his head toward the legs. The combined pull and head swing should be forceful and abrupt, to gain maximal momentum. With each pull, the patient drags his supporting elbow further toward his legs. This step is repeated until the torso has reached the desired position. (The torso's target position will depend on the method that will be used to move the trunk into an upright position.)

During initial practice, the therapist can assist the patient with the motion to give him a feel for the maneuver. The therapist should emphasize that the motions need to be abrupt and forceful. The patient should progress quickly to practicing without assistance.

Independent Work: Once an individual is able to walk his supporting elbow toward his trunk with at least minimal success, he can practice the skill independently.

From Forearm-Supported Side Lying, Push/Pull into Sitting Position. Before practicing this skill, a patient must be able to extend one elbow, using either his triceps or muscle substitution.

This maneuver begins with the person propped on one elbow in side lying with his hips flexed beyond 90 degrees (Fig. 12–8**F**). The other arm is hooked behind his knees or thighs.

The patient pulls on his legs to unweight the supporting elbow. He then internally rotates the shoulder of the supporting arm, stabilizing his palm on the mat. The shoulder should be internally rotated enough that the elbow points toward the ceiling (Fig. 12–8G). Once his hand is planted on the mat, he extends his elbow to push his torso up and over his legs. At the same time he pulls with the other arm. He can also throw his head toward his legs, using momentum to assist in the motion.

The most difficult part of this maneuver is the beginning, when the person starts pushing and pulling to move his trunk. As the trunk moves up and over the legs, the task becomes easier.

Functional training should begin in the end position, where the skill is easiest. Practice should start with the patient sitting, propped to the side on an arm with its elbow extended. The other arm should be hooked around his legs (Fig. 12–19A). From this position the patient practices lowering his trunk to the side and returning to sitting. He should start with small motions, lowering his trunk slightly and pushing/pulling back up (Fig. 12–19B and C). He can lower his trunk further as his skill increases, gradually building to the point where he can raise his trunk from forearm-supported side lying. During practice, the motions should be small enough that the patient is able to retain control yet large enough to be a challenge.

Independent Work: Once the patient has developed the ability to lean slightly from and return to sitting, he can practice this skill independently.

Sitting Skills

Dynamic Shoulder Control In Sitting, Propped Back on One Hand. A cord-injured person performing this activity sits, propped on one extended arm, and pivots his trunk on the supporting shoulder. He must maintain his balance while moving the supporting shoulder forward and back. To keep his trunk balanced over his base of support, he pivots his trunk in the direction opposite the supporting shoulder's movements: as the shoulder moves forward, his trunk rotates back. (Fig. 12–20 illustrates the motions involved.) Motions of the free arm and head are used to augment balance.

The first step in developing this skill is learning to balance while sitting, propped back on one hand. The therapist can assist the patient into position and ask him to maintain the position. The patient uses his head and free arm to balance, using them to keep his center of gravity over his base of support: when he starts to fall in one direction, he moves his head and arm in the opposite direction.

Once the patient is able to maintain his balance in this position, he is ready to practice dynamic shoulder control. He should start by moving his shoulder forward and back through small arcs of motion. The therapist may first move him passively to give him a feel for the motion involved. The patient should then perform the motions with assistance and spotting.

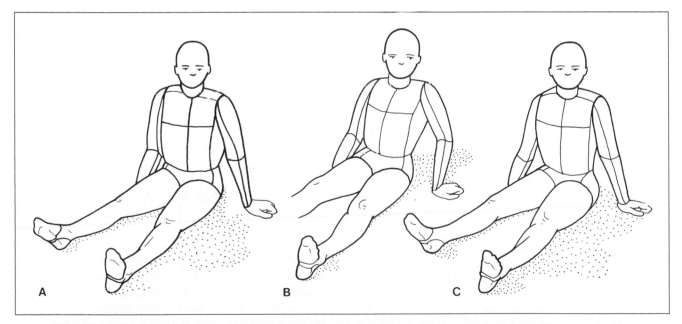

Figure 12–19. In long-sitting, practice lowering the trunk to the side. **A.** Starting position: long-sitting, propped to the side on one arm, other arm hooked around legs. **B.** The patient lowers trunk to the side. **C.** Push/pull back to starting position.

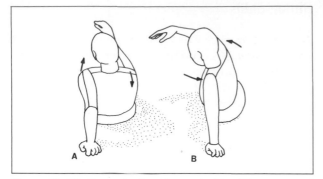

Figure 12–20. Dynamic shoulder control in sitting, propped back on one hand (*Viewed from behind*). **A.** As the supporting shoulder moves forward, the trunk rotates back. **B.** As the supporting shoulder moves back, the trunk rotates forward.

As the patient's skill develops, he can increase the forward and back motions of his supporting shoulder until he is able to move through large arcs. He should always practice moving through an arc that is large enough to be a challenge but small enough for him to control.

The patient should also practice abducting the scapula of his supporting shoulder when his trunk is rotated to a position vertically over this shoulder. This scapular abduction raises the trunk, increasing the distance between the free shoulder and the mat. This skill is important in the technique of coming to sitting, which involves rolling and throwing the arms.

Dynamic shoulder control is most difficult when the supporting shoulder is positioned in extreme hyperextension. Control should be developed first in easier positions with the trunk relatively upright.

Independent Work: Once a patient is able to balance while moving his supporting shoulder through small arcs, he should be able to practice independently.

From Sitting Propped Back On One Hand, Throw Free Arm Back. To practice this skill, a patient must have balance and dynamic shoulder control in this position. He should also have good shoulder range of motion, without any limitation of extension or horizontal abduction.

While sitting propped back on one hand, the patient throws his free arm back. As the arm moves, the trunk pivots on the supporting shoulder and moves past the balance point, falling toward the moving arm. When the hand lands, the swinging arm needs to be positioned so that it can accept weight: palm against the mat medial to the shoulder with the elbow extended, the shoulder externally rotated and hyperextended, and the scapula adducted.

If the hand lands before the upper extremity reaches a stable position, the elbow will flex, and the patient will fall to the mat. To increase the likelihood of success, the throw should be forceful and initiated with the shoulder of the swinging arm as high as possible. A more thorough explanation is given above, in the section entitled "From Forearm-Supported Side Lying, Throw Free Arm Back."

During early practice, the therapist can move the patient's trunk and free arm passively. While doing so the therapist can demonstrate how the supporting shoulder collapses forward as the trunk falls and the free arm swings back. The patient can then practice the technique. He is likely to have many failed attempts as he learns the skill. Verbal feedback from the therapist at this point can help him perfect his technique.

Independent Work: Once a patient has developed some ability in this maneuver, he can practice alone. He is likely to need frequent assistance at first.

Weight Shift While Sitting, Propped Back on Two Hands. Before practicing this skill, a patient must be able to tolerate an upright sitting position. It is not necessary to be able to extend the elbows, since they are placed in a position of passive locking.

In this activity the patient shifts his weight laterally while sitting, propped back on two locked arms. During early training the therapist can place the patient in position and ask him to shift to the side. He should shift a short distance, return to upright, and shift in the opposite direction. The therapist may assist the weight shifts by placing a hand against the patient's shoulder and having him push against it.

Independent Work: Once the patient can shift his weight to the right and left through small arcs, he can work independently. As his skill improves, he can increase the distance of his weight shifts. He should work in a range that is challenging, yet within his capabilities.

From Sitting Propped Back on Two Hands, Walk Hands Forward. A patient must be able to tolerate an upright sitting position to practice this skill and must be able to weight shift in this position.

To perform this maneuver, the cord-injured person shifts his weight laterally and moves his unweighted hand forward slightly by elevating and protracting the scapula. He then shifts his weight in the opposite direction and moves the other hand. By repeating these steps, he walks his hands forward toward his buttocks.

The hands must move over short distances and should move straight forward. If a hand is moved too far forward, the trunk can tilt excessively onto the other arm. This makes it difficult to weight shift in the opposite direction. If the person moves his hand laterally instead of forward, this arm will not be in a stable position for accepting weight.

During early practice, the therapist should instruct the patient to lean to one side, then shrug the unweighted shoulder up and forward. If the patient has difficulty moving the unweighted upper extremity, he can add power to the attempt by throwing his head forward and toward the supporting arm.

Independent Work. Once a patient can perform this skill with some success, he can practice independently. As an advanced activity for independent work, the patient can walk his hands forward until he reaches an upright sitting position, balance briefly in sitting, throw his arms back, catch himself on his hands, and walk his hands forward again.

With One Arm Through Overhead Loop, Throw Free Arm Back. To practice this skill, a patient must be able to tolerate an upright sitting posture.

The endpoint of this maneuver is illustrated in Figure 12–10F. The patient starts in a semireclined position, supporting his trunk with a forearm hooked through a loop that is hanging from overhead. He throws his free arm back, landing with his palm located medial to his shoulder. The thrown arm must land in a position that will enable it to accept weight: elbow extended, shoulder externally rotated and hyperextended, and scapula adducted. To ensure that the arm ends in a proper position, it should be thrown forcefully and in the direction of shoulder horizontal abduction rather than extension.

A patient holding an overhead loop is in a stable position; he does not need to concern himself with maintaining his center of gravity over his base of support. For this reason, throwing an arm while hanging from an overhead loop is not as difficult as doing so while propped on an elbow or hand. Practice should emphasize the force and direction of the throw.

In Sitting, Propped Back on One Hand, Pull On Suspended Loop And Walk Supporting Hand Forward. A patient must be able to tolerate an upright sitting posture to practice this skill.

To perform this skill, the patient sits in a semireclined posture with one forearm placed through a suspended loop. The other arm is in a locked po-

sition behind him, supporting his trunk (Fig. 12–10G).

The patient must unweight his supporting arm to walk the hand forward. To do so, he pulls forcefully on the loop and throws his head forward. At the same time he moves his supporting hand forward toward his buttocks. This maneuver is repeated until the patient has walked his hand as far as he can with that loop.

During initial practice, the therapist can assist the patient with the motions to give him a feel for the maneuver. The therapist should emphasize that the motions need to be abrupt and forceful.

Independent Work: Once the patient is able to walk his supporting hand forward with at least minimal success, he can practice the skill independently.

In Long-Sitting, Move Buttocks Forward and Back. To perform this skill, a patient must be able to tolerate an upright sitting position, propping on his arms with his elbows extended.

The head-hips relationship is used in these maneuvers. To move his buttocks forward, the cord-injured person starts in long-sitting, propped forward on his arms. He then pushes into the mat to lift or unweight his buttocks and throws his head back forcefully. To move his buttocks back, he starts with his arms behind and slightly lateral to his buttocks. From this position he pushes into the mat while throwing his head forward forcefully.

During early practice the therapist can help the patient get a feel for the maneuvers by assisting him with the motions. Once the patient has a feel for the motion, he can practice on his own.

In Long-Sitting, Prop to the Side on One Extended Arm. A patient must be able to tolerate upright sitting before practicing this skill. In the absence of functioning triceps, he must be able to lock his elbows.

During early practice, the therapist can assist the patient into position and ask him to help hold the elbow straight. As the patient's ability to support himself improves, the therapist's support is reduced.

Once the patient is able to support his trunk's weight on his arm, he can practice balancing on that arm. The therapist should assist him into position and ask him to stay upright. The patient balances using his head and free arm: when his trunk starts to fall, he moves his head and free arm in the direction opposite the fall.

The patient can work on his balance with spotting at first. To prepare for more advanced activities, he can practice holding the position as the therapist pushes his shoulders in various directions.

Dynamic Stability in Long-Sitting, Propped to the Side on One Extended Arm. To practice this skill, a patient must be able to tolerate upright sitting and prop to the side on one arm with the elbow extended.

While propping to the side in long-sitting, the patient practices maintaining his balance while he rotates his trunk, shifts it laterally, and moves his head and free arm in various directions.

Independent Work: The activities described above can be performed alone, long-sitting on a mat. The patient should be far enough from the mat's edge to allow him to fall safely.

Sitting Propped to the Side on One Extended Arm, Use Free Arm to Move Lower Extremity. Before practicing this skill, a patient must have dynamic stability in long-sitting while propped to the side on one extended arm.

When positioning his legs in long-sitting, the patient moves one lower extremity at a time. He props to the side on one arm, leaning in the direction toward which he plans to move his leg. He pulls the leg using his free arm, at the same time moving his head and torso forcefully in the direction of the pull.

The therapist should emphasize the coordination of the head and trunk motions with the pull. The motions' force should also be emphasized. During early practice, the therapist can assist the patient with the maneuver to give him a feel for the motions involved.

Independent Work: Once the patient can move a leg with at least minimal success, he can practice the skill independently.

PROGRAM DESIGN

When using this text as a resource to assist in working toward a functional goal, the therapist should first read the text's description of that functional activity. Based on that description, the corresponding charts, or both, the therapist can determine what physical and skill prerequisites are required to perform the skill. Taking into consideration the patient's evaluation results, the therapist can determine where the patient has deficits relevant to the functional goal. The program should then be designed to address these deficits, developing the needed physical and skill prerequisites.

Many strategies are available for increasing

strength and range of motion; the field of physical therapy has a variety of approaches for accomplishing these ends. The program may include any combination of the following: proprioceptive neuromuscular facilitation, progressive resistive exercises (concentric and eccentric), strengthening through functional tasks, isokinetic exercise, prolonged stretching, and electrical stimulation. Strengthening and stretching will also occur with increased activity. The patient can exercise independently, in groups, and one on one with the therapist.

This chapter presents functional training strategies for each prerequisite skill. The therapist can use these suggestions, coupled with his own imagination, clinical expertise, and problem solving, to design a functional training program. The program should aim first at developing the most basic prerequisite skills and build to more advanced skills as the patient's abilities develop.

In most cases a patient will have many functional goals. The therapeutic program must progress him toward all of these goals. Fortunately there is much overlap of prerequisites between skills. Thus a person working on rolling from supine is potentially progressing toward independence in rolling, assuming prone on elbows, and coming to sitting without equipment. Furthermore, work aimed at developing one ability can benefit other, seemingly unrelated, activities. For example, the strengthening and motor learning that results from practicing mat skills may benefit a patient's transfers or basic wheelchair skills.

Example: Coming to Sitting Without Equipment by Walking on Elbows. To assume a sitting posture using this method, a cord-injured person needs adequate strength in his deltoids, elbow flexors, and shoulder internal rotators. He must also possess adequate range in elbow flexion and shoulder flexion, abduction, internal rotation, and horizontal abduction. He must be able to assume a prone on elbows posture, weight shift and walk his elbows to the side in this position, move into forearm-supported side lying, walk his supporting elbow toward his legs in this position, push-pull into a sitting position, push with his arms to lift his trunk from a forward lean in sitting, and tolerate an upright sitting posture. If he lacks innervated triceps, he must be able to extend his elbows using muscle substitution.

An individual's program design will depend on his unique needs. If he has any deficits in prerequisite strength or range, the program should include exercises to address these deficits. Most patients benefit from hamstring stretching and strengthening of all innervated upper extremity musculature, with emphasis on muscles used in elbow extension and shoulder flexion and horizontal adduction.

If the patient has none of the needed skill prerequisites, functional training should start with the most basic skills: ability to extend the elbows using muscle substitution (if the triceps are not innervated), tolerate an upright sitting position, and weight shift in prone on elbows once placed in that posture. When he has developed these abilities, he can work on more challenging skills, such as walking the elbows to the side in prone on elbows, moving from this position to forearm-supported side lying, and lifting his trunk from a forward lean in sitting. As his strength and motor control develop, he can work on walking his elbow in forearm-supported side lying and moving from this position to a sitting posture. As prerequisite skills are mas-

tered, they can be practiced in combination. By building his skill in this manner, the patient progresses to independence in coming to sitting without equipment by walking on his elbows.

SUGGESTED READINGS

For additional information on functional mat techniques used by people with spinal cord injuries, the reader is referred to the following books:

Ford, J. & Duckworth, B. (1987). *Physical Management for the Quadriplegic Patient* (2nd ed.). Philadelphia: F. A. Davis.

Nixon, V. (1985). *Spinal Cord Injury: A Guide to Functional Outcomes in Physical Therapy Management.* Rockville, MD: Aspen.

13

Wheelchair Skills

Most people with spinal cord injuries use wheelchairs as their sole means of locomotion. This is true even for those who learn to walk with knee-ankle-foot orthoses (KAFOs) and assistive devices during their rehabilitation (Heinemann, Magiera-Planey, Schiro-Geist, & Gimines (1987). If ambulation is impaired, a wheelchair provides a faster and more energy-efficient means of mobility than does walking. Even people who have such low lesions that they retain active hip flexion and knee extension and are able to walk with ankle-foot orthoses (AFOs) and assistive devices find wheelchair mobility to be faster and to require less energy than walking (Waters & Lunsford, 1985). Thus almost all people who sustain spinal cord injuries should develop wheelchair skills during their rehabilitation.

Someone who uses a wheelchair for mobility must possess a variety of skills to function independently. These skills include propulsion of the wheelchair over even surfaces and negotiation of obstacles, as well as the more basic skills of pressure reliefs, positioning one's trunk and buttocks within the wheelchair, and handling the chair's parts. Chapter 11 addresses the skills required for positioning and the management of wheelchair parts.

Wheelchair skills can provide freedom and mobility. In addition, independent wheelchair propulsion can be good exercise, resulting in cardiovascular conditioning and muscle strengthening. The increased strength gained through manual wheelchair propulsion can benefit other areas of function, such as transfers and mat skills.

This chapter presents a variety of wheelchair skills,[1] as well as suggestions on how to teach them. The descriptions of techniques and training presented here should be used as a guide, not as a set of hard-and-fast rules. The motions used to perform any functional task vary among people. This variability is due to differences in body build, skill level, range of motion, muscle tone, and patterns of strength and weakness. During functional training, the therapist and patient should work together to find the exact techniques that best suit that particular patient.

PRACTICE IN DEPARTMENT AND "REAL WORLD"

The physical therapy department in a rehabilitation center should be equipped with curbs of varying heights, stairs, and a ramp. This equipment is useful for initial practice of obstacle negotiation. However, practice should not end with mastery of these artificial obstacles. Many obstacles that a wheelchair user will encounter outside of the department will be more difficult to negotiate. For example, ascending a cement curb from a street is likely to be more difficult than ascending a wooden curb from a linoleum floor. The "real world" is full of uneven sidewalks, long and steep staircases, heavy doors, elevators that snap shut with a death grip, and uneven surfaces such as grass and sand. Functional training should include practicing wheelchair skills outside of the department so that the individual will be better prepared to function in the "real world" after rehabilitation.

EQUIPMENT

Improper fit or adjustment of a wheelchair can contribute to the development of postural abnormalities and pressure ulcers and can limit a person's ability to propel his chair and negotiate obstacles. For this reason a properly fit and adjusted wheelchair should be provided as soon as the cord-injured person begins out-of-bed activities.

A variety of options are available when selecting wheelchairs. The therapist and prospective

---

[1] This chapter does not attempt to present all possible wheelchair skills. An individual who is unable to master a skill described in this chapter may fare better with a variation of that technique or an altogether different method.

wheelchair user have numerous choices to make when selecting a chair, ranging from armrest style to power versus manual propulsion. In fact, even the seemingly minor details can be important; a wheelchair's components can have a significant impact on functional ability. Thus wheelchair selection should be a matter of careful consideration.[2]

SITTING POSTURE

Following spinal cord injury, mild tightness in the lower back will make independent transfers easier. A patient whose low back has been overstretched is likely to have difficulty lifting his buttocks for a transfer: when he pivots forward on his arms, his back will lengthen and his buttocks will not lift as high.

Poor sitting posture is a prime source of overstretched low backs. A cord-injured person who habitually sits with his buttocks forward on the wheelchair seat is likely to stretch his lumbar area (Fig. 13–1A). Sitting with the buttocks well back on the seat will help to protect the low back (Fig. 13–1B).

It can be tempting for a therapist to place a patient in a poor sitting posture, especially if the

---

[2] Chapter 19 addresses wheelchair fit, adjustment, options, and selection in greater depth.

individual has a high lesion and has not yet developed the ability to maintain an upright sitting posture. By pulling the patient's buttocks out (forward) in the seat, the therapist places him in a more stable position and enables him to stay upright more easily. Although this practice may seem to be sensible in the short run, it is likely to damage the patient's back. In addition, it can encourage the habit of sitting with poor posture. To preserve lower back tightness, the therapist and patient should work together to develop the patient's ability to sit (and habit of sitting) upright with his buttocks well back on the seat.

PHYSICAL AND SKILL PREREQUISITES

Each method of performing a functional activity involves a particular set of skills. Each activity also has strength, joint range of motion, and muscle flexibility requirements. A deficiency in any of these skills or physical requirements will impair a person's performance of the activity.

The descriptions of functional techniques presented below are accompanied by charts that summarize the physical and skill prerequisites. Exact values for the physical prerequisites are not given because the requirements vary among individuals.

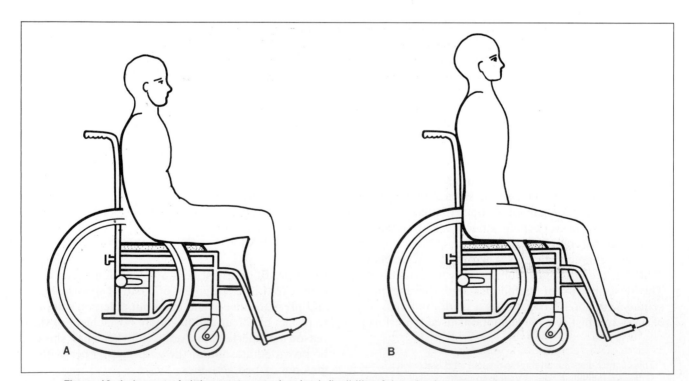

Figure 13–1. Impact of sitting posture on low back flexibility. **A** Low back overstretched by sitting with buttocks forward on seat. **B** Low back protected by positioning buttocks well back on wheelchair seat.

For example, someone who is very skillful in curb negotiation will require less strength for this activity than another person who is less skillful and must use sheer strength rather than momentum.

WHEELCHAIR SKILLS

Positioning in the Chair

The ability to position one's self and to maintain that position within a wheelchair is one of the most basic requirements for the independent use of a wheelchair. To use a wheelchair independently, a cord-injured person needs to be able to maintain an upright sitting posture.[3] He should also be able to reposition his trunk and buttocks in the chair so that he can adjust his posture in the event that his position shifts during the day.

With Functioning Biceps and Deltoids. Chapter 11 presents techniques for stabilizing the trunk in a wheelchair and for moving the trunk and buttocks. These techniques require functional strength in the deltoids and biceps.

In the Absence of Functioning Biceps and Deltoids. Without functioning biceps and deltoids, the potential for stabilizing and moving the trunk is limited. However, a person with high quadriplegia can gain some skills in this area. Through motions of his head and scapulae, he can exercise some control over his position in the wheelchair.

To maintain an upright sitting posture, a person with a high lesion can hold his head upright and his scapulae adducted. This posture can be a useful adjunct to trunk stability for anyone with a spinal cord injury.

A person with functioning trapezius, sternocleidomastoid, and cervical paraspinal musculature (present with C4 quadriplegia) can also make limited adjustments in his trunk's position, tilting his trunk laterally by throwing the head and shoulders. For example, he can tilt his trunk to the left by repeatedly throwing his head to the left while simultaneously elevating his right scapula. These neck and scapular motions are performed forcefully to maximize momentum. This technique can be used to tilt to the side from an upright position or to return to upright from a slight lateral tilt.

The physical and skill prerequisites required for positioning in the chair in the absence of functioning biceps and deltoids are presented in Charts 13–1 and 13–2.

Pressure Reliefs

In terms of survival value, the ability to perform pressure reliefs is probably the most important functional skill that a cord-injured person can acquire. When someone with a complete spinal cord injury sits for more than a few minutes, he requires peri-

Chart 13—1 High-Lesion Skills: Positioning in Wheelchair and Electric Wheelchair Propulsion—Physical Prerequisites

	Positioning in wheelchair	Hand-control wheelchair	Chin-control wheelchair	Mouth-control wheelchair	Breath-control wheelchair
Strength					
Cervical paraspinals	√	√	√		
Sternocleidomastoid	√		√		
Trapezius	√	√ −	√		
Anterior deltoids	●	●			
Middle deltoids	●	●			
Posterior deltoids	●	●			
Serratus anterior	●	●			
Oral musculature				√	√
Biceps, brachialis, and/or brachioradialis		√ −			
Range of Motion					
Cervical Lateral flexion	√ −				
Rotation			√ −		
Flexion			√ −		
Extension	√ −		√ −		
Scapular Elevation	√ −				
Abduction		√ −			
Adduction		√ −			

√ − = At least 2 − /5 strength is needed for this activity, or severe limitations in range will inhibit this activity.

● = Not required, but helpful.

√ = At least 3/5 strength is needed for this activity.

---

[3] An individual who is unable to do so without equipment may use a strap, but this will inhibit independent pressure reliefs.

Chart 13–2 High-Lesion Skills: Positioning in Wheelchair and Electric Wheelchair Propulsion—Skill Prerequisites

	Positioning in wheelchair	Hand-control wheelchair	Chin-control wheelchair	Mouth-control wheelchair	Breath-control wheelchair
Sitting in wheelchair, move trunk using head and scapular motions	✓				
Place hand on joystick		✓			
Move joystick in all directions using arm and scapular motions		✓			
Move joystick in all directions using chin or tongue motions			✓	✓	
Signal wheelchair by sipping and puffing in appropriate pattern					✓
Propel electric wheelchair over even surfaces		✓	✓	✓	✓

odic relief of pressure over his buttocks to prevent decubiti. A cord-injured person who cannot perform pressure reliefs independently must depend upon expensive and heavy cushions or assistance or both from others throughout the period of sitting.

The purpose of a pressure relief is to reduce the pressure on tissues that have been bearing weight, allowing circulation in areas that have been ischemic during weight bearing. When sitting with good posture, the bulk of weight bearing occurs on the ischial tuberosities. It is the skin over these boney prominences that must be relieved during a pressure relief.

People vary in their requirements for pressure relief. During rehabilitation, each must discover his skin's requirements for the duration of each pressure relief and the length of time that can pass between reliefs.[4]

Pushup. Perhaps the quickest and most effective method of pressure relief is the sitting pushup. Someone with adequate strength in his triceps can eliminate pressure over his ischial tuberosities by lifting his buttocks completely off the supporting surface. To do so, he places his hands lateral to his buttocks on the wheelchair's seat, armrests, or wheels. He then lifts his body by pushing down, extending his elbows and depressing his shoulders.

Weight Shift. Pressure reliefs do not require complete elimination of pressure on the ischial tuberosities. Adequate relief can be obtained by redistributing weight bearing, reducing pressure on the ischial tuberosities by moving the pressure to different areas (Swarts, Krouskop, & Smith, 1988). A cord-injured person can perform a pressure relief by leaning forward enough to unweight his ischial tuberosities. He can also perform a pressure relief

---

[4] Additional information on skin care is presented in Chapters 3 and 8.

Chart 13–3 Comparison of Wheelchair Propulsion Options

Power wheelchair	Advantages:	Makes independent mobility possible for people who cannot propel manual wheelchairs. When daily activities necessitate propulsion over long distances, conserves time and energy for other tasks.
	Disadvantages:	No cardiovascular or muscular conditioning occurs with propulsion. Wheelchair restricted to accessible environments; cannot be transported in car.
Manual wheelchair with handrim projections	Advantages:	Not restricted to wheelchair-accessible environments. Cardiovascular conditioning and muscle strengthening occur with propulsion. Can be transported in car.
	Disadvantages:	Handrim projections make wheelchair wider and interfere with efficient propulsion rhythm. Strengthening limited to shoulder and elbow flexion. Some people with high lesions are unable to propel manual wheelchairs.
Manual wheelchair with standard handrims	Advantages:	Not restricted to wheelchair-accessible environments. Can be transported in car. Cardiovascular conditioning and muscle strengthening occur with propulsion. Muscle strengthening optimal for enhancement of transfer skills.
	Disadvantages:	Some people with high lesions are unable to propel manual wheelchairs with standard handrims.

by leaning to one side and then the other, unweighting one side at a time. Chapter 11 presents techniques for moving the trunk forward or laterally in a wheelchair.

Wheelchair Propulsion Over Even Surfaces

Independence in propulsion over even surfaces brings the freedom to move about within a wheelchair-accessible environment. The functional use of a wheelchair requires the ability to propel forward and backward and to turn.

The methods used for propulsion depend upon the type of wheelchair used; different techniques are used to propel manual wheelchairs with standard or pegged handrims and the various types of electric wheelchairs. One task of the rehabilitation therapist involves working with the patient to determine the propulsion mode that is most appropriate for that individual. This analysis involves weighing the advantages and disadvantages of the different options for the individual concerned. Chart 13–3 presents a comparison of some of the advantages and disadvantages of power wheelchairs and manual chairs with pegged and standard handrims.

Propulsion Over Even Surfaces Using Manual Wheelchair With Standard Handrims

A person with functioning finger flexors can propel his wheelchair by grasping the handrims and pulling forward or backward. The techniques described below are appropriate for people who lack functional finger flexors. In these techniques friction is used to move the handrims. Adequate strength is required in the deltoids and biceps.

The physical and skill prerequisites required to propel a manual wheelchair with standard handrims are summarized in Charts 13–4 and 13–5.

Forward. To propel forward without grasping the wheelchair's handrims, a cord-injured person starts by placing his palms against the lateral surface of the handrims. His elbows are flexed and his shoulders are internally rotated slightly. Using elbow extension and combined shoulder adduction, external rotation, and flexion, he stabilizes his palms against the handrims and pushes forward. In the absence of functioning triceps, the anterior deltoids are used to extend the elbows.

Efficient propulsion requires long strokes. The wheelchair user starts with his hands well back on the handrims and pushes until they are well forward (Fig. 13–2). As he reaches back to start another stroke, the wheelchair continues to glide forward.

Backward. Backward propulsion without innervated finger flexors can be accomplished by re-

Chart 13–4 Propulsion of Manual Wheelchair With Standard Handrims—Physical Prerequisites

	Forward	Backward pulling handrims	Backward pushing tires	Turning
Strength				
Trapezius	✓	✓	✓	✓
Anterior deltoids	☑	✓	✓	✓
Middle deltoids	✓	✓	✓	✓
Posterior deltoids	✓	✓	✓	✓
Infraspinatus, teres minor	✓		✓	✓
Pectoralis major, teres major	●	●		●
Biceps, brachialis, and/or brachioradialis	✓	✓	✓	✓
Serratus anterior	●			●
Triceps	●		●	●
Hand musculature (active grasp)	●	●	●	●
Range of Motion				
Scapular Elevation			✓	
Depression			✓	
Abduction	✓			
Adduction	✓	✓	✓	✓
Shoulder Flexion	✓	✓		✓
Extension	✓	✓	✓	✓
Internal rotation	✓	✓		✓
External rotation	✓		☑	✓
Abduction			✓	
Elbow Flexion	✓	✓		✓
Extension	✓	✓	✓	✓

✓ = Some strength is needed for this activity, or severe limitations in range will inhibit this activity.

☑ = A large amount of strength or normal or greater range is needed for this activity.

● = Not required, but helpful.

Chart 13–5 Propulsion of Manual Wheelchair With Standard Handrims—Skill Prerequisites

	Forward	Backward pulling handrims	Backward pushing tires	Turning
Maintain upright sitting position[a]	√	√	√	√
Place palms against standard handrims	√	√		√
Push standard handrim(s) forward	√			√
Pull standard handrim(s) backward		√		
Place palms on tires, behind seat			√	
With palms on tires behind seat, propel wheelchair backwards using elbow extension and scapular depression *or* using only scapular depression			√	
Propel manual wheelchair over even surfaces	√			

[a] Refer to Chapter 11 for a description of this skill and therapeutic strategies.

Chart 13–6 Propulsion of Manual Wheelchair With Pegged Handrims—Physical Prerequisites

	Forward	Backward	Turning
Strength			
Trapezius	√	√	√
Anterior deltoids	√	√	√
Middle deltoids	√	√	√
Posterior deltoids	√	√	√
Biceps, brachialis, and/or brachioradialis	√	√	√
Pectoralis major, teres major		√	
Range of Motion			
Scapular adduction		√	
Shoulder Flexion	√	√	√
Extension	√	√	√
Internal rotation		√	
Elbow Extension	√	√	√

√ = Some strength is needed for this activity, or severe limitations in range will inhibit this activity.
☑ = A large amount of strength or normal or greater range is needed for this activity.
● = Not required, but helpful.

versing the technique for forward propulsion. The person places his palms on the outer surface of the handrims, squeezes in, and pulls back (Fig. 13–3**A**).

Figure 13–4**B** illustrates an alternate method of backward propulsion. The person places his palms on top of the tires, just posterior to his buttocks. With his hands facing backward and his shoulders externally rotated, he pushes backward on the tires by extending his elbows, using either triceps or anterior deltoids.

Someone who is unable to extend his elbows against the resistance supplied by his chair's wheels may be able to propel backward using a third method, illustrated in Figure 13–3C. When using this method the person starts by placing his palms against the medial-superior surfaces of his tires, posterior to his buttocks. His shoulders should be externally rotated and elevated and his elbows

locked[5] in extension. By depressing his scapulae, he then pushes the wheels backward.

Turning. The technique used to turn will depend upon the turning radius desired. Turning in a long arc simply involves pushing harder with one hand than the other, or pushing one wheel while applying resistance to the other wheel. To turn sharply, the wheelchair user can pull one wheel backward while he pushes the other one forward. The techniques for pushing the wheels forward and backward are described above.

Propulsion Over Even Surfaces Using Manual Wheelchair With Pegged Handrims

Inadequate strength or range of motion can make propulsion with standard handrims impossible or

---

[5] Elbow locking is addressed in Chapter 11.

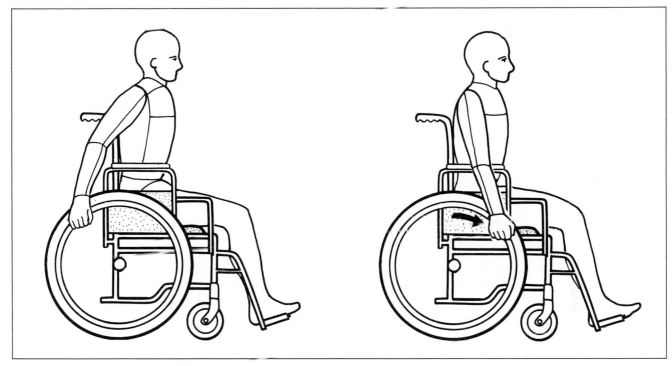

Figure 13–2. Efficient wheelchair propulsion using long strokes.

prohibitively difficult. Handrim projections, also called pegs, may make propulsion easier in these instances. Functional deltoids and biceps are required.

The physical and skill prerequisites required to propel a manual wheelchair with pegged handrims are summarized in Charts 13–6 and 13–7.

Forward. To propel forward using pegged handrims, each palm or forearm is placed behind a peg. Using

Chart 13–7 Propulsion of Manual Wheelchair With Pegged Handrims—Skill Prerequisites

	Forward	Backward	Turning
Place palms or forearms against handrim projections	√	√	√
Pull handrim projections forward	√		√
Pull backward on handrim projections		√	√
Propel manual wheelchair over even surfaces	√		

shoulder and elbow flexion, the wheelchair user pulls forward on the pegs. Propulsion will be more efficient if he uses long strokes, starting with his hands on pegs which are posterior to his buttocks (Fig. 13–4).

Backward. Backward propulsion can be accomplished by pulling back on the handrim projections. With his shoulders internally rotated, the cord-injured person places his hands or forearms against the front aspects of anteriorly located pegs. He then pulls back using glenohumeral extension and scapular adduction.

An individual who is strong enough may be able to propel backward by pushing against the backs of his tires, as described above.

Turning. Turning is accomplished in the same manner as turning a wheelchair with standard handrims. Using the techniques described above, the person pushes one wheel harder than the other or pushes one wheel forward while pulling the other backward.

Propulsion Over Even Surfaces Using Electric Wheelchair

Manual wheelchair propulsion requires the presence of functioning deltoids and biceps. An individual who lacks innervation or adequate strength in

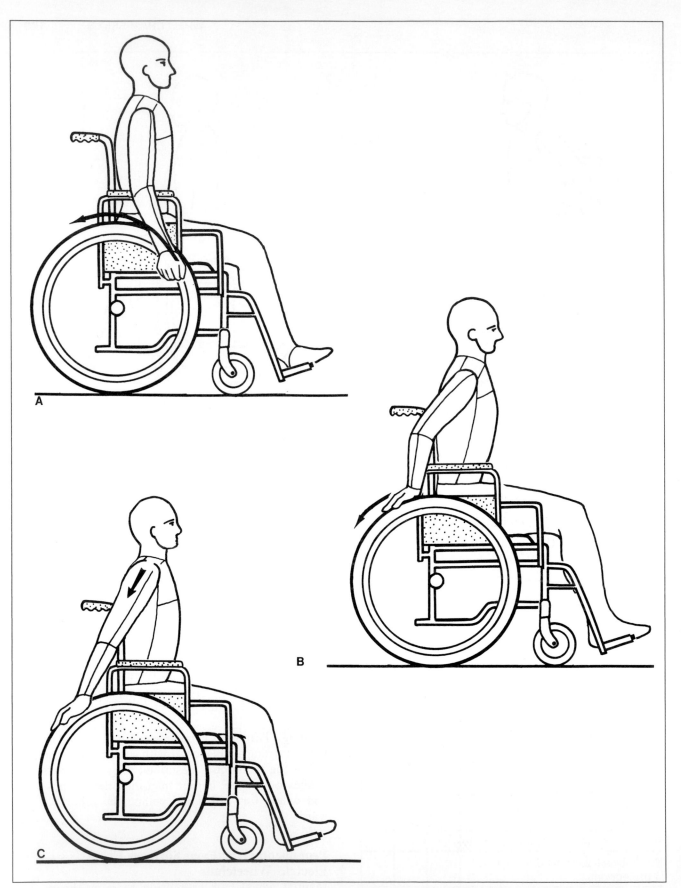

Figure 13–3. Backward propulsion without innervated finger flexors, using standard handrims. **A.** Squeezing in and pulling back on handrims. **B.** Pushing back on tires using elbow extension. **C.** Pushing back on tires using scapular depression.

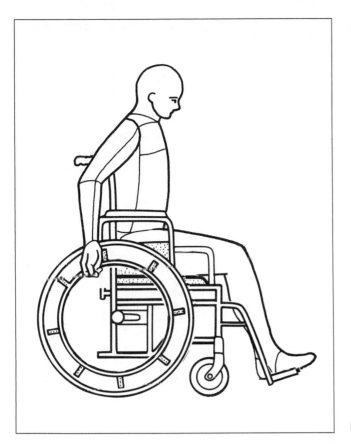

Figure 13–4. Foward propulsion using pegged handrims.

this musculature will require an electric wheelchair for independent mobility. Various control options are available for powered wheelchairs. The types of control most commonly used by cord-injured people with power wheelchairs are hand, chin, mouth, and breath (sip and puff) control.

The physical and skill prerequisites required to

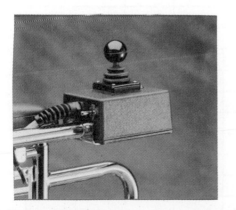

Figure 13–5. Joystick mounted for hand control. (Reproduced with permission from Invacare Corporation, 899 Cleveland Street, Elyria, OH 44036.)

propel an electric wheelchair are summarized in Charts 13–1 and 13–2.

Hand, Chin, and Mouth Control. With a hand- chin- or mouth-controlled wheelchair, the chair's motions are controlled using a joystick (Fig. 13–5). The direction in which the person pushes the stick determines the direction of the chair's motion. Moving the joystick on a hand-controlled wheelchair forward, back, or at any angle between will cause the chair to move forward or back or to turn in a like direction. The directional control with chin or mouth control is the same, except that the plane of the stick's motion is more vertical. If a wheelchair has proportional control, the magnitude of the joystick's motions determines the speed: larger motions of the stick will result in faster speeds.

To drive a hand-controlled wheelchair, the cord-injured person places his hand on the joystick and pushes it in the desired direction. If he is unable to hold the stick, it can be adapted to make it easier to maneuver. If necessary, a strap can be added to hold the hand in place. People with quadriplegia as high as C4 have the potential to drive electric wheelchairs using hand controls (McClay, 1983).

Chin-controlled wheelchairs are driven using neck motions. With his chin on a cup attached to the joystick, the wheelchair user directs the chair through cervical flexion, extension, and rotation. People with C3 and lower quadriplegia have the musculature required for these motions.

Driving in a mouth-controlled wheelchair involves holding the joystick in the mouth and moving it with the tongue. Since the musculature used for these actions is innervated by cranial nerves, people with quadriplegia as high as C1 can use mouth-controlled wheelchairs.

Breath Control. With a sip-and-puff wheelchair, the chair's motion is directed using a tube that is held in the mouth. By sucking air in (sipping) or blowing air out (puffing) through the tube and moving the tube laterally with his tongue, the wheelchair user controls the chair's speed and direction.

Dependence upon a respirator does not pre-

Chart 13—8 Negotiation of Ramps and Uneven Terrain—Physical Prerequisites

	Ascend ramp	Descend ramp on four wheels	Descend ramp in wheelie position	Negotiate uneven terrain on four wheels	Negotiate uneven terrain in wheelie
Strength					
Trapezius	√	√	√	√	√
Anterior deltoids	☑	√	√	☑	☑
Middle deltoids	√	√	√	√	√
Posterior deltoids	√	√	√	√	√
Infraspinatus, teres minor	√			√	
Pectoralis major, teres major	●	●	√	●	√
Biceps, brachialis, and/or brachioradialis	√	√	√	√	√
Serratus anterior	●			●	√
Triceps	●		√	●	√
Hand musculature (active grasp)	●	●	√	●	√
Range of Motion					
Scapular Abduction	√		√	√	√
Adduction	√		√	√	√
Shoulder Flexion	√		√	√	√
Extension	√	√	√	√	√
Internal rotation	√	√	√	√	√
External rotation	√			√	
Elbow Flexion	√	√	√	√	√
Extension	√		√	√	√
Finger Flexion			√		√

√ = Some strength is needed for this activity, or severe limitations in range will inhibit this activity.
☑ = A large amount of strength or normal or greater range is needed for this activity.
● = Not required, but helpful.

clude the use of an electric wheelchair equipped with this type of control. Sipping and puffing are accomplished using oral musculature, controlled by cranial nerves. Thus people with even the highest cord lesions can use breath-controlled wheelchairs.

Negotiation of Obstacles

Independent wheelchair propulsion over even surfaces will enable a person to be mobile indoors within the confines of a single-level home or work environment, provided that there are no narrow doorways or elevated thresholds in the doors. For independent mobility within a greater variety of environments, obstacle negotiation skills are necessary.

Techniques for negotiation of ramps, curbs, uneven terrain, stairs, and narrow doorways are presented below. The descriptions apply to manual wheelchairs with standard handrims but can be adapted to pegged handrims.

Charts 13–8 through 13–15 summarize the physical and skill prerequisites for independent negotiation of obstacles.

Ramps

Training in ramp negotiation often focuses on ascending, since this is the more difficult part of the task. However, skill in descending ramps should also be developed. To be safe descending a ramp in a wheelchair, the wheelchair user should maintain control of the chair for the entire length of the ramp. He should be able to steer to the right or left and stop at will. If he does not have this level of control, he may eventually collide with someone or something that gets in the way. There is no guarantee that a clear ramp will stay clear as a wheelchair descends.

Practice in ramp negotiation should not be limited to the gentle 1:12 grade of a standard public incline. Many, if not most, ramps found in the community are far steeper than this. People undergoing rehabilitation should develop the skills to ascend and descend ramps as steep as possible within their potentials.

Ascending. Fully innervated upper extremities make ramp ascension easier but are not required for this activity. Someone with C5 quadriplegia should be able to negotiate gentle slopes. More and stronger innervated musculature will make it possible to negotiate steeper ramps.

Propulsion up a ramp is accomplished on four wheels, using variations of the techniques described above for forward propulsion. The techniques are

Chart 13—9 Negotiation of Ramps and Uneven Terrain—Skill Prerequisites

	Ascend ramp	Descend ramp on four wheels	Descend ramp in wheelie position	Negotiate uneven terrain on four wheels	Negotiate uneven terrain in wheelie
Propel wheelchair over even surfaces	✓			✓	
Propel wheelchair up a slope	✓				
Descending slope on four wheels, control wheelchair by applying friction to handrims		✓			
Assume wheelie position			✓		✓
Maintain balance point in wheelie position			✓		✓
Descending slope in wheelie, control wheelchair by applying friction to handrims			✓		
Negotiate uneven terrain on four wheels				✓	
Propel wheelchair forward (glide) in wheelie position			✓		✓
Turn in wheelie position					✓
Propel backward in wheelie position					✓
Negotiate uneven terrain in wheelie position					✓

Chart 13–10 Negotiation of Curbs—Physical Prerequisites

	Ascend from stationary position	Ascend using momentum	Descend backwards	Descend in wheelie
Strength				
Trapezius	√	√	√	√
Anterior deltoids	☑	☑	√	√
Middle deltoids	√	√	√	√
Posterior deltoids	√	√	√	√
Infraspinatus, teres minor	√	√		
Pectoralis major, teres major	●	●	●	√
Biceps, brachialis, and/or brachioradialis	√	√	√	√
Serratus anterior	●	●	●	●
Triceps	●	●	●	√
Hand musculature (active grasp)	●	●	●	√
Range of Motion				
Scapular Abduction	√	√	√	√
Adduction	√	√	√	√
Downward rotation	√	√		
Shoulder Flexion	√	√		
Extension	√	√	√	√
Internal rotation	√	√	√	√
External rotation	√	√		
Elbow Flexion	√	√		√
Extension	√	√	√	√
Finger Flexion				√

√ = Some strength is needed for this activity, or severe limitations in range will inhibit this activity.
☑ = A large amount of strength or normal or greater range is needed for this activity.
● = Not required, but helpful.

altered to enable the wheelchair user to propel up the ramp without tipping over backward or rolling backward between pushes. To ascend a ramp without tipping over backward, the wheelchair user pushes forward forcefully but avoids jerking the wheels abruptly. A forward lean of the head and (when possible) trunk will also help prevent backward tipping. To avoid rolling backward between pushes, he uses shorter strokes and moves his hands back rapidly between pushes.

Descending on Four Wheels. When a wheelchair descends a ramp, gravity provides the force that moves the chair. The wheelchair user *controls* the chair rather than propels it. During the descent, he keeps the chair under control by resisting its motion.

Chart 13–11 Negotiation of Curbs—Skill Prerequisites

	Ascend by muscling up	Ascend using momentum	Descend backwards	Descend in wheelie
Position trunk in wheelchair[a]	√	√	√	
Propel manual wheelchair over even surfaces	√	√	√	
From stationary position, lift casters from floor	√			
Pop casters onto curb from stationary position	√			
Position casters at edge of curb	√			
Ascend curb from stationary position	√			
Lift casters off floor while chair moves forward		√		
Pop casters onto curb while chair moves forward		√		
Ascend curb using momentum		√		
Backing down curb, control rear wheels' descent			√	
Lower casters from curb by turning wheelchair			√	
Assume wheelie position				√
Glide forward in wheelie				√
Descend curb in wheelie position				√

[a] Refer to Chapter 11 for a description of this skill and therapeutic strategies.

Chart 13—12 Negotiation of Stairs—Physical Prerequisites

	Ascend on buttocks	Ascend in wheelchair	Descend on buttocks	Descend in wheelchair holding rail	Descend in wheelie
Strength					
Fully innervated upper extremities	●	☑	●	●	✓
Anterior deltoids	☑	☑	☑	☑	✓
Middle deltoids	✓	✓	✓	✓	✓
Posterior deltoids	✓	✓	✓	✓	☑
Biceps, brachialis, and/or brachioradialis	☑	✓	☑	☑	☑
Serratus anterior	☑	☑	☑		✓
Latissimus dorsi	☑	☑	☑		
Triceps	☑	☑	☑	●	✓
Hand musculature (active grasp)	✓	●	✓	●	✓
Range of Motion					
Scapular Abduction	✓	✓	✓	✓	✓
Adduction	✓	✓	✓		✓
Downward rotation	✓	✓	✓		
Upward rotation	✓	✓	✓	✓	
Shoulder Flexion	✓	✓	✓	✓	
Extension	☑	☑	☑	✓	✓
Internal rotation	✓	✓	✓	✓	✓
External rotation				✓	
Elbow Flexion	✓	✓	✓	✓	✓
Extension	✓	✓	✓	✓	✓
Finger Flexion	✓		✓		✓

✓ = Some strength is needed for this activity, or severe limitations in range will inhibit this activity.

☑ = A large amount of strength or normal or greater range is needed for this activity.

● = Not required, but helpful.

He can slow or turn the chair while descending by applying resistance to the wheel rims.

A cord-injured person with functioning hand musculature can control the chair by gripping the handrims loosely and allowing them to slide through his hands. His grip should provide enough resistance to the handrims to slow and control the chair's descent.

An individual who lacks functioning finger flexors can control the chair's descent by pressing his palms against the handrims. The palms should be slightly in front of the hips, with the elbows slightly flexed and the shoulders internally rotated.

Descending In a "Wheelie" Position. Many ramps are steep, with an abrupt angle at the bottom where the ramp meets the street or sidewalk. When someone descends such a ramp on four wheels, the footplates may "bottom out," striking the street or sidewalk. The chair comes to an abrupt stop, and the rider may be thrown out of the chair. This problem can be avoided by descending ramps in a wheelie (balanced on the rear wheels).

Descending a ramp in a wheelie is an easy skill to master for anyone who can glide on two wheels. The wheelchair user approaches the ramp in a wheelie, then grips the chair's handrims loosely and allows them to slide through his hands as he descends the ramp. His grip should provide just enough resistance to slow and control the chair's descent. Good hand function is required for this skill.

Curbs

Although ramps and curb ramps have become fairly common, many public places remain inaccessible to wheelchairs. Certainly most private residences are inaccessible. Thus it is likely that many places where an individual wants to go will not have ramps or will have ramps that are obstructed or placed in inconvenient locations.

Curb negotiation skills can be used to get over

Chart 13-13 Negotiation of Stairs—Skill Prerequisites

	Ascend on buttocks	Ascend in wheelchair	Descend on buttocks	Descend in wheelchair holding rail	Descend in wheelie
Transfers between wheelchair and floor[a]	✓		✓		
Position buttocks and legs on step[a]	✓		✓		
Sitting on step or floor, tilt wheelchair back to position to ascend or descend stairs	✓		✓		
Sitting on step, stabilize wheelchair by pushing down through push handles	✓		✓		
Transfer up a step while stabilizing wheelchair	✓				
Sitting on step, position buttocks and legs while stabilizing wheelchair	✓		✓		
Sitting on step or landing, pull wheelchair up	✓				
Sitting on floor, pull wheelchair to upright position	✓		✓		
Belt self into wheelchair		✓			
Lower chair into position to ascend stairs in wheelchair		✓			
Sitting in wheelchair tilted back onto steps, reposition hands		✓			
Sitting in wheelchair, push on step to lift wheelchair up a step		✓			
Return wheelchair to upright		✓			
Sitting on a step, lower wheelchair down a step			✓		
Sitting on a step, transfer down a step while stabilizing wheelchair			✓		
Sitting in wheelchair holding stair handrail(s), lower chair down stairs				✓	
Assume wheelie position					✓
Glide forward, back, and turn in wheelie					✓
In wheelie, position wheels at top of step					✓
In wheelie, stabilize wheels against step					✓
Descend step, remaining in wheelie position					✓

[a] Refer to Chapter 11 for a description of this skill and therapeutic strategies.

Chart 13—14 Negotiation of Narrow Doorways—Physical Prerequisites

	Sitting on armrest	Remaining on the seat
Strength		
Fully innervated upper extremities	√	√
Range of Motion		
Scapular — Abduction	√	
Adduction	√	
Downward rotation	√	
Upward rotation	√	
Shoulder — Flexion	√	
Extension	√	
Internal rotation	√	√
Elbow — Flexion	√	√
Extension	√	
Finger — Flexion	√	√

√ = Some strength is needed for this activity, or severe limitations in range will inhibit this activity.
☑ = A large amount of strength or normal or greater range is needed for this activity.
● = Not required, but helpful.

a variety of obstacles that block a wheelchair's path with a vertical obstruction. Examples of such obstacles include curbs at the junctures between streets and sidewalks, irregularities in sidewalks, elevated thresholds or weatherstripping in doorways, and entranceways in which the floor on one side of the doorway is higher than on the other side.

Ideally someone who uses a wheelchair for mobility in the community will be able to negotiate tall curbs—the taller the better. However, any skill in curb negotiation, no matter how limited, will be helpful. Even the ability to negotiate a 1-inch curb will be useful, making it possible to get over weather stripping or an irregularity in the sidewalk.

The height of curb that an individual will be able to master will be influenced by his lesion level as well as his strength and skill. It is possible for people with quadriplegia as high as C6 to ascend 2-inch, even 4-inch, curbs using either of the methods de-

scribed below. However, curb negotiation is challenging with such a high lesion. It is more readily accomplished by people with fully innervated upper extremities. For someone with paraplegia, independent negotiation of 6-inch or higher curbs is a reasonable goal.

Ascending From Stationary Position. This curb ascension technique utilizes strength more than momentum. It requires less space than ascending using momentum, since it does not involve a running start. It also requires less skill than ascending using momentum; the timing of motions is not as critical. However, this technique is more limited: higher curbs can be negotiated using momentum.

To ascend a curb from a stationary position, the wheelchair user approaches the curb front on and stops a few inches shy of the curb (Fig. 13–6A). From this position he pops his casters onto the curb: starting with his hands well back on the handrims, he pulls forward forcefully and abruptly (Fig. 13–6B). To lift his casters, he may need to throw his head back simultaneously with the pull.

Once the casters are on the curb, the person backs his chair until the casters are at the edge (Fig.

Chart 13—15 Negotiation of Narrow Doorways—Skill Prerequisites

	Sitting on armrest	Remaining on the seat
Transfer to armrest	√	
Maintain balance while sitting on armrest	√	
Narrow wheelchair while sitting on armrest	√	
Sitting on armrest, pull doorjamb to move narrowed wheelchair through door *or* Sitting on armrest, propel narrowed wheelchair	√	
Transfer from armrest to wheelchair seat	√	
Narrow wheelchair by rocking side-to-side		√
Propel wheelchair over even surfaces		√

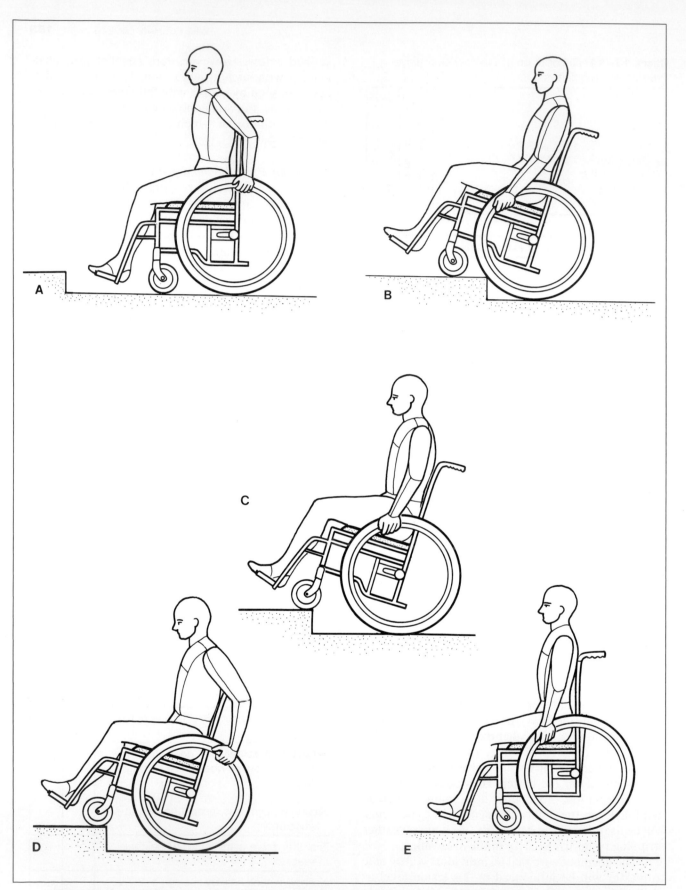

Figure 13–6. Ascending curb from stationary position. **A.** Starting position: facing the curb, a few inches from curb. **B.** Casters popped onto curb. **C.** Casters backed to edge of curb. **D.** Hands placed well back on handrims. **E.** Curb ascended.

13–6C). Positioning the chair in this manner makes it possible to gain some momentum in the next step.

When the casters are positioned appropriately, the wheelchair user places his hands well back on the handrims (Fig. 13–6D). He then pulls forward forcefully and throws his head and trunk forward. If the wheels hit the curb with enough force, the chair will ascend (Fig. 13–6E). During this step, the trunk may fall forward. This should not pose a problem; the person can return to an upright sitting position once the chair is past the curb.

Ascending Using Momentum. Ascending a curb using momentum involves finesse rather than sheer muscle power. It is faster than ascending from a stationary position, since the wheelchair user does not stop in front of the curb before ascending. Taking advantage of momentum also makes it possible to get up higher curbs than can be ascended from a stationary position.

Using this method, people with C6 quadriplegia can ascend low curbs. An exceptionally skillful person with fully innervated upper extremities can ascend 10-inch or higher curbs.

To ascend a curb using momentum, the wheelchair user approaches the curb head on, with speed. At the last moment he pops his casters up onto the curb: without slowing the chair, he reaches back and pulls forward on the wheel rims abruptly and forcefully. He may need to throw his head back at the same time to lift the casters. The caster pop should be timed so that the casters lift over the curb and land just before the rear wheels hit the curb. Momentum will carry the chair up the curb if the maneuver is timed correctly and the curb is approached with adequate speed.

Descending Backwards. This method of descending curbs does not involve a wheelie. Thus it is the method of choice for people who cannot glide in a wheelie.

Like ascending from a stationary position, descending backwards is most appropriate for lower curbs. On higher curbs, the chair may tip over backwards.

To descend a curb backwards, the wheelchair user first backs his chair to the edge of the curb (Fig. 13–7A). After the wheels pass the curb's edge, he controls the chair's descent by resisting the handrims' motion. Leaning the trunk and head forward will reduce the likelihood of the chair tipping over backward when the wheels hit the ground (Fig. 13–7B).

After lowering the chair's rear wheels, the wheelchair user removes the casters from the curb. He can roll the casters straight back off of the curb

only if the curb is a very low one. If he rolls his chair straight back from too high a curb, the footplates will catch on the curb. Once the footplates are caught, it will be difficult to free the chair from the curb.

Most curbs are high enough that backing the casters off is not possible. To avoid catching his footplates on the curb, the wheelchair user lowers the casters by turning the chair rather than backing up (Fig. 13–7C). He should turn his chair in a tight arc, pushing one wheel forward while pulling the other back. Once the casters move past the curb, they will drop safely to the lower surface.

Descending in a "Wheelie" Position. Descending curbs in a wheelie is faster than descending backwards. To descend backwards, the individual must interrupt his chair's forward motion to turn around and approach the curb backwards and must turn again after descending the curb. Descending in a wheelie does not require this interruption of forward motion. Good hand function is required for this method.

To descend a curb using this method, the wheelchair user pops his chair into a wheelie position as he approaches the curb. He glides toward the curb in a wheelie and maintains that position as the chair descends the curb (Fig. 13–8). The curb descent itself simply involves letting the handrims slide through the hands as the chair descends. The wheelie may be maintained after the curb has been descended, but that is not necessary for safe curb negotiation.

Uneven Terrain
Slightly uneven terrain, such as bumpy asphalt or a well-groomed lawn, may be negotiated using the same techniques as are used for propulsion over even surfaces. Propulsion on these surfaces will be more difficult, requiring more strength. Someone who is only marginally functional pushing on even surfaces will not be able to propel on uneven terrain.

Very uneven terrain is more challenging. A wheelchair's casters tend to get caught in ruts or bog down in deep gravel or sand. Because the greatest difficulty in propelling over uneven terrain involves catching or sinking of the casters, uneven surfaces are often easier to negotiate with the casters off the ground. The wheelchair user assumes a wheelie position and maintains it as he propels over the rough surface.

Stairs
Why should a disabled person learn to negotiate stairs in this day and age? Most public buildings

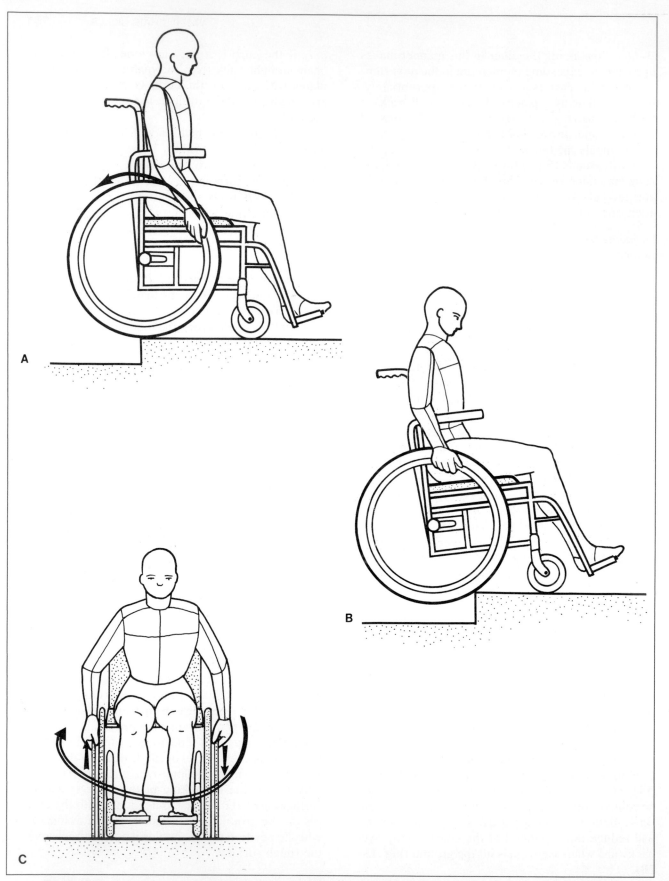

Figure 13–7. Descending curb backwards. **A.** Starting position: chair backed to edge of curb. **B.** Controlling chair's descent. **C.** Turning the wheelchair in a tight arc to lower casters from curb.

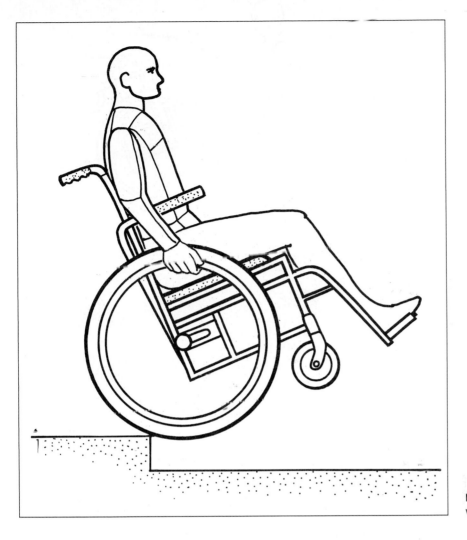

Figure 13–8. Descending curb in a wheelie.

have elevators. However, most private buildings don't. Someone who wants to visit friends and relatives, or his own second floor, is likely to have to negotiate stairs. And even public buildings with elevators *don't* have functioning elevators when there is a power outage or a fire.

Independent stair negotiation is more convenient than assisted stair negotiation; someone capable of helping may not always be available. Independent stair negotiation is also safer. An attendant, family member, or helpful stranger can slip or lose his grasp. A wheelchair user who can ascend and descend stairs without help will be in control, rather than dependent on the skill, strength, and sobriety of another.

Ascending on Buttocks. This method of ascending stairs is slow but requires less strength than ascending in a wheelchair. It may be possible for someone with C8 quadriplegia to perform this skill, but it is more feasible for people with fully inner-

vated upper extremities. To ascend stairs on his buttocks, an individual must be able to transfer independently between his wheelchair and the floor.

The first task in ascending stairs on the buttocks is a transfer from the wheelchair to a low step (Fig. 13–9A). The transfer can be to the lowest step or to the one above it, depending on the individual's ability. Once on the step, the person positions his buttocks and legs. His buttocks should be securely on the step, with the legs facing down the steps and the knees bent. The step-to-step transfers that follow will be easiest to perform if the legs are aligned with the body's midline, instead of leaning to the side. To maintain this alignment, the cord-injured person can position his feet laterally and lean his knees against each other.

After aligning his buttocks and legs on the step, the person positions his chair. Maintaining his balance by propping on one arm, he grasps the chair with the other hand. He then turns the chair so that it faces away from the stairs, with the rear wheels

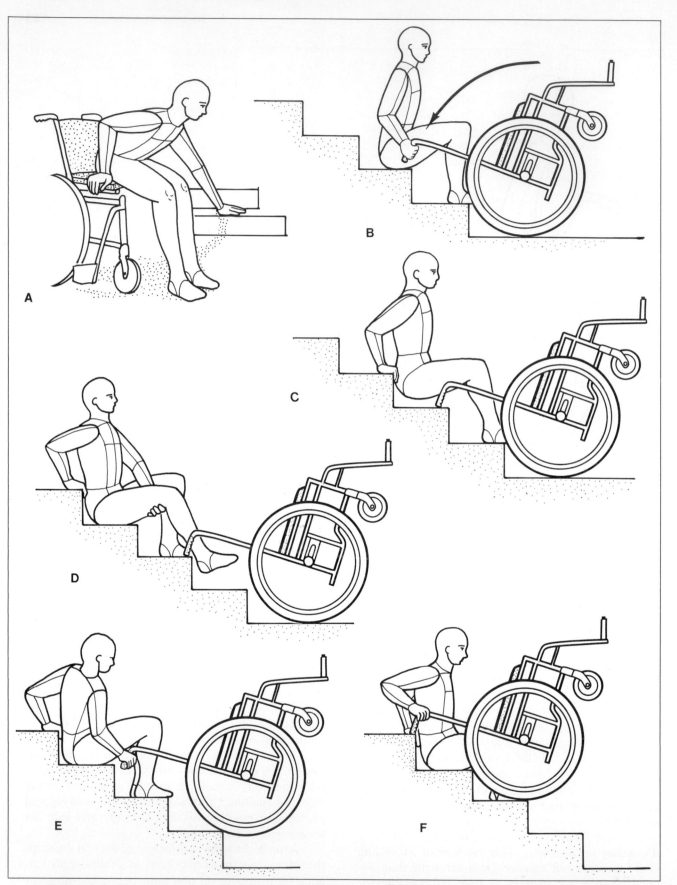

Figure 13–9. Ascending stairs on buttocks. **A.** Transferring to step. **B.** Tilting wheelchair back onto step. **C.** Transferring up a step. **D.** Repositioning legs, **E.** Pulling wheelchair up a step. **F.** Transferring up a step while stabilizing wheelchair.

against the lowest step. Tilting the chair back, he places the push handles on the highest step that they will reach (Fig. 13–9B).

From this point the individual ascends the stairs by transferring up one step at a time and pulling the chair along. To transfer up a step, he places both hands on the higher step and leans back while pushing down (Fig. 13–9C). As his buttocks clear the edge of the higher step, he lifts them onto the step by depressing his shoulders and tipping his head forward.

Once the person has transferred up a step, he moves his legs. He should place them with the knees flexed and the feet flat on a lower step (Fig. 13–9D). Positioning the legs in this manner will make it easier to transfer to the next step.

It may be possible to transfer up a step before moving the chair. As the individual moves further up the stairs, he must bring the chair along. The chair will remain beside him as he ascends. To pull the wheelchair up a step, he first places his buttocks well back on the step and positions his legs as described above. He then places his free hand (the one farthest from the chair) on the step above the one on which he sits. The hand should be slightly lateral to his trunk. Propping on this arm, he leans back and pulls the chair up a step, placing the push handles on the step above the one on which he sits (Fig. 13–9E and F).

Once a person has brought his wheelchair up onto the steps so that the wheels rest on a step, he must hold the chair to keep it from falling. If he lets go even briefly, it will fall. Maintaining a hold on the chair while transferring from step to step is most easily accomplished by bearing weight through the push handle when transferring. The force on the push handle must be directed straight downward.

Ascending stairs involves repeating the process of pulling the wheelchair up a step, transferring up, and repositioning the legs. Once the person has reached the landing at the top of the stairs, he pulls the wheelchair onto the landing. He then rights the chair (Away from the edge, please!) and transfers into it.

Ascending in a Wheelchair. Ascending stairs in a chair is faster than ascending on the buttocks. In addition, when ascending in his chair, a person does not risk traumatizing the skin over his ischial tuberosities or sacrum on the stairs and will not get his clothes wet or dirty. Unfortunately not everyone can ascend stairs in this manner. Strong, fully innervated upper extremities are required.

The wheelchair user first belts himself into the wheelchair, placing the belt so that it encircles his thighs and the wheelchair seat (Fig. 13–10A). He then backs up to the stairs, grasps the rail(s), and pulls on the rail(s) to tip the chair back. He lowers himself until the push handles rest on a step (Fig. 13–10B). From this position he pulls himself up the stairs, one step at a time.

To ascend a step, the person first places his hands on the step above the one on which the push handles rest (Fig. 13–10C). He then lifts his buttocks and the wheelchair by pushing down forcefully (Fig. 13–10D). He will feel the chair's resistance reduce substantially as the wheels get up over the edge of the step.

Once an individual has lifted his wheelchair up a step, he moves his hands to the next step. To keep the chair from falling back down the stairs, he must move his hands one at a time. This involves balancing first on one arm and then the other and moving the free hand up a step.

The stairs are ascended one step at a time by the repeated process of pulling the wheelchair up a step and repositioning the hands to the next step. Once an individual has reached the landing at the top of the stairs, he pulls the wheelchair well onto the landing. After pulling his chair a safe distance from the top of the stairs, he can right the chair while remaining in it. Alternatively, he can get out of the wheelchair, return it to an upright position, and perform a floor-to-chair transfer.

Descending Stairs on Buttocks. To descend stairs on his buttocks, the wheelchair user performs in reverse the sequence of maneuvers used to ascend stairs on his buttocks.

Descending in a Wheelchair, Holding Rail. Using this technique to descend stairs, a wheelchair user holds the rail and lowers himself backwards. Since he stays in his wheelchair, he does not risk traumatizing his skin on the stairs or getting his clothes dirty. This skill would be very helpful in the event of an emergency, since it enables a person to descend stairs safely and quickly without assistance.

Virtually anyone with fully innervated upper extremities should be able to master this technique. However, full use of the upper extremities is not required.

To descend stairs using this method, the wheelchair user positions his chair close to one rail at the top of the stairs, facing away from the stairs (Fig. 13–11A). He grasps the rail firmly with both hands.[6] The hand of the arm closest to the rail should be

---

[6] On a narrow stairway, it may be possible to reach both rails. A person may then choose to position his chair in the center of the stairs and hold both rails as he lowers himself.

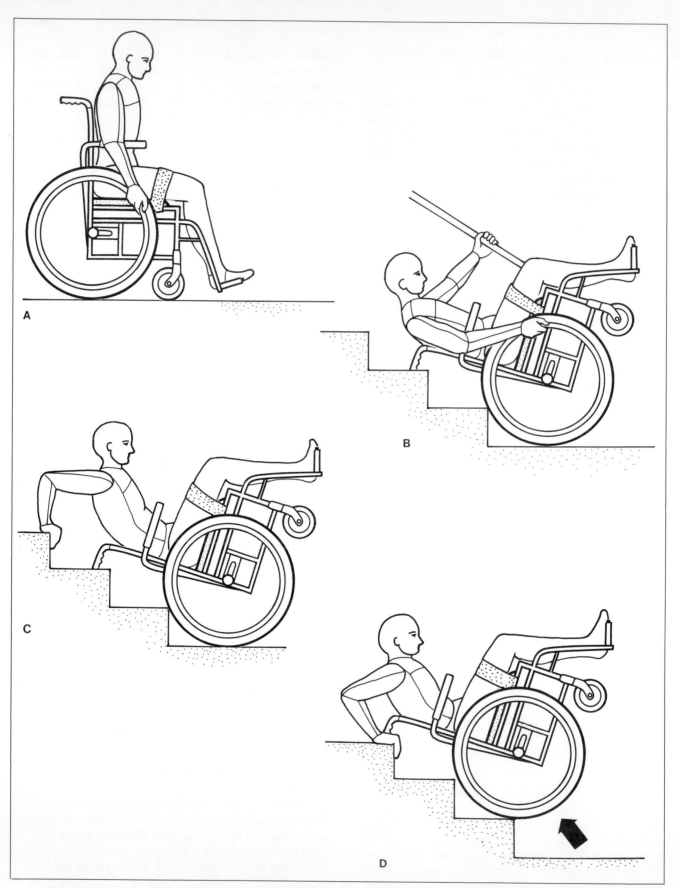

Figure 13–10. Ascending stairs in wheelchair. **A.** Belted into wheelchair. **B.** Chair lowered onto step. **C.** Hands positioned for ascending step. **D.** Ascending step.

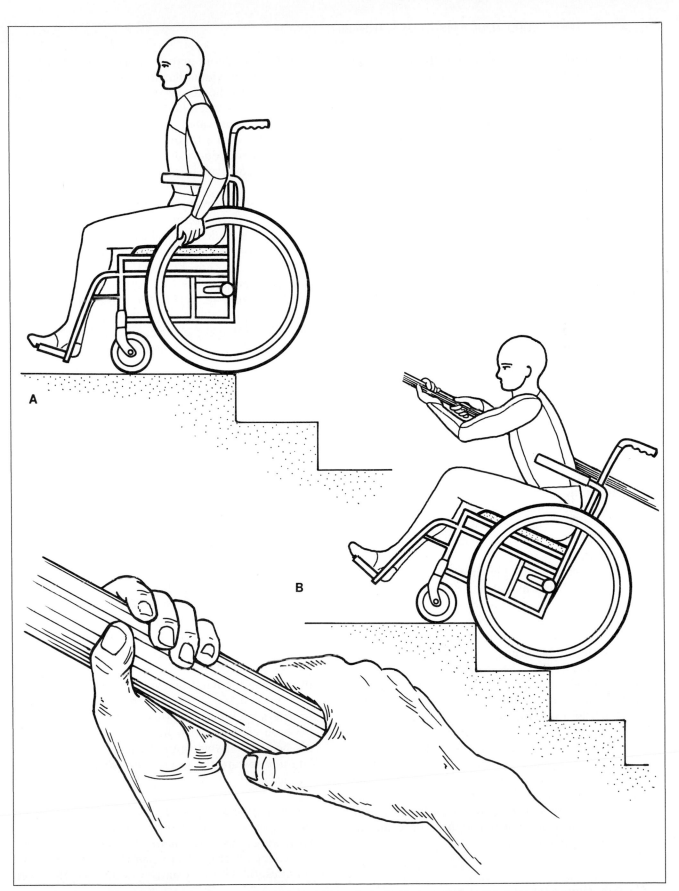

Figure 13–11. Descending stairs in wheelchair, holding rail. **A.** Starting position: chair backed to top step. **B.** Lowering wheelchair down stairs. **C.** Hand positions.

positioned lower on the rail than the other hand. Figure 13–11**C** illustrates the hand positions.

Pulling on the rail, the person moves his chair to the edge of the top step. As the wheels move past the edge, he leans his trunk forward. Once the tires move past the step's edge, gravity provides the force to move the chair. The wheelchair user's task is to control the chair's descent. He does so by maintaining his grasp on the rail and lowering the chair (Fig. 13–11**B**). As the chair progresses down the stairs, he moves his hands down the rail, sliding one hand at a time.

Descending in a Wheelie. This stair negotiation technique involves maintaining the chair in a wheelie position during the descent. The wheelchair user faces down the stairs and holds the wheelchair's handrims rather than the stair rails. This technique is safest when the steps have large horizontal surfaces and small vertical rises. It is also safer with a small series of stairs rather than a long flight.

Like descending holding a rail, descending stairs in a wheelie is fast and does not require the person to leave the chair. However, descending in a wheelie is more difficult and involves a greater risk of falling. This maneuver can be performed only by people with fully innervated upper extremities who are exceptionally proficient in wheelchair skills. Its greatest advantage is that it enables people to descend stairs quickly in wheelchairs when rails are absent.

When descending stairs in a wheelie, the person maintains a wheelie as he lowers the chair down one step at a time. He first approaches the stairs in a wheelie and positions the wheels at the edge of the top step (Fig. 13–12**A**). From this position he pushes forward on the handrims until the tires move over the edge and he feels the chair begin to descend. At this point he stops pushing forward and works to control the chair's descent as gravity pulls it down the step (Fig. 13–12**B**). He maintains control by gripping the handrims loosely and allowing them to slide through his grasp. When the wheels reach the next step, he can stabilize the chair by pulling back on the handrims until the wheels press against the vertical surface of the higher step (Fig. 13–12**C**). He is then ready to repeat the process on the next step. In this manner the wheelchair user descends the stairs one step at a time.

Narrow Doorways

Many doorways in private homes are too narrow for wheelchairs to pass through. This is especially true of bathroom doors and of doors in mobile homes. Even if an individual has the financial resources to adapt his own home, he is likely to encounter narrow doorways when he leaves his home.

Fully innervated upper extremities (and a wheelchair with a folding frame) are needed to negotiate narrow doorways using the techniques described below.

Sitting on an Armrest. In preparation for getting his wheelchair through a narrow doorway, the person positions his chair. If possible, his footplates should extend into the doorway and the doorjamb should be within reach (Fig. 13–13**A**). After positioning the chair, he removes his foot from one footplate and folds the footplate up (Fig. 13–13**B**). (Otherwise the footplates will collide as the chair narrows, limiting the amount that the chair can be narrowed.)

Once the chair is positioned, the person places his hands on the armrests so that he can transfer onto an armrest. The hand toward which he plans to transfer should be well forward, to leave room for his buttocks.[7] The transfer is achieved by pushing down forcefully and throwing the head down and away from the armrest (Fig. 13–13**C**).

After the transfer to the armrest, balance is maintained by propping with one arm on the opposite armrest. With his free hand, the wheelchair user reaches to the opposite side of the seat. Grasping a loop (if present) or the seat itself, he pulls upward forcefully and abruptly (Fig. 13–13**D**). As he does so, he shifts his weight off of his supporting hand. When he pulls on the chair in this manner, it narrows slightly. Repeated pulls will narrow the wheelchair to the desired width.

Once he has narrowed his chair sufficiently, the wheelchair user is ready to move through the doorway. Still balancing on one arm, he pulls on the doorjamb (Fig. 13–13**E**) or propels through the door by pushing the handrims with his free hand.

After passing through the door, the person transfers back into the wheelchair's seat. With one hand on each armrest, he pushes down and tucks his head to lift his buttocks and swings his head laterally toward the armrest on which he has been sitting.

Remaining on the Seat. This method of negotiating tight spaces enables people to remain seated while narrowing their wheelchairs. A chair's width cannot be reduced a great deal using this technique, so it is not useful with very narrow doorways. However,

---

[7] When sitting on an armrest, the person actually balances on his proximal thighs.

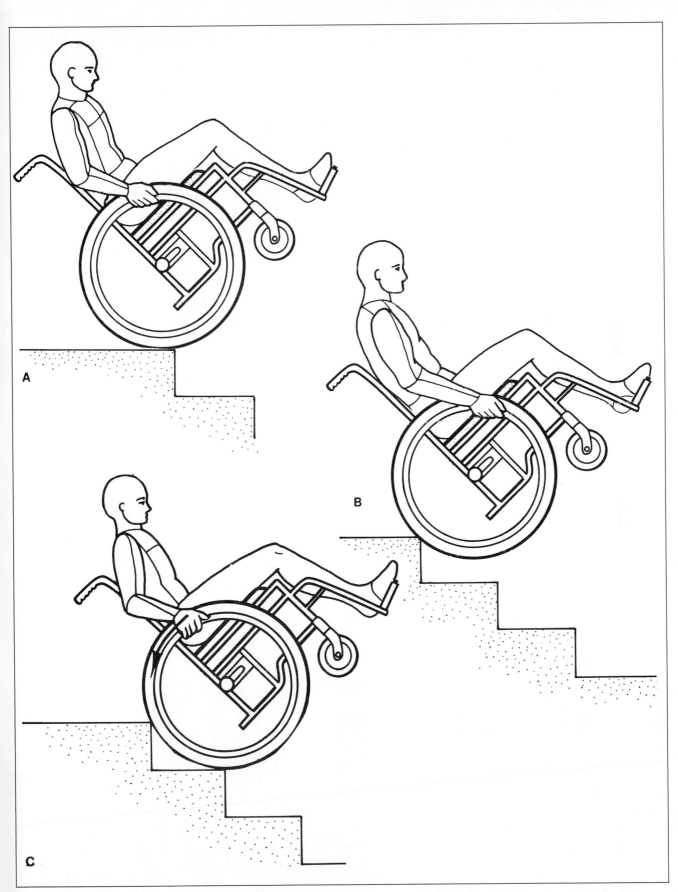

Figure 13–12. Descending stairs in a wheelie. **A.** Starting position: in wheelie, wheels positioned at edge of top step. **B.** Controlling chair's descent. **C.** Stabilizing wheelchair by pulling wheel against stair.

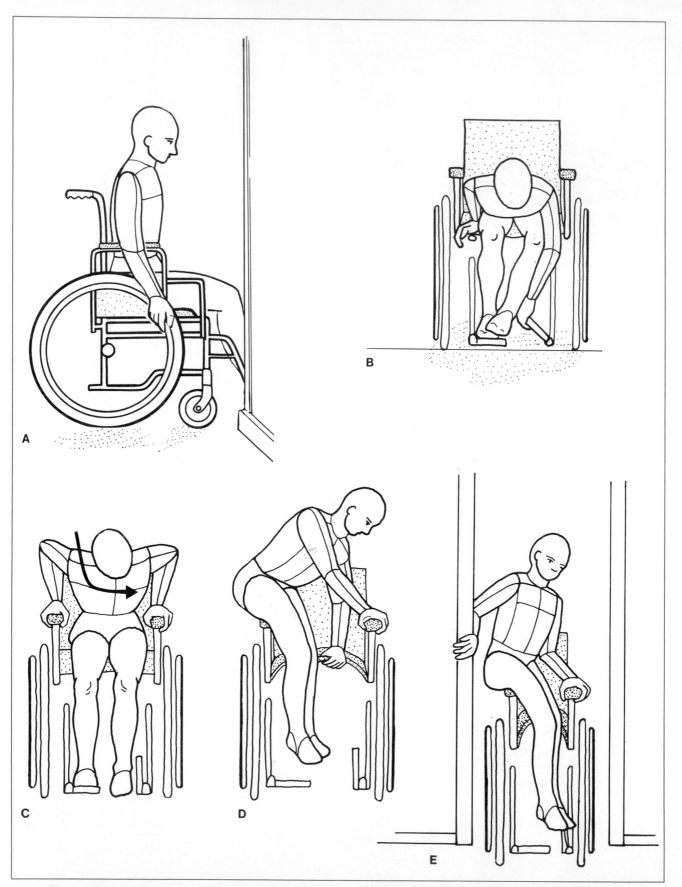

Figure 13–13. Negotiating narrow doorway, sitting on an armrest. **A.** Initial position of wheelchair. **B.** Folding footplate after removing foot. **C.** Transferring onto armrest. **D.** Narrowing wheelchair by pulling upward on the seat. **E.** Pulling on doorjamb to pull wheelchair through doorway.

this technique provides a means of narrowing a chair for the many who choose not to use armrests on their chairs.

Reducing a wheelchair's width while remaining seated involves rocking the chair side to side while pulling up on the sides of the seat. The wheelchair user initiates the process by throwing his head to one side, simultaneously pulling up on the opposite side of the seat. (If rocking to the left, he throws his head to the left and pulls up on the right side of the seat.) The head motions and pulls on the seat must be performed forcefully and abruptly. As this maneuver is repeated, the chair rocks to one side and then the other. With each rock and pull, the chair narrows slightly. Once the chair's width has been reduced sufficiently, it can be propelled through the doorway.

Falling Safely

Many advanced wheelchair skills involve propelling the chair with the casters lifted off the ground. These activities involve a risk of falling. A person who negotiates curbs independently or propels his chair in a wheelie is likely to fall eventually. While performing the maneuver, he will inadvertently move past his balance point, and the wheelchair will tip over backward. To minimize the risk of injury, anyone who learns to lift his casters off the ground should learn to fall safely.

Falling backward safely in a wheelchair simply involves tucking the head and holding the wheels. When a person falls in this manner, he is not likely to injure himself or even experience discomfort. The chair's push handles, not the person's back or head, take the brunt of the force when the chair lands.

When the wheelchair lands, the legs' momentum may cause the person's knees to hit his face. An alternate method of falling can prevent this. Using this method, the wheelchair user tucks his head and maintains his hold on one wheel. He quickly crosses his free arm across his legs and grasps the opposite armrest or seat. This arm blocks his thighs as they fall, keeping his knees from hitting his face (Fig. 13–14).

Returning to Upright After Fall

After someone has fallen safely in his wheelchair, he faces the task of getting back up and into his chair. One option is to get out of the chair, place it in an upright position, and transfer back into it. A faster alternative involves staying in the chair while pushing it back to upright. Fully innervated upper extremities are required to perform this maneuver.

Righting a wheelchair while remaining in it requires proper positioning: buttocks on the seat, legs looped over the front edge of the seat (Fig. 13–15A). If the wheelchair user has held on during his fall, he should be fairly well positioned already. If he has slid out slightly or if his legs have fallen forward,

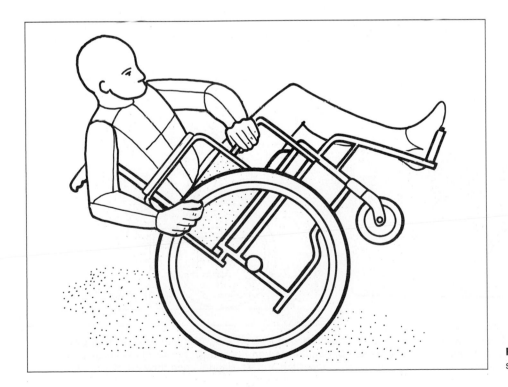

Figure 13–14. Falling backward safely.

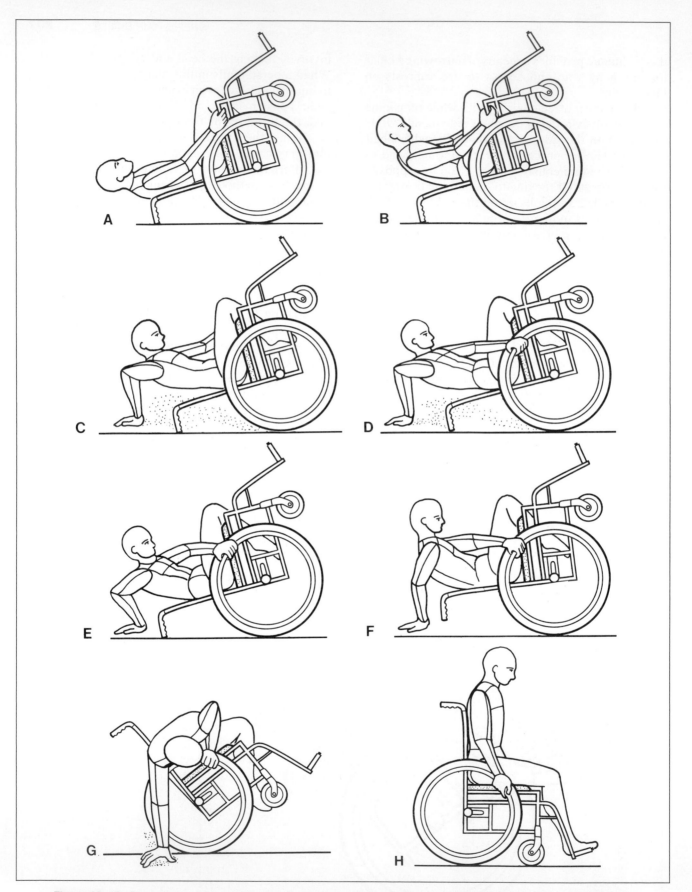

Figure 13–15. Returning to upright after fall. **A.** Starting position: buttocks on seat, legs looped over front edge of seat. **B.** Trunk lifted by pulling on front of wheelchair. **C.** Hand placed on floor. **D.** Opposite wheel grasped. **E. and F.** Rocking wheelchair toward upright by pushing with supporting arm. **G.** Hand inched forward. **H.** Upright.

he will need to position himself in the chair before righting it. To move his buttocks back onto the seat, he pulls on the wheels. He can then grasp his legs and position them, looping them over the seat.

Once positioned appropriately, the person locks the chair's brakes. He then lifts his upper trunk from the floor by pulling on the front of the chair (Fig. 13–15**B**). Once he has lifted his trunk, he releases one hand, turns, and places this hand on the floor (Fig. 13–15**C**). For simplicity, this hand will be called "the supporting hand" for the rest of this description. The other hand will be called "the free hand."

Chart 13–16 Falling Safely and Returning to Upright—Physical Prerequisites

		Falling safely	Block lower extremities while falling safely	Return to upright while remaining in wheelchair
Strength				
	Fully innervated upper extremities	●	√	√
	Sternocleidomastoid		√	
	Biceps, brachialis, and/or brachioradialis		√	
	Hand musculature (active grasp)	●		
Range of Motion				
Scapular	Abduction		√	√
	Adduction			√
	Upward rotation			√
Shoulder	Flexion			√
	Extension			√
	Internal rotation		√	√
	External rotation			√
	Abduction			√
Elbow	Flexion	√	√	√
	Extension	√	√	√

√ = Some strength is needed for this activity, or severe limitations in range will inhibit this activity.
☑ = A large amount of strength or normal or greater range is needed for this activity.
● = Not required, but helpful.

Chart 13–17 Falling Safely and Returning to Upright—Skill Prerequisites

	Falling safely	Return to upright while remaining in wheelchair
While falling backward in wheelchair, tuck head and hold wheels *or* Tuck head and block legs	√	
After falling backward in wheelchair, position self in chair		√
Sitting in overturned wheelchair, lock brakes		√
Sitting in overturned wheelchair, lift upper trunk from floor		√
Sitting in overturned wheelchair, balance on one hand		√
Sitting in overturned wheelchair, rock chair to upright		√

The supporting hand should be positioned directly beneath the trunk, so that weight can be shifted onto it. Balancing on the supporting hand, the person releases the chair. He then reaches his free hand across his body and grasps the opposite wheel (Fig. 13–15**D**).

Righting the chair from this position involves rocking it forward repeatedly and walking the supporting hand around to the side. Rocking the chair is accomplished by bending the elbow of the supporting arm and then extending it (Fig. 13–15**E** and **F**). The push against the floor should be forceful and abrupt enough to thrust the chair toward an upright position. Each time the chair rocks forward, the supporting hand is inched forward around the side of the chair.[8] When the chair falls back from its forward rock, the person balances on his supporting arm and repeats the process.

As the wheelchair user rocks the chair and inches his supporting hand forward, his chair gradually assumes a more upright position (Fig. 13–15**G**). Eventually he will reach a position from which he can thrust hard enough to rock the chair forward past its balance point, returning it to an upright position (Fig. 13–15**H**).

---

[8] This maneuver will be easier if the armrest has been removed, particularly if the wheelchair user is short.

THERAPEUTIC STRATEGIES

General Strategies

To accomplish a functional goal, a patient must acquire both the physical and skill prerequisites for that activity. For example, when working on propelling a hand-controlled power wheelchair, a cord-injured person must develop adequate strength in his shoulder girdle, as well as developing the ability to push the chair's joystick in various directions.

When developing skill prerequisites for a functional goal, the patient should start with the most basic prerequisite skills and progress toward more challenging activities. (A person had best develop skill in maintaining a wheelie before attempting to negotiate stairs in this position.)

Before asking a patient to attempt a new skill, the therapist should explain and demonstrate the technique. The demonstration should provide a clear idea of the motions involved, as well as the timing of these motions. The therapist should also demonstrate how the new skill will be used functionally.

During functional training, the therapist should remember that every cord-injured person will perform a particular activity differently. Each has a unique combination of body build, coordination, strength and flexibility, and these characteristics influence the manner in which he performs functional tasks. As a result of these individual variations, each person is unique in the exact motions that he uses and the timing of these motions as he ascends a curb or rights his wheelchair after a fall. What works for one patient may be a total disaster for the next. The challenge of functional training is finding the timing and maneuvers that best suit the individual involved.

As a therapist and patient work together on a skill, they can learn from failed attempts by analyzing the problem. Is the patient strong enough to perform the maneuver? Did he drop his casters too early or too late as he attempted to ascend the curb? Did he approach the curb with adequate speed? Strategies for addressing the various prerequisite skills are presented below.

Specific Strategies

Sitting in a Wheelchair, Move Trunk Using Head and Scapular Motions. Training in this skill will be easiest if the patient is able to tolerate upright sitting.[9] In a reclined sitting position, weight bearing through the back makes it more difficult to move the trunk laterally.

During initial practice of this skill, the patient can work on moving laterally from a midline sitting position. The therapist can demonstrate the technique and then manually guide him through the motions. The patient then practices throwing his head and shoulder vigorously and repeatedly in one direction at a time. In this manner he can practice moving laterally past his balance point in one direction and then the other.

Early training should also include practice in returning upright from a lateral lean. This practice should start with the patient sitting with a *slight* lean, in a position barely lateral to midline sitting. The therapist should encourage him to move his trunk back to upright using vigorous head and scapular motions.

Once the patient is able to move both toward and away from an upright position, he can combine practice of the two skills, shifting a short distance to the side and returning to upright. As his ability improves, he can gradually increase the arc of motion. He should practice moving laterally toward and away from upright over increasing arcs until he achieves his maximal capability.

Independent Work: Once able to move laterally in and out of upright sitting over small arcs, the patient can practice alone. He should be encouraged to shift as far as he can while maintaining control over the motion; he should move far enough to make the activity challenging but not so far that he cannot return to upright independently.

Place Palms Against Standard Wheelchair Handrims. This prerequisite skill rarely requires much, if any, training. Most people who have the physical potential to propel a manual wheelchair are able to place their palms against their chairs' handrims without practice. However, a few have difficulty recognizing when their palms are in contact with the handrims. These patients require training in this prerequisite skill.

When training is required, the patient should be encouraged to focus on alternative sensory cues to recognize when his hands are placed appropriately. He can concentrate on proprioceptive and tactile sensations from his hands and arms while the therapist places his hands passively on the chair's handrims. He can progress to placing his hands with assistance and finally practice placing his hands without help.

Push Standard Wheelchair Handrim(s) Forward. To practice this skill, a patient should be able to place his palms against the wheelchair's handrims.

---

[9] Training can be initiated in slightly reclined positions before the individual can tolerate fully upright sitting. The therapist and patient should be aware that the task will be easier when the patient sits upright.

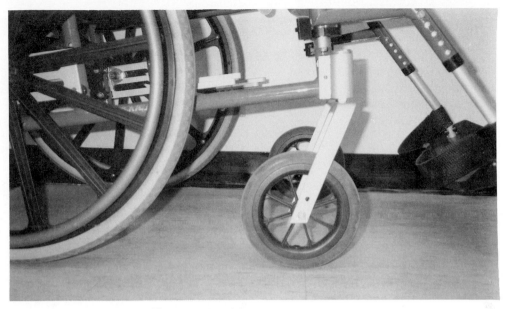

Figure 13–16. Caster in trailing position.

Most people with intact upper extremity musculature are able to push their wheelchair handrims forward without extensive training. At most they may require brief instruction and practice.

People who lack functioning finger flexors require more training to acquire this skill. They must learn to compensate for their lack of active grasp, moving the handrims by pressing their palms inward against the rims and pushing forward. During early practice, therapists may move their patients' hands passively to give them a feel for the motions involved. The patients can then assist with the motions and progress to pushing without assistance.

Since moving a wheelchair's handrims involves moving the wheelchair, a fair amount of upper extremity strength is required. Initially an individual with impaired upper-extremity function may not be strong enough to move his handrims. When this is the case, the therapist can make the task easier by placing the chair's casters in a trailing position (Fig. 13–16). If an individual remains unable to move his handrims despite this positioning, the therapist can assist with the chair's motion. While the patient attempts to push the handrims forward, the therapist pushes the chair, providing just enough force to enable him to move the wheelchair. As his ability and strength improve, the assistance should be decreased.

The functional training strategy described above is appropriate if the individual is on the verge of being able to propel without assistance. This approach has the advantage of enabling the patient to develop propulsion skills using the type of handrims that he will ultimately use. Unfortunately this training strategy does not allow for independent practice.

A different approach may be needed for weaker individuals. When a patient lacks the strength to propel his wheelchair without assistance, the therapist can make the task easier by wrapping the chair's handrims with rubber tubing (Fig. 13–17). The tubing provides small handholds for the patient, making it easier to push the handrims. Since the handholds are small, he must use the same motions to propel the chair as he would without the tubing: he squeezes in and pushes forward. Thus while he practices pushing his chair with his handrims wrapped, he develops the musculature and skills required for propulsion without tubing.[10]

Some people initially lack the strength to push a chair even with the handrims wrapped in tubing. When this is the case, the therapist may resort to placing pegged handrims on the patient's chair. Handrim projections can enable a weak individual to propel his chair, making practice possible. The patient should grow stronger with practice and may eventually build his strength enough to enable him to propel with standard handrims. The disadvantage of practicing with pegged handrims is that the motions used are different from those used to propel

---

[10] One nice thing about rubber tubing is that it deteriorates. Thus as the patient's strength and skill are improving, the tubing is gradually disintegrating. Often the individual's readiness to progress to propulsion without tubing coincides with the tubing's deterioration. This can make the transition to propulsion without tubing easier.

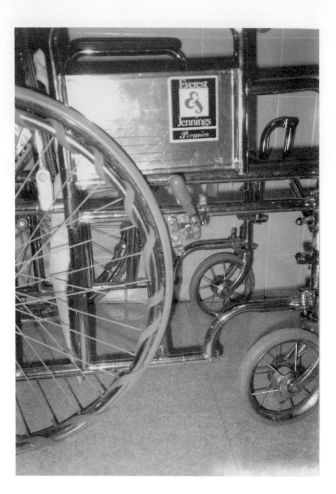

Figure 13–17. Wheelchair handrim wrapped in rubber tubing.

with standard handrims. Instead of squeezing in and pushing forward, the wheelchair user simply pulls forward on the handrim projections. Because the musculature and skills involved are different, the transition from pegged to standard handrims will be more difficult than a transition from wrapped to unwrapped standard handrims.

If a cord-injured person's upper extremity strength is impaired, propulsion will be slow and laborious at first. Therapists should resist the temptation to alter the handrims to make the task easy. A patient will gain maximal benefit from practice in pushing his wheelchair handrims if he practices at the point where the activity is challenging but possible with effort. If a patient can propel his chair, albeit slowly, with unwrapped standard handrims, then he should practice with the handrims unwrapped. If he is unable to do so, wrapping the handrims with rubber tubing is appropriate. If the individual remains unable to push his handrims, a period of practice and strengthening with pegged handrims is indicated.

Pull Standard Wheelchair Handrim(s) Backward. Before working on this skill, a patient should be able to place his palms against the wheelchair's handrims.

Most people with intact upper extremity musculature are able to pull their wheelchair handrims backward without extensive training. At most they may require brief instruction and practice.

People who lack functioning finger flexors require more training to acquire this skill. They must learn to compensate for their lack of active grasp, moving the handrims by pressing their palms inward against the rims and pulling backward. During early practice, therapists may move their patients' hands passively to give them a feel for the motions involved. The patients can then assist with the motions and progress to pulling their handrims backward without assistance.

Since moving a wheelchair's handrims involves moving the wheelchair, a fair amount of upper extremity strength is required. Initially an individual with impaired upper extremity function may not be

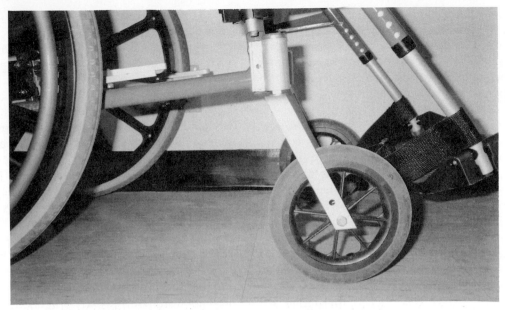

Figure 13–18. Caster positioned anteriorly.

strong enough to move his handrims. When this is the case, the therapist can make the task easier by positioning the chair's casters anteriorly (Fig. 13–18). If an individual remains unable to move his handrims despite this positioning, the therapist can assist. While the patient attempts to pull the handrim(s) backward, the therapist helps move the chair, providing just enough force to enable him to move the wheelchair. As his ability and strength improve, the assistance should be decreased.

Independent Work: Once an individual is able to pull his handrims backward without assistance, he can develop his skill by practicing alone.

Place Palms on Tires, Behind Seat. A patient must be able to place his arms behind his chair's push handles before he begins work on this skill.[11] Once he has acquired that prerequisite skill, learning to place his palms on the tires should require only demonstration and a brief period of practice.

With Palms on Tires Behind Seat, Propel Wheelchair Backwards Using Elbow Extension and Scapular Depression. To practice this skill, a patient should be able to place his palms on his wheelchair's tires, behind the seat. An individual who lacks functional

strength in his triceps must be able to extend his elbows using muscle substitution.[12]

The therapist should first demonstrate the skill, pushing the tires backward using elbow extension and scapular depression. During initial practice, therapists may move their patients' arms passively to give them a feel for the motions involved. The patients can then assist with the motions and progress to pushing their wheels backward without assistance.

Initially a person with impaired upper extremity function may not be strong enough to push his chair backwards. When this is the case, the therapist can make the task easier by positioning the casters anteriorly (Fig. 13–18). If an individual remains unable to propel his chair backwards despite this positioning, the therapist can assist. While the patient attempts to push the chair, the therapist provides just enough force to enable him to move the wheelchair. As his ability and strength improve, this assistance should be decreased.

Independent Work: Once a patient is able to push his handrim backwards without assistance, he can develop his skill by practicing alone.

With Hands on Tires Behind Seat, Propel Wheelchair Backwards Using Scapular Depression. People who are unable to propel their wheelchairs backward using combined elbow extension and scapular

---

[11] Strategies for developing this skill are described in Chapter 11.

[12] Strategies for developing this skill are described in Chapter 11.

depression may learn to do so using scapular depression alone. To practice this skill, a patient should be able to place his palms on the wheelchair's tires, behind the seat. Training can be done using the strategy described above for backward propulsion using elbow extension and scapular depression.

Place Palms or Forearms Against Handrim Projections.

This prerequisite skill rarely requires much, if any, training. Most people who have the physical potential to propel a manual wheelchair are able place their palms or forearms against their chairs' handrim projections without practice. However, a few have difficulty recognizing when their palms or forearms are in contact with the pegs. These individuals require training in this prerequisite skill.

When training is required, the patient should be encouraged to focus on alternative sensory cues to recognize when his arms are placed appropriately. The wheelchair user can concentrate on proprioceptive and tactile sensations from his hands and arms while the therapist places his palms or forearms passively on the chair's handrims. He can progress to placing his hands with assistance and finally practice placing his hands without help.

Pull Handrim Projections Forward.

Once a patient has developed the ability to place his palms or forearms against the posterior aspects of his hair's handrim projections, he can work on pulling these projections forward.

Training in this skill should begin with a demonstration of how a wheelchair can be propelled by placing the hands or forearms behind posteriorly located handrim projections and pulling forward. During early practice, therapists may move their patients' arms passively to give them a feel for the motions involved. Patients can then assist with the motions and progress to pushing without assistance.

Since moving a wheelchair's handrims involves moving the wheelchair, a fair amount of upper extremity strength is required. Initially an individual with impaired upper extremity function may not be strong enough to move his chair's handrims. When this is the case, the therapist can make the task easier by placing the casters in a trailing position (Fig. 13–16). Propulsion will also be easier if the handrim projections are positioned symmetrically on the two sides of the chair. If an individual remains unable to move his handrims despite this positioning of the casters and pegs, the therapist can assist with the chair's motion. While the patient attempts to push the handrims forward, the therapist pushes the chair, providing just enough force to enable him to move the wheelchair. As the patient's ability and

strength improve, this assistance should be decreased.

If a patient is able to propel his wheelchair forward easily, he is probably ready to work with standard handrims.

Independent Work: Once a patient is able to pull his handrim projections forward without assistance, he can develop his skill by practicing alone.

Pull Backward on Handrim Projections.

Before practicing this skill, a person should be able to place his palms or forearms against the anterior aspects of his chair's handrim projections.

Training in this skill should begin with a demonstration of how a wheelchair can be propelled backward by placing the hands or forearms in front of anteriorly located handrim projections and pulling backward. During early practice, therapists may move their patients' arms passively to give them a feel for the motions involved. Patients can then assist with the motions and progress to pushing without assistance.

Initially an individual with impaired upper extremity function may not be strong enough to move his chair's handrims. When this is the case, the therapist can make the task easier by positioning the casters anteriorly (Fig. 13–18). Propulsion will also be easier if the handrim projections are positioned symmetrically on the two sides of the chair. If a patient remains unable to move his handrims despite this positioning of the casters and pegs, the therapist can assist with the chair's motion. While the patient attempts to pull the handrims backward, the therapist pushes the chair, providing just enough force to enable him to move the wheelchair. As his ability and strength improve, this assistance should be decreased.

Propel Manual Wheelchair Over Even Surfaces.

Once an individual is able to push his handrims forward, with or without assistance, he is ready to begin work on forward wheelchair propulsion. The training strategy is the same whether the patient uses pegged or standard handrims.

For people who can push their handrims forward easily, efficient propulsion is readily achieved. The therapist should demonstrate, showing how long strokes make propulsion less energy consuming. The patient should be encouraged to start each push with his hands well back, then push through and allow the chair to glide between strokes. During early practice, the therapist should give the patient feedback on his propulsion technique. The patient can then practice on his own.

Wheelchair propulsion training is more time consuming for people who have difficulty pushing their handrims forward. Before learning the finer points of efficient propulsion, these patients must learn to propel. This takes practice, practice, and more practice. Propulsion is likely to be painfully slow at first, but the patient should grow stronger and faster with practice. He should be encouraged to push wherever he goes in the course of each day. As his ability improves, he can work on developing a more efficient pattern of propulsion.

The therapist and patient should remember that wheelchair propulsion will be difficult initially if upper extremity musculature is impaired. Pushing is likely to be too slow to be functional at first, but the patient should keep at it. The only way to become more proficient is to practice.

Independent Work: Once an individual is able to propel his chair forward and turn without assistance, he can practice independently. He should be encouraged to push to therapies and meals during the day, and can propel during his free time in the evenings.

Place Hand on Joystick. A person who has enough strength in his deltoids and biceps to move well against gravity should be able to learn to place his hand on his wheelchair's joystick without difficulty. He may require only a demonstration and brief practice.

Someone with limited ability to move against gravity in elbow flexion and shoulder flexion and abduction may be able to learn this skill but will require more practice. An individual with such pronounced upper-extremity weakness places his arm on the joystick using a combination of scapular, shoulder, and elbow motions. The maneuvers used are determined by the arm's starting position. If the arm is initially positioned hanging down outside of the armrest, the person elevates his scapula to lift his arm. By partially abducting and internally rotating his shoulder, he places his elbow in a gravity-reduced position for elbow flexion. He can then place his hand on the joystick by flexing his elbow.

If the person's arm is positioned in his lap, he first moves the arm to the outside of his armrest. This is accomplished through a combination of scapular elevation and retraction, shoulder abduction and external rotation, and elbow flexion. Once his arm is positioned outside of the armrest, he can lift it onto the joystick using the maneuver described above.

When an individual has limited ability to move his shoulder and elbow against gravity, practice of the required motions may begin with the arm suspended in a sling or supported by a skateboard placed on a board (Fig. 13–19). Using this equipment, the patient can practice moving repeatedly through gravity-eliminated arcs. As his strength and skill improve, he can progress to moving up a slight slope and increase the slope as appropriate. With different positions of the sling or board, he can work on moving his shoulder and elbow through the various motions required to place his hand on a joystick. In this manner he can build the strength required for this skill.

Skill training can begin with the patient working on moving his hand onto the joystick from a position just lateral to the stick. As his ability improves, he can move his hand from positions progressively lateral and inferior to the joystick. In this manner he can gradually develop the ability to lift his hand onto the joystick, starting with his arm hanging at his side lateral to the armrest. The ability to perform this skill with the arm initially positioned in the lap can be developed using the same strategy: the patient begins by repeatedly placing his hand from a position just medial to the joystick. As his skill builds, he works from progressively medial and inferior starting positions.

Independent Work: The strengthening and skill practice described above are ideal independent exercises.

Move Joystick In All Directions Using Arm and Scapular Motions. When a joystick is mounted for hand control, it is mounted vertically. To control his wheelchair, the person must be able to move his hand in all directions in the horizontal plane. Independent placement of the hand on the joystick is not necessary for practicing this skill.

Practice in moving a joystick should be done with the wheelchair's motor disconnected. The patient can then work on pushing the stick in various directions without having the chair whirl about uncontrollably.

People with good scapular and shoulder control are not likely to need much training to master this skill. They may require only a demonstration and brief period of practice.

Individuals with weaker proximal musculature require more extensive training. Before learning to push a joystick, they must develop the ability to perform the necessary motions. Practice may begin with the arm suspended in a sling or supported by a skateboard placed on a board (Fig. 13–19). Using this equipment the patient can practice moving his hand in all directions in the horizontal plane. Back-

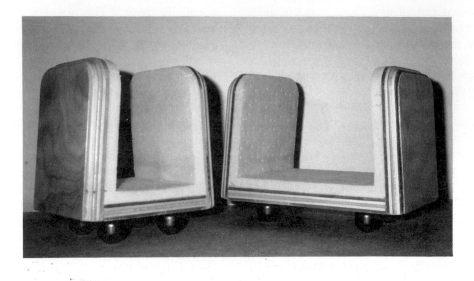

Figure 13–19. Skateboards.

ward and forward motion can be accomplished using scapular adduction and abduction.[13] Glenohumeral horizontal adduction and abduction are used for lateral motions. Diagonal motions are performed by combining these glenohumeral and scapular motions.

Once able to move his hand well with his arm supported by a sling or skateboard, the patient can practice using a joystick. If he remains unable to move the joystick, the therapist can facilitate practice by making the task easier. This can be done by suspending the arm in a sling, splinting the elbow and wrist, and strapping the hand to the joystick. As the patient's skill improves with practice, these "crutches" can be removed.[14]

Independent Work: The strengthening and skill practice described above are ideal independent exercises.

Move Joystick in all Directions Using Chin or Tongue Motions. When a joystick is mounted for chin or mouth control, it is placed in a position close to horizontal; the end of the joystick moves in a nearly vertical plane. To control his wheelchair, the person moves the end of the joystick in all directions within this plane. With chin control, neck and jaw motions are used to move the stick up, down, laterally, and diagonally. With mouth control, the patient uses his tongue to push the joystick.

This skill should not require much training to achieve. The therapist should explain and demonstrate the motions and allow the patient to practice pushing the stick in all directions. Practice moving the joystick should be done with the wheelchair's motor disconnected.

Signal Wheelchair by Sipping and Puffing in Appropriate Pattern. This skill should not require extensive training to achieve. The therapist should explain and demonstrate the sipping and puffing pattern and allow the patient to practice. Initial practice should be done with the wheelchair's motor disconnected.

Propel Electric Wheelchair Over Even Surfaces. Before practicing propulsion of an electric wheelchair, a person must be able to operate the controls. He must be able to signal his wheelchair either by pushing a joystick in all directions (hand, chin, or mouth control) or by sipping and puffing.

Unlike practice in manipulating an electric wheelchair's controls, practice in propulsion begins

---

[13] In the absence of active scapular abduction, the patient can adduct actively using the middle trapezius and allow passive abduction upon relaxation of the trapezius.

[14] The "crutches" should be removed one at a time as skill increases. With each removal, the patient's performance can be expected to deteriorate temporarily until his skill improves.

with the motor connected. Training should begin in a large area that is free of obstacles and potential victims. The chair should be set to operate at a low speed, and a therapist should be present to override the controls when necessary.

During early work on propulsion, emphasis should be placed on gaining *control* of the chair. The patient should practice starting, stopping, and maneuvering in all directions. Once he has mastered these tasks, he can progress to propelling over greater distances and maneuvering around obstacles.

For people with C4 quadriplegia, learning to use hand controls for wheelchair propulsion can be a challenging task. During early practice, the patient may require added equipment to make the task easier. A sling to suspend the arm, splints to stabilize the elbow and wrist, and a strap to hold the hand on the joystick may facilitate practice. These "crutches" can be removed, one at a time, as skill and strength improve with practice.[15]

Independent Work: Once an individual has gained some ability to control his chair, he can practice without constant supervision. He may first practice within the department, where assistance is available when needed. As his skill and confidence improve, he can practice in other areas, further removed from assistance.

Propel Manual Wheelchair up a Slope. To practice this skill, a person must be able to propel a manual wheelchair independently over even surfaces. Since ascending a slope takes greater strength and skill than does propelling on a horizontal surface, the patient should be fairly skillful in wheelchair propulsion prior to beginning ramp negotiation practice.

Before attempting to ascend a ramp, the patient should be shown proper technique: each push is forceful but not abrupt, and the hands are repositioned rapidly between pushes. When pushing and repositioning, he should move his hands simultaneously and symmetrically. The strokes are shorter than those used for propulsion over even surfaces. Forward flexion of the head, and, if possible, trunk can help prevent backward tipping.

Practice in ramp negotiation should begin on a ramp with a very gentle slope. Initially the patient may not be able to push the chair forcefully enough to ascend. When this is the case, the therapist can assist, applying just enough force to the chair's push handles to enable the patient to push up the ramp with maximal effort. The assistance should be reduced as his ability improves with practice.

People learning to push their wheelchairs up ramps often reposition their hands too slowly between pushes, allowing their chairs to roll backward excessively. Guarding is required to ensure safety at this point. While guarding, the therapist should allow a slight backward roll between pushes. The chair's motion, combined with verbal cueing, can provide feedback to the patient regarding his technique.

As a patient's skill in ascending slopes increases, the assistance given should be reduced. Once the individual masters a slope of a particular grade, he should progress to steeper slopes. Training in ramp negotiation can continue in this manner until the patient has reached his maximal potential.

Descending Slope on Four Wheels, Control Wheelchair by Applying Friction to the Handrims. When descending a slope on four wheels, the wheelchair user controls his chair's descent by applying friction to the handrims as they slide past his hands. He does this by gripping the handrims loosely or by pressing his palms inward against the rims, depending on whether or not his finger flexors are innervated.

During functional training, emphasis should be placed on *controlling* the chair's descent. To negotiate a ramp safely, a person must be able to stop the chair or to turn while descending. This is possible only if he maintains control throughout the descent rather than releasing the handrims and trying to regain control when the need arises.

Practice in descending ramps should begin on gentle slopes at low speeds. Once an individual has developed the ability to slow, stop, and turn a manual wheelchair while slowly descending a gentle slope, he can progress to practicing at higher speeds and on steeper inclines.

Even on a mild incline and at a slow speed, a patient may be unable to control his chair's descent at first. When this is the case, the therapist can help to slow the chair. The therapist should apply just enough force to the push handles (resisting the chair's downhill motion) to enable the person to control the chair with maximal effort. This assistance can be reduced as the patient's ability improves.

Maintain Balance Point in Wheelie Position. The balance point in a wheelie is the position in which a wheelchair is balanced on its rear wheels. A chair at its balance point is in equilibrium, falling neither forward nor backward. A patient need not be able

---

[15] For additional training strategies, the reader is referred to "Power Wheelchair Training for Patients With Marginal Upper Extremity Function" (O'Neil & Seelye, 1990).

to assume his balance point independently before beginning practice in maintaining this position.

The first step in teaching a person how to maintain his balance point in a wheelie is showing him where that point is located. If the individual has an inaccurate understanding of where his balance point is located, he will be unable to maintain the correct position. (If his notion of the balance point is tilted forward from the correct position, he will resist tipping back his chair far enough. As a result he will constantly fall forward.) To teach a person where his balance point is located, the therapist can demonstrate in his own chair and then tip the patient back[16] and allow him to feel the position (Fig. 13–20A).

After showing the patient his balance point, the therapist should teach him how to control his chair in a wheelie. With the therapist guarding closely, the patient can pull his handrims forward and back while in a wheelie position, paying attention to the effects that these maneuvers have on the chair's position (Fig. 13–20B and C). Gross motions are acceptable at this point; the purpose of this exercise is to familiarize the patient with the control motions.

Once the patient has learned how to tip his chair forward and back in a wheelie, he is ready to begin working on maintaining his balance point. The therapist can assist the patient to the balance point and encourage him to keep the chair balanced. The therapist should spot closely while the patient makes adjustments in his position. The patient is likely to overcorrect at first. He should be encouraged to maintain his balance with smaller corrections.

From this point on in the functional training, hands-off guarding is best (Fig. 13–20D). If the therapist's hands remain on the push handles while the patient works to maintain his balance, the therapist is likely to make corrections for him. This will deprive the patient of practice and can make it difficult for him to discern when he has moved off his balance point. The therapist should allow the chair to fall a short distance when it moves out of the balance point, so the patient can feel that he has lost his balance and needs to make corrections.

Fear is often the largest barrier to learning this skill. Someone who is afraid of falling over back-

wards is unlikely to allow himself to remain tipped far enough back to balance. He will attempt to maintain the chair's wheelie in a position tilted too far forward and as a result will not be able to balance. This tendency is compounded by the fact that wheelchairs balance at a point that is tilted further back than most would expect. A patient may feel as though he is about to fall backward when he is at his balance point. Therapists can aid the process of learning to maintain a balanced wheelie by attending to their patients' feelings during functional training. The therapist should remain reassuring and calm and should encourage the patient to relax. When assisting a fearful patient to his balance point, the therapist should avoid quick, jerky motions that may increase the patient's fear. In addition, the therapist can assure the patient that he will catch him if he starts to fall.

Independent Work: If a patient is able to get into a balanced wheelie position without assistance, he can practice maintaining that position independently. Figure 13–21 illustrates a setup in which the wheelchair's push handles are secured to suspended straps. The straps are attached with enough slack to allow the patient to move slightly past his balance point but without enough slack to allow him to fall to the floor.

Assume Wheelie Position. In a wheelie, the wheelchair rests on its rear wheels with the casters off the ground. To assume a wheelie position, the wheelchair user essentially tips his chair over backwards. This skill may be easier to acquire if the patient has initiated (not necessarily completed) training in maintaining his balance in a wheelie. This prior exposure to wheelies can give him an understanding of how far back he must tip his chair, and it can make him less fearful about falling over backwards.

A wheelchair's construction influences the difficulty of this task. An ultralight wheelchair with its axles positioned relatively anteriorly is easy to tip backwards. With a heavier wheelchair or more posteriorly located axles, the task is more difficult.

With intact upper extremities, and an ultralight wheelchair, the wheelie position can be attained easily from a stationary position. The wheelchair user grasps[17] the handrims posteriorly and pulls them forward abruptly and forcefully. If an individ-

---

[16] The therapist should take care to show the patient his true balance point. The balance point is easily found if the therapist pays attention to the force that he must exert on the chair to keep it tipped back on the rear wheels. At the balance point the chair will remain in position (briefly) without any assistance from the therapist. If the chair is tipped too far back or forward, the therapist will have to apply force to keep the chair from tipping further back or forward, respectively.

---

[17] An individual who lacks functioning finger flexors moves his handrims using friction, pressing in on the rims instead of grasping them.

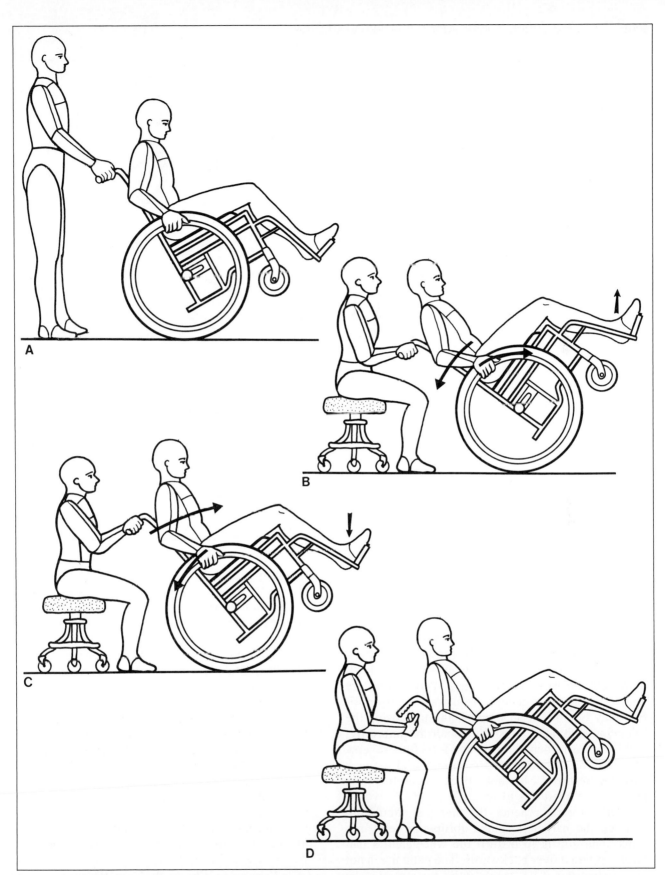

Figure 13–20. Instruction in maintaining balance point in wheelie. **A.** Therapist places patient in balanced wheelie position. **B.** Chair tips further back when wheels are pushed forward. **C.** Chair tips toward upright when wheels are pulled back. **D.** Noncontact guarding for wheelie practice.

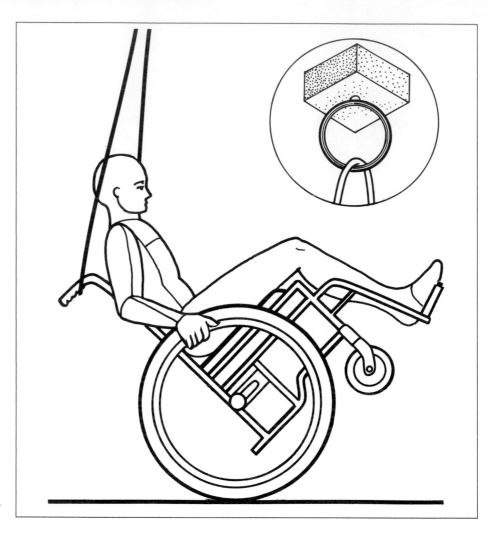

Figure 13–21. Safety rigging for independent practice of achieving and maintaining wheelie position.

ual is unable to lift his casters in this manner, he may be able to do so by throwing his head back forcefully when he pulls his handrims.

Impaired upper extremity function, a heavy wheelchair, or posteriorly located axles make it more difficult to tilt a chair back. People who are unable to "pop a wheelie" from a stationary position may be able to accomplish the task using the following technique: grasp the handrims anteriorly, pull backward, then abruptly and forcefully reverse the direction of pull. The person may find the task easier if he throws his head back forcefully when he pulls the handrims forward.

During early practice the therapist should encourage the patient to make abrupt, forceful motions. The aim is to disturb the wheelchair's balance, tipping it over backwards. The patient will not accomplish this if he "eases into" his motions. To gain enough momentum to tilt his chair, he may need to exaggerate his motions at first. He can refine his motions as he develops a feel for the maneuver.

An individual who is unable to lift his casters may be pulling his handrims, in the wrong direction, throwing his head in the wrong direction, or timing his maneuvers inappropriately. The therapist should observe him closely as he makes his attempts and give him feedback on his technique.

Independent Work: For some, this skill takes a good deal of practice to achieve. Independent work will make this extensive practice feasible. Safety rigging, described above and illustrated in Figure 13–21, is required to keep the patient from falling backwards. With this safety rigging, an individual who has been instructed and has received some initial practice and feedback can independently practice attaining his balance point.

Glide Forward in Wheelie Position. Before beginning training in this skill, a person should be able to assume and to maintain his balance point in a wheelie.

To initiate a forward glide in a wheelie, the

wheelchair user positions his chair at its balance point (Fig. 13–22A) and tips the chair forward slightly. The forward tilt will make the chair start to fall forward (dip); (Fig. 13–22B). The person counteracts this fall and propels the chair forward by pushing forward on the handrims (Fig. 13–22C). He should allow the rims to slide through his hands as his chair glides forward in its balance point (Fig. 13–22D). From the balance point he can repeat the dip and push. By repeating this sequence of actions, the wheelchair user glides forward in a wheelie.

After demonstrating and explaining how to glide in a wheelie, the therapist should allow the patient to practice with spotting.[18] The chair's motions are likely to be jerky at first, with exaggerated up and down motions. As the patient gains skill and confidence, the therapist should encourage him to smooth out the motion. The patient should also work to gain *control* of his glide; to use a glide functionally, he will need to be able to glide at various speeds, turn, and stop his chair at will. With practice, he should gain the capacity to glide faster, with greater control, and with less vertical motion of the casters.

Independent Work: A patient should practice this skill independently *only after he has learned to fall safely.* Once he can fall safely and has developed some initial skill in a wheelie glide, he can practice on his own.

Turn in Wheelie Position. Before initiating practice of this skill, the patient should be able to assume and to maintain his balance point in a wheelie.

Turning while balanced on two wheels can be accomplished by pushing one handrim forward while pulling the other back. As he does this, the wheelchair user must make adjustments as necessary to keep his chair in a balanced position. To turn while propelling forward or backward in a wheelie, he can push or pull one handrim more forcefully than the other.

After demonstrating and explaining how to turn in a wheelie, the therapist should allow the patient to practice with spotting.[19] At first, the chair's motions are likely to be jerky, with excessive vertical motions of the casters. As the patient gains skill and confidence, the therapist should encourage him to smooth out the motion.

---

[18] As was explained above, the therapist should avoid touching the wheelchair while spotting. His hands should be poised under the push handles, ready to catch if needed.

[19] As was explained above, the therapist should avoid touching the wheelchair while spotting. His hands should be poised under the push handles, ready to catch if needed.

Independent Work: A patient should practice this skill independently *only after he has learned to fall safely.* Once he can fall safely and has developed some initial skill in turning in a wheelie, he can practice on his own.

Propel Backward In Wheelie Position. To practice this skill, a patient should be able to assume and to maintain his balance point in a wheelie.

Propelling backward in a wheelie is like gliding forward, with the actions performed in reverse. From a balanced wheelie position, the wheelchair user tips his chair back slightly. The backward tilt will make the chair start to fall backward. The person counteracts this fall and propels the chair backward by pulling back on the handrims.

After demonstrating and explaining how to propel backward in a wheelie, the therapist should allow the patient to practice with spotting.[20] At first, the chair's motions are likely to be jerky. As the patient gains skill and confidence, the therapist can encourage him to smooth out the motion.

Independent Work: A patient should practice this skill independently *only after he has learned to fall safely.* Once he can fall safely and has developed some initial skill in backward propulsion in a wheelie, he can practice on his own.

Descending Slope on Two Wheels, Control Wheelchair by Applying Friction to Handrims. When descending a slope in a wheelie, the wheelchair user controls the chair's descent by applying friction to the handrims as he allows them to slide through his hands. The force applied to the handrims should be light, giving slight resistance to the rims' forward motion.

This skill can be taught using the functional training strategies used to teach descending a ramp on four wheels. Before beginning training, the patient should be skillful in gliding forward and turning in a wheelie.

From Stationary Position, Lift Casters From Floor. Before learning to lift his casters from the floor, the patient should be proficient in forward propulsion over even surfaces. He need not be able to assume or to maintain a balanced wheelie position.

Lifting a wheelchair's casters from the floor is a lesser version of assuming the wheelie position; the same maneuvers are used, but they are performed less forcefully. To teach a patient to lift his

---

[20] As was explained above, the therapist should avoid touching the wheelchair while spotting. His hands should be poised under the push handles, ready to catch if needed.

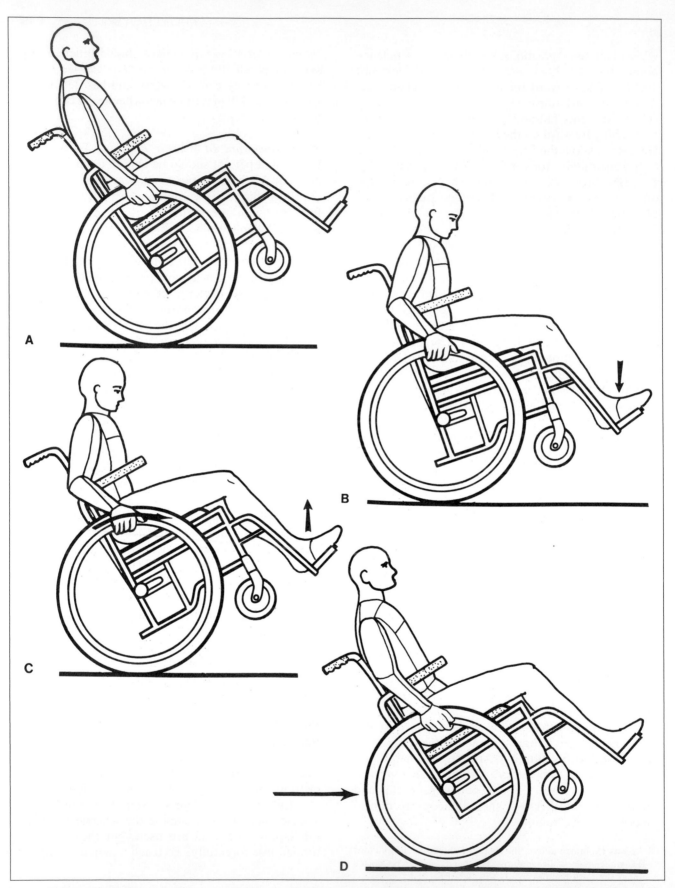

Figure 13–22. Forward glide in a wheelie. **A.** Starting position: balanced wheelie position. **B.** Wheelchair falls forward slightly. **C.** Forward push on handrims propels chair forward and lifts casters. **D.** Glide in balance point.

casters, the therapist can use the training strategies presented above for teaching a patient to assume a balanced wheelie position.

Pop Casters onto Curb From Stationary Position. Training in this skill should begin after the patient has acquired the ability to lift his wheelchair's casters from the floor from a stationary position. Once an individual can lift his casters consistently, he can practice popping his casters onto small (1-inch) curbs. As his skill develops, he can progress to taller curbs.

Independent Work: A patient who is independent in lowering his chair's casters from a curb and has developed some initial skill in popping his casters onto a curb can practice alone. If his skill level is such that he is likely to tip his chair over backward and if he has not learned to fall safely, he can practice while using safety rigging as shown in Figure 13–21.

Position Casters at Edge of Curb. When a cord-injured person ascends a curb from a stationary position, he first pops his chair's casters onto the curb and then backs them to the edge of the curb. This repositioning requires proficiency in backward propulsion and turning. Training in repositioning the casters on the curb will be easier if the patient is able to place his casters on the curb.

A person with the physical potential to ascend curbs should be able to master this prerequisite skill with minimal practice. During training, the therapist should emphasize placing the casters right at the edge of the curb (Fig. 13–23A). Placing the casters in this position maximizes the distance between the curb and the chair's rear wheels (Fig. 13–23B). This increased distance makes it possible to gain more momentum for ascending the curb.

Independent Work: This skill can be practiced concurrently with placing the casters on and lowering them from a curb if the patient has developed some

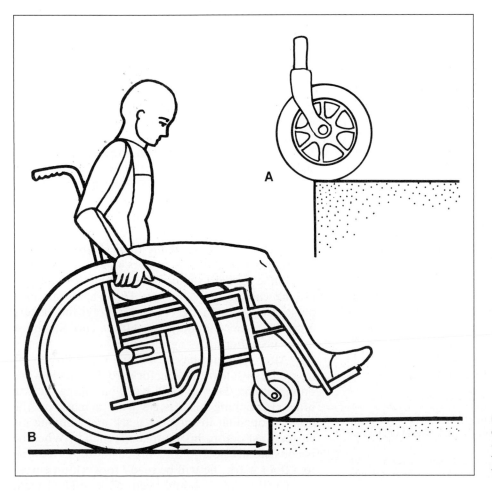

Figure 13–23. Positioning casters at edge of curb. **A.** Correct caster position. **B.** Caster position maximizes distance between curb and rear wheels.

ability in each of these maneuvers. If his skill level is such that he is likely to tip his chair over backward and if he has not learned to fall safely, the patient can practice using safety rigging, as shown in Figure 13–21.

Ascend Curb From Stationary Position. To practice ascending a curb from a stationary position, a patient must be proficient in forward propulsion. Training will be easier if he can place his casters on the curb and position them at the curb's edge.

Once a wheelchair user has positioned his casters appropriately to ascend a curb, he grasps[21] the chair's handrims posteriorly and pulls forward forcefully. To add to the chair's forward momentum, he throws his head and (if possible) trunk forward as his chair approaches the curb. This added momentum is especially important with higher curbs or when the individual's upper extremity musculature is impaired.

Training should start on a small (1-inch) curb. As the person's skill improves, he can progress to taller curbs. The curb height should be increased in small increments, with the patient progressing only when he is able to ascend a curb of a given height consistently.

Independent Work: A patient should practice this skill independently *only after he has learned to fall safely.* Once he can fall safely and has developed some initial skill in curb negotiation, he can practice on his own.

Lift Casters Off of Floor While Chair Moves Forward. Lifting a wheelchair's casters while propelling forward is more difficult than doing so from a stationary position. Impaired upper extremity function, a heavy wheelchair, or posteriorly located axles will make it difficult to accomplish this task. However, these factors will not necessarily prevent acquisition of this skill.

This maneuver requires appropriate timing rather than the application of brute force. To lift his casters while propelling forward, a wheelchair user grasps[22] his handrims posteriorly and pulls them forward abruptly and forcefully. If he is unable to lift his casters in this manner, he may be able to do so by throwing his head back forcefully when he pulls his handrims.

---

[21] A person who lacks functioning finger flexors moves his handrims using friction, pressing in on the rims instead of grasping them.

[22] A person who lacks functioning finger flexors moves his handrims using friction, pressing in on the rims instead of grasping them.

With intact upper extremities and an ultralight wheelchair, many patients are able to master this skill without excessive difficulty. During early practice the therapist should encourage the patient to make abrupt, forceful motions. The aim is to disturb the wheelchair's balance, tipping it backwards. The patient will not accomplish this if he "eases into" his motions. To gain enough momentum to lift his casters, he may need to exaggerate his motions at first. He can refine his technique as he develops a feel for the maneuver.

An individual who is unable to lift his casters may be pulling his handrims in the wrong direction throwing his head in the wrong direction, or timing his maneuvers inappropriately. The therapist should observe him closely as he makes his attempts and give him feedback on his technique.

Fear is a potential roadblock to acquiring this skill; someone who is afraid that he will fall over backward may not pull on the handrims forcefully enough. For this reason this skill may be easier to acquire if the patient has initiated (not necessarily completed) training in maintaining his balance in a wheelie. This prior exposure to wheelies can give him an understanding of how far back he must tip his chair to fall, and it can make him less fearful about falling over backward when lifting his casters from the floor.

During early practice lifting his casters while propelling his chair forward, the patient can work at low speeds. As his skill develops, he can increase his speed.

Independent Work: A person should practice this skill independently *only after he has learned to fall safely.* Once he can fall safely and has developed some initial skill in lifting his casters while propelling forward, he can practice on his own.

Pop Casters onto Curb While Chair Moves Forward. Popping a wheelchair's casters onto a curb while propelling forward requires more than the ability to lift the casters high enough. The wheelchair user must time the maneuver appropriately: the casters must lift before the footplates hit the curb and must lower just after crossing the curb.

After a patient has developed the ability to lift his casters while propelling forward, he should work on his timing. During early work on timing, he can practice popping his casters over a mark on the floor, propelling toward the mark and popping his casters just before his footplates reach it. When he is consistently able to time his caster lift in relation to a floor mark, he will be ready to work on curbs.

Curb training should begin on a small (1-inch)

curb, with the patient progressing to higher curbs as his skill develops. Once he has developed some skill in popping his casters onto a curb of a given height, he can practice this maneuver concurrently with ascending the curb using momentum.

Independent Work: When a patient performs this maneuver with improper timing, he may fall forward out of his chair or tip the chair over backward. For this reason this skill should be practiced independently only after the patient has had a good deal of practice and is not likely to fall. In addition, he should practice this skill independently *only after he has learned to fall safely.*

Ascend Curb Using Momentum. Before initiating practice in ascending curbs using momentum, a patient must be able to lift his casters off of the floor while propelling forward. He must also have developed some skill in popping his casters onto a curb while his chair moves forward, but he need not have perfected this maneuver.

To ascend a curb using momentum, a wheelchair user approaches the curb front on and pops his casters onto the curb at the last moment. Timing

is crucial; the casters should lift over the curb and land just before the rear wheels hit the curb. If the maneuver is timed correctly and the wheelchair has approached the curb with enough speed, momentum will carry the chair up the curb. During functional training, the therapist should carefully observe the patient's timing so that he can provide feedback. He should also encourage the patient to be aware of the timing.

For most people a good deal of practice is required to learn this skill. Training should start on a small (1-inch) curb. As the patient's skill improves, he can progress to taller curbs. The curb height should be increased in small increments, with the patient progressing only when he is able to ascend a curb of a given height consistently.

Close spotting is required as the patient works on ascending curbs using momentum. If the chair is not tipped back enough or if it drops too early as it approaches the curb, the casters will hit the curb's vertical surface (Fig. 13–24A). The chair will stop abruptly, and the rider may be thrown forward out of the chair. If the casters drop too late, the rear wheels will hit first while the chair is still tipped back (Fig. 13–24B). Again, the chair is likely to stop ab-

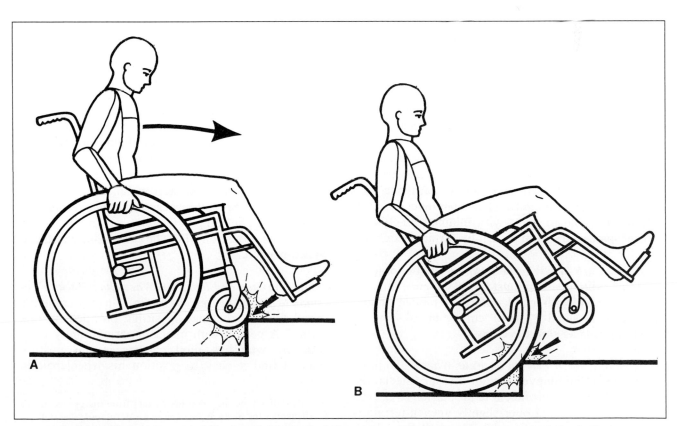

Figure 13–24. Problems resulting from improper technique when ascending curb using momentum. **A.** Caster strikes curb's vertical surface. **B.** Rear wheel strikes curb while chair still tipped back.

ruptly. On a tall curb, an abrupt stop can cause the chair to fall over backward.

Since a patient can fall forward or backward during curb negotiation practice, the therapist must be prepared to catch in either direction. The therapist can guard from behind, following closely as the patient propels toward the curb. Alternatively the therapist can guard from the front. This involves standing beside the curb, prepared to catch when the patient reaches it.

Practice in curb ascent and descent can be combined: after an individual succeeds in popping his casters onto the curb or ascending the curb, he can practice getting back down.

Independent Work: This skill should be practiced independently only after the patient has had a good deal of practice and is not likely to fall. In addition, he should practice this skill independently *only after he has learned to fall safely*. He should also be able to descend curbs without assistance.

Backing Down Curb, Control Rear Wheels' Descent. Backing a wheelchair down a curb under control requires the ability to apply a strong forward force on the wheels. A patient should be skillful in forward manual wheelchair propulsion before beginning practice backing down a curb.

Functional training in this skill should emphasize developing control. The patient should practice backing just past the curb's edge and resisting the chair's motion as gravity pulls it downward. Training should begin on small (1-inch) curbs, progressing to higher curbs as skill develops. Curb descent can be practiced concurrently with curb ascent.

Lower Casters From Curb by Turning Wheelchair. To perform this maneuver, a person need only be able to turn his wheelchair in a tight arc. Anyone who is able to propel a manual wheelchair independently should be able to learn with minimal practice to lower his casters from a curb by turning his chair.

Descend Curb in a Wheelie Position. Before practicing this skill, a patient must be able to glide forward in a wheelie with good control. Training should begin with small (1-inch) curbs, progressing to higher curbs as skill develops.

Negotiate Uneven Terrain on Four Wheels. To practice negotiating uneven terrain on four wheels, the patient should be proficient in propulsion over even surfaces. Propelling over slightly uneven terrain is primarily a matter of pushing hard. If the wheelchair's progress is impeded by a tough spot, such

as a clump of grass, the person may be able to get past it by backing up and ramming the obstacle.[23]

Practice should start with slightly uneven terrain, such as a level sidewalk that is in good condition. As the patient's strength and skill improve, he can progress to more challenging surfaces such as grass, sand, gravel, and sidewalks in disrepair. The patient should practice propelling over the various surfaces that he is likely to encounter after his rehabilitation.

Independent Work: A patient can work on this skill independently once he has gained some ability. He should practice where he can obtain assistance when needed, in case he gets stuck.

Negotiate Uneven Terrain In a Wheelie. The challenge of negotiating uneven terrain in a wheelie is maintaining one's balance. While pushing hard to propel his chair over irregularities in the supporting surface, the wheelchair user must compensate for the effects that these irregularities have on the chair's equilibrium.

Before beginning work on this skill, a patient should be proficient in propulsion forward, backward, and turning in a wheelie on even surfaces. Once skillful on even surfaces, he can begin work on a slightly uneven surface such as a sidewalk that is in good condition. As his strength and skill improve, he can progress to more challenging surfaces, such as grass, sand, gravel, and sidewalks in disrepair. The patient should practice propelling over the various surfaces that he is likely to encounter after his rehabilitation.

Independent Work: A patient should practice this skill independently *only after he has learned to fall safely*. Ideally he should also be able to right his chair after a fall. Once he can fall safely and has developed some skill in negotiating uneven terrain in a wheelie, he can practice on his own. He should practice in a location where he can obtain assistance when needed.

Sitting on Step or Floor, Tilt Wheelchair Back to Position to Ascend or Descend Stairs. This skill requires good dynamic balance in sitting propped on one arm.[24] A person with intact upper extremity musculature who has good balance in this posture should find it easy to position his wheelchair in

---

[23] Alternatively he may pop his casters from the ground to lift them over the obstacle. Strategies for developing this skill are described above.

[24] This skill is addressed in Chapter 11.

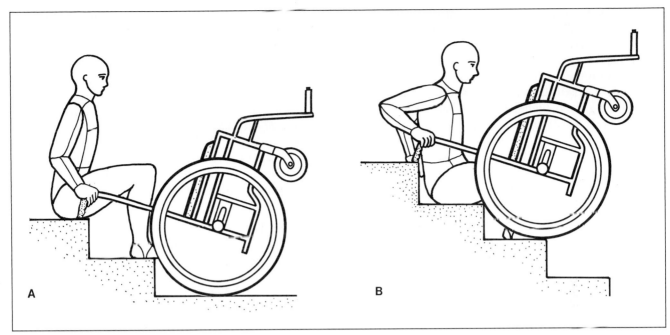

Figure 13–25. Stabilizing wheelchair while ascending stairs. **A.** Early practice on lower step, with rear wheel on floor. **B.** Practice on higher step, wheelchair's rear wheel resting on stairs.

preparation to ascend or to descend stairs on his buttocks. He simply grasps a push handle and pulls on it to turn and tip the chair. A brief period of practice should be sufficient to master this maneuver.

Sitting on Step, Stabilize Wheelchair by Pushing Down Through Push Handles. Before beginning work on this skill, a patient must have good balance when positioned in short-sitting propped forward on two arms.[25] People with the physical potential to ascend stairs on their buttocks should learn without difficulty to stabilize their wheelchairs.

During functional training, the patient should be encouraged to push straight downward through the chair's push handle. An obliquely directed push may cause the chair to slide on the step. Practice should start with the patient sitting on a step that is close to the base of the stairway. A wheelchair is easier to stabilize in this location, since it is supported by the floor (Fig. 13–25**A**). After brief practice at the base of the stairs, the patient can progress to practicing on higher steps, where the chair is not supported by the floor (Fig. 13–25**B**).

Transfer up a Step While Stabilizing Wheelchair. Training in this skill should begin after the patient can stabilize his wheelchair while sitting on stairs.

He must also be proficient in using the head-hips relationship and performing step-high, back-approach, uneven transfers from the floor.[26]

Before an individual becomes skillful in this maneuver, he may have difficulty stabilizing his chair while transferring. While concentrating on the transfer between stairs, the inexperienced patient may apply an obliquely directed force to the chair's push handle, causing it to slide. The therapist should encourage him to push straight downward through the push handle as he transfers.

Practice should begin on a low step, where the chair is supported by the floor. As the patient's skill develops, he should progress to transferring from higher steps, where the chair is not supported by the floor (Fig. 13–25). After he has developed some skill in transferring up a step while stabilizing his chair, he can practice this skill concurrently with the skill of pulling the chair up a step.

Sitting on Step, Position Buttocks and Legs While Stabilizing Wheelchair. Training in this skill should begin after the patient can stabilize his wheelchair while sitting on stairs. He should also be independent in gross mat mobility and leg management.[27]

---

[25] This skill is addressed in Chapter 11.

[26] Training strategies for the head-hips relationship and transfer skills are presented in Chapter 11.

[27] Training strategies for gross mat mobility and leg management are presented in Chapter 12.

A cord-injured person who has the required prerequisite skills should learn without difficulty to position his buttocks and legs while stabilizing his wheelchair on stairs. Practice should begin on a low step, where the chair is supported by the floor. As the patient's skill develops, he should progress to transferring from higher steps, where the chair is not supported by the floor (Fig. 13–25).

Sitting on Step or Landing, Pull Wheelchair up. A patient must have good dynamic balance in one-hand–supported short-sitting before beginning training in this skill.[28] If he has good balance, he should learn to pull his wheelchair up a step or onto a landing with minimal practice. The patient is likely to find the task easier if he leans away from the chair as he pulls it up.

Sitting on Floor, Pull Wheelchair to Upright Position. To right a wheelchair while sitting on the floor, a cord-injured person first gets into long-sitting. Propping on one arm, he pulls upward on one of the wheelchair's push handles to right the chair.

A patient must have good dynamic balance in one-hand–supported long-sitting to practice this skill.[29] If he has good balance, he should learn to right his wheelchair with minimal practice.

Belt Self into Wheelchair. A person who has the physical potential to ascend stairs in a wheelchair should be able to learn to belt himself into his wheelchair with minimal practice. Before attempting this maneuver, he should have mastered basic wheelchair skills: dynamic balance and the ability to move his trunk to and from upright.[30]

Lower Chair into Position to Ascend Stairs in Wheelchair. Someone who has the physical potential to ascend stairs in a wheelchair should learn with minimal practice to lower his chair into position. If a patient has difficulty at first, he can practice lowering and raising himself through a small arc of motion, gradually increasing the arc as his skill and confidence develop (Fig. 13–26).

Sitting in Wheelchair Tilted Back onto Steps, Reposition Hands. In this maneuver a person who is sitting in a wheelchair that is tilted back onto a step moves his hands from one step to another. This maneuver is made challenging by the fact that he must support himself and the chair while he does so. To do this he supports himself on one hand at a time, repositioning his free hand to the step above.

Practice should start at the base of the stairway. A wheelchair is easier to stabilize in this location, since it is supported by the floor. After brief practice at the base of the stairs, the patient can progress to practicing on higher steps, where the chair is not supported by the floor (Fig. 13–25).

Once an individual has developed some skill in repositioning his hands, he can practice this skill concurrently with pulling his chair up a step.

Sitting in Wheelchair, Push on Step to Lift Wheelchair up a Step. Lifting a wheelchair up a step while sitting in the chair is more a matter of strength than skill. This maneuver will be easier to learn if the patient is skillful in back-approach uneven transfers[31] and can reposition his hands between steps.

Training should start at the base of a stairway, with the patient belted into a wheelchair that is tilted back onto the stairs. If the patient is both strong and able to reposition his hands between steps, he may practice pulling himself up the stairs without prior preparation. He is likely to find the maneuver easier if he lifts one wheel at a time up the step. A patient who has difficulty pulling his chair up the steps may first practice raising and lowering his chair over a single step at the base of the stairs.

Sitting on a Step, Lower Wheelchair Down a Step. A patient must have good dynamic balance in one-hand–supported short-sitting before beginning training in this skill.[32] If he has good balance in this position, he should learn to lower his wheelchair down a step with minimal practice. The patient should be encouraged to lean away from the chair as he lowers it to avoid losing his balance forward.

Sitting on a Step, Transfer Down a Step While Stabilizing Wheelchair. Training in this skill should begin after the patient can stabilize his wheelchair and reposition his hands while sitting on stairs. He must also be proficient in using the head-hips relationship and performing step-high back-approach uneven transfers to the floor.[33]

Before a patient becomes skillful in this maneuver, he may have difficulty stabilizing his wheelchair while transferring. While concentrating on the

---

[28] This skill is addressed in Chapter 11.

[29] Long-sitting skills are addressed in Chapter 12.

[30] Functional training strategies for these skills are presented in Chapter 11.

[31] These transfers are presented in Chapter 11.

[32] This skill is addressed in Chapter 11.

[33] Training strategies for the head-hips relationship and transfer skills are presented in Chapter 11.

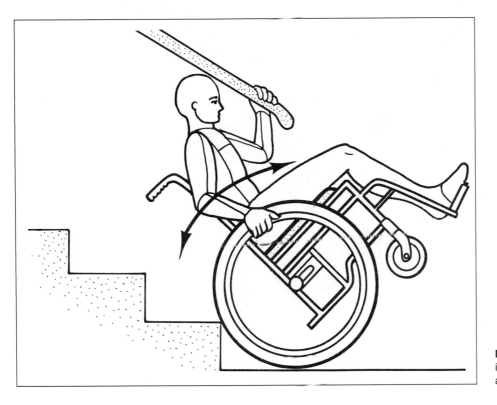

Figure 13–26. Practice lowering wheelchair into position to ascend stairs in wheelchair.

transfer between stairs, the inexperienced person often applies an obliquely directed force to the chair's push handle, causing it to slide. The therapist should encourage the patient to push straight downward through the push handle as he transfers.

Practice should begin on a low step, where the chair is supported by the floor. As the patient's skill develops, he should progress to transferring from higher steps, where the chair is unsupported by the floor. After he has developed some skill in transferring down a step while stabilizing his chair, the patient can practice this skill concurrently with lowering the chair.

Sitting in Wheelchair and Holding Stair Handrail(s), Lower Wheelchair Down Stairs. This maneuver is very easy to learn, requiring great amounts of neither strength nor skill. The greatest obstacle to overcome during functional training is fear: understandably, many people are afraid at first that they will lose control of the chair and fall down the stairs.

To reduce a patient's fear during functional training, the therapist should stress the maneuver's safety and make a point of modeling comfort while demonstrating the technique. The therapist should also make it clear to the patient that he is spotting carefully during practice. The patient may feel more secure during initial practice if it takes place on a short (2- or 3-step) stairway. He can progress to

working on longer stairways as his comfort level increases.

In Wheelie, Position Wheels at Top of Step. Before working on this skill, a patient must be proficient in gliding forward, backward, and turning in a wheelie. Functional training then simply involves demonstration and practice. A patient who has difficulty positioning his chair at the top edge of a step may start with practice positioning the chair relative to a mark on the floor. He can progress to positioning his chair at the top edge of a low (1-inch) curb, then practice on higher curbs, and finally work on positioning his chair at the top of a stairway.

In Wheelie, Stabilize Wheelchair Against Step. To practice this skill, a patient should be proficient in maintaining a balanced wheelie position.

During initial practice, the patient should work on stabilizing his chair against a curb rather than against a step, as this will make spotting easier. After demonstrating the technique, the therapist can position the patient in a wheelie with the back of the chair's wheels resting against a curb. Once positioned, the patient can practice stabilizing the chair by pulling back on the wheels' handrims. He can work on maintaining the chair's position and lowering and raising (tilting) the chair through small arcs of motion (Fig. 13–27).

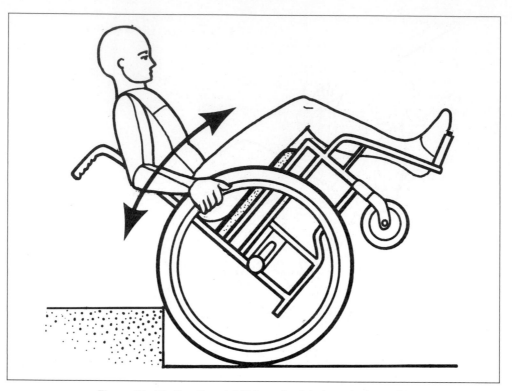

Figure 13–27. Practice stabilizing wheelchair against a curb.

Once an individual is able to stabilize his chair well, he should learn to get his chair into position. Starting positioned in a wheelie with the chair a small distance (a few inches) from the curb, he should practice backing until the wheels make contact with the curb, then practice stabilizing the wheels. Once he can perform these maneuvers well at a curb, he can practice on the bottom step of a stairway.

When a patient has developed skill in stabilizing his chair against a curb and descending a curb while remaining in a wheelie, he can practice the two skills concurrently.

Independent Work: A patient who has good control in a wheelie, can fall safely, and is independent in propelling backward in a wheelie can practice stabilizing his chair against a curb.

Descend Step, Remaining in Wheelie Position. A patient should be able to stabilize his wheelchair against a step in a wheelie position before beginning practice in this skill. He should also be skillful in balancing, gliding, and descending curbs in a wheelie.

When descending a curb in a wheelie, one does not have to remain in the wheelie position; once the chair's rear wheels have reached the base of the curb, the casters can drop without threat to the

rider's safety. In contrast, one *must* remain in a wheelie when descending steps forward. If the chair tips forward before it has reached the bottom of the stairway, it and the rider will fall down the stairs. It is this risk of falling that makes descending stairs in a wheelie hazardous to all but the most skillful riders.

During functional training, the patient should develop the ability to descend a step under control, remaining in a wheelie during and after the descent. He should develop his skill on curbs first, since practice there will be safer than on stairs. The patient may start on low curbs, progressing to higher curbs as his skill develops. Once he is consistently able to remain in a wheelie while and after descending a step-high curb, and can stabilize his wheelchair against the step, he can practice on stairs. When first practicing on stairs, it may be best to start on a small flight of stairs. The patient can also start on stairs with a small vertical rise per step, progressing to higher steps and longer stairways as his skill improves.

Independent Work: A patient who can independently descend a curb in a wheelie can practice remaining in a wheelie after descending.

Transfer to Armrest. To practice transferring to an armrest, a patient should be adept in even and slightly uneven transfers without a sliding board and in using the head-hips relationship to move his buttocks.[34]

The therapist should demonstrate and then have the patient practice transferring from his wheelchair seat to the armrest. The patient should be encouraged to push down hard and throw his head and upper trunk forcefully down and to the side to lift his buttocks. Emphasis should be placed on exaggerated motions of the head and upper trunk.

During initial practice many patients will be able to get onto their armrests with only spotting. These individuals can develop their skill by practicing with spotting until they become independent. Other patients have more difficulty learning the transfer. When this is the case, the therapist can make the task easier to placing cushions on the wheelchair's seat, reducing the distance that must be traversed in the transfer. As the patient's skill increases with practice, he can reduce the number of cushions on the seat, transferring from progressively lower levels until he can transfer directly from the seat to the armrest.

Maintain Balance While Sitting on Armrest.
Before working on this skill, the patient should have good dynamic balance while propped forward on one extended arm in short-sitting.[35]

Practice should start with the patient sitting on an armrest, with one hand on each armrest (Fig. 13–28A). From that position he shifts his weight and lifts the hand that is propped next to his buttocks (Fig. 13–28B). Once he can maintain this position, the patient can begin working on dynamic balance, shifting his weight while propping on one arm. Finally he can practice maintaining his balance while reaching in all directions (Fig. 13–28C).

Initial functional training in this skill will be most practical if the patient works on it concurrently with transfers to the armrest: he can alternate transferring onto the armrest and balancing there. Once he has become skillful in maintaining his balance while sitting on an armrest, he should practice this skill with the chair narrowed. This can be done concurrently with practice narrowing the chair.

Narrow Wheelchair While Sitting on Armrest.
To practice narrowing his wheelchair while sitting on an armrest, a patient must first be able to maintain his balance while sitting on an armrest, propped on one arm. Once he has dynamic balance in that position, narrowing the chair is not particularly difficult.

The therapist should demonstrate narrowing the wheelchair, then have the patient practice with spotting. The patient should be encouraged to pull forcefully and abruptly upward on the wheelchair seat while maintaining his balance. The chair will be easier to narrow if he shifts his weight off his supporting arm each time he pulls on the seat. He should be encouraged to regain his balance between pulls.

In preparation for negotiating narrow doorways, the patient can combine practice narrowing the chair with practice balancing on the narrowed wheelchair. To reopen the chair, he can transfer from the armrest onto the seat.

Sitting on Armrest, Pull on Doorjamb to Move Narrowed Wheelchair Through Door.
This skill requires the ability to maintain dynamic balance while sitting on the armrest of a narrowed wheelchair, propped on one arm. A patient who can maintain his balance in this position should learn without difficulty to pull the chair through a doorway. After demonstrating the maneuver, the therapist should spot the patient while he practices grasping the doorjamb and pulling himself through the doorway.

Sitting on Armrest, Propel Narrowed Wheelchair.
This skill requires the ability to maintain dynamic balance while sitting on an armrest of a narrowed wheelchair, propped on one arm. A patient who can maintain his balance in this position should learn without difficulty to propel his chair through a doorway. After demonstrating the maneuver, the therapist should spot the patient while he practices propelling the chair by pushing on one handrim at a time with his free hand.

Transfer From Armrest to Wheelchair Seat.
This maneuver is initiated with the wheelchair user sitting on an armrest, with one hand on each armrest. From this position, he pushes down hard on the armrests and tucks his head to lift his buttocks. As his buttocks lift, the person twists his head and shoulders laterally away from the seat.

Before practicing this skill, a patient should be adept in even and slightly uneven transfers without a sliding board and in using the head-hips relationship to move his buttocks.[36] A patient who has these prerequisite skills should be able to transfer from an armrest to the wheelchair seat without difficulty after a brief period of practice with spotting. During initial practice, the wheelchair should remain open. As his skill develops, the patient can progress to transferring into the seat of a narrowed wheelchair.

---

[34] These skills are addressed in Chapter 11.
[35] This skill is covered in Chapter 11.
[36] These skills are addressed in Chapter 11.

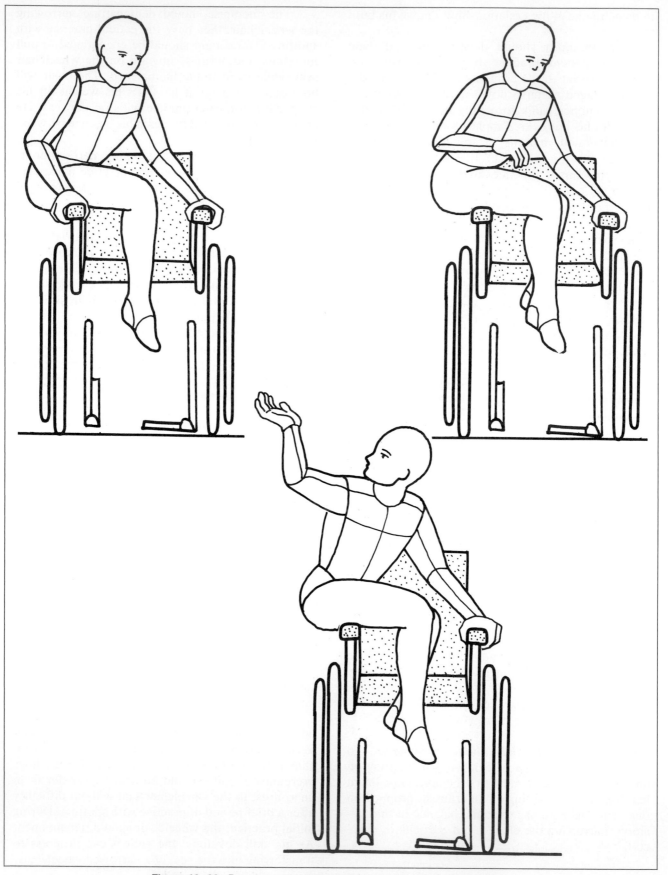

Figure 13–28. Practice maintaining balance while sitting on armrest.

Narrow Wheelchair by Rocking Side to Side. The therapist should demonstrate this technique and have the patient practice with spotting. The patient should be encouraged to use forceful and abrupt motions, synchronizing his head throws with upward pulls on the seat.

While Falling Backward in Wheelchair, Tuck Head and Hold Wheels. For most people the automatic reaction when tipping over backward in a wheelchair is to turn and reach out a hand, with the elbow extended. A person who reaches in this manner when falling lands on his palm, taking the force of the fall through his upper extremity. In the process he may injure himself. During functional training, this automatic reaction must be replaced by a safer falling technique.

Falling safely is a simple ability, without any true skill prerequisites. Functional training in this instance is more a matter of developing a new habit than of acquiring a new skill.

Fear can be a barrier to developing the habit of falling safely. To reduce a patient's fear, the therapist should model comfort with falling and demonstrate that it does not hurt. The therapist can also help the patient overcome his fear by introducing the fall gradually. The patient can first practice the appropriate actions to take when falling, tucking his head and holding the chair's wheels. He can then perform these maneuvers while the therapist simulates a fall, lowering the chair backward from a balanced wheelie position (Fig. 13-29**A**). At first these simulated falls can be slow, with warning, and over a small arc. As the patient's tolerance to this activity increases, the therapist can increase the speed and distance of the chair's "fall" and finally omit the warning.

In the activity described above, the therapist should remain in control of the wheelchair, preventing a true fall. Once the patient develops some tolerance to falling and demonstrates the ability to respond appropriately, he can practice true falls. A fearful patient can develop his tolerance to falling by building up the distance over which he falls. Starting with a short fall onto a pile of floor mats, he can fall over progressively larger distances as his tolerance and habit develop (Fig. 13-29**B**).

Independent Work: Following initial practice, a patient who is able to return to upright after a fall can practice falling onto floor mats without spotting.

While Falling Backward in Wheelchair, Tuck Head and Block Legs. This skill can be taught using the strategies described above for developing the habit of tucking the head and holding the wheels during a fall.

After Falling Backward in Wheelchair, Position Self in Chair. This skill involves pulling on the chair's wheels to slide the buttocks back onto the seat, grasping the legs, and placing them so that they hang over the front edge of the seat. A cord-injured person who has the physical potential to right his chair after a fall should be able to master this prerequisite skill with minimal practice.

Independent Work: Once a patient has been shown this technique and has had some initial practice, he can practice independently. The maneuver can be practiced concurrently with the other skill prerequisites for returning a chair to upright after a fall.

Sitting in Overturned Wheelchair, Lock Brakes. To lock his brakes while sitting in an overturned wheelchair, the cord-injured person simply grasps his brakes and locks them. He will probably need to move his trunk by pulling on an armrest or the frame of his wheelchair to reach the brakes. These maneuvers may be awkward when sitting in an overturned chair, but they should be readily accomplished with practice.

Independent Work: Once a patient has been shown this technique and has had some initial practice, he can practice independently. This maneuver can be practiced concurrently with the other skill prerequisites for returning a chair to upright after a fall.

Sitting in Overturned Wheelchair, Lift Upper Trunk From Floor. A person who has the physical potential to right his chair after a fall should be able to master this prerequisite skill with minimal practice.

Independent Work: Once a patient has been shown this technique and has had some initial practice, he can practice independently. The maneuver can be practiced concurrently with the other skill prerequisites for returning a chair to upright after a fall.

Sitting in Overturned Wheelchair, Balance on One Hand. Before beginning training in this skill, a patient must have good dynamic balance when sitting propped back on one arm.[37]

Appropriate hand placement is the key to balancing on one hand while sitting in an overturned wheelchair. The hand should be positioned directly behind the trunk, so that the person can support his weight on it. The patient should practice placing his hand, shifting his weight onto it, and releasing the other hand's grasp on the chair. When he has developed the ability to release the chair and balance

---

[37] This skill is addressed in Chapter 12.

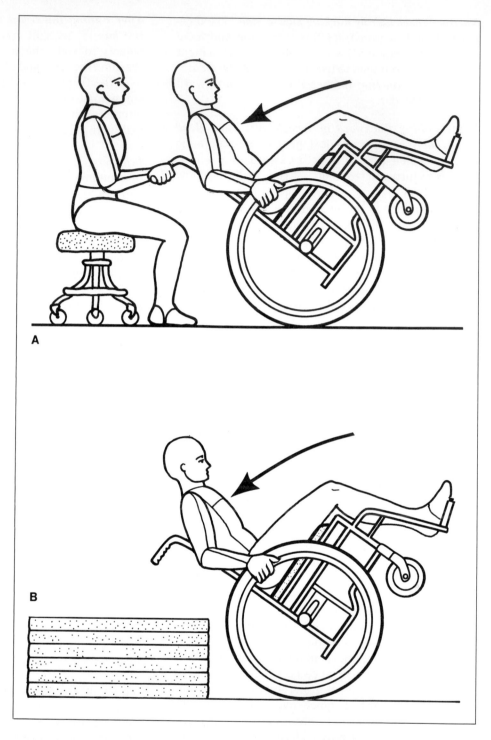

Figure 13–29. Practice safe falling technique. **A.** With therapist assisting. **B.** Onto floor mats.

ance on one hand, he should practice reaching his free hand toward the opposite wheel.

Independent Work: Once a patient has been shown this technique and has had some initial practice, he can practice independently. This skill can be practiced concurrently with the other skill prerequisites for returning a chair to upright after a fall.

Sitting in Overturned Wheelchair, Rock Chair to Upright. Before beginning training in this skill, a patient must have good dynamic balance when sitting in an overturned wheelchair propped back on one arm.

Starting in the position shown in Figure 13–15D, the patient should practice rocking the chair toward upright. The therapist should encourage him to use forceful and abrupt motions to thrust the chair upward from the floor. When the patient has rocked the chair forward enough to unweight his supporting hand, he should inch this hand forward around the side of the chair. He should reposition the hand rapidly and over short distances, so that he can support himself and maintain his balance when the chair rocks back. The therapist can facilitate practice at first by assisting with the chair's forward rock, pulling up on the chair's push handles while the patient pushes. The therapist can also help support the chair if the patient does not regain his one-hand support quickly enough when the chair rocks back. As the patient's skill develops, this assistance should be withdrawn.

Independent Work: Once a patient has been shown this technique and has had some initial practice, he can practice independently. He can practice rocking his wheelchair to upright concurrently with the other skill prerequisites for returning a chair to upright after a fall.

PROGRAM DESIGN

When using this text as a resource to assist in working toward a functional goal, the therapist should first read the text's description of that functional activity. Based on that description, the corresponding charts, or both the therapist can determine what physical and skill prerequisites are required to perform the skill. Taking into consideration the patient's evaluation results, the therapist can determine where the patient has deficits relevant to the functional goal. The program should then be designed to address these deficits, accomplishing the needed physical and skill prerequisites.

Many strategies are available for increasing strength and range of motion; the field of physical therapy has a variety of approaches for accomplishing these ends. The program may include any combination of the following: proprioceptive neuromuscular facilitation, progressive resistive exercises (concentric and eccentric), strengthening through functional tasks, isokinetic exercise, electrical stimulation, and prolonged stretching. Strengthening and stretching will also occur with increased activity. The patient can exercise independently, in groups, and one on one with the therapist.

This chapter presents functional training strategies for each prerequisite skill. The therapist can use these suggestions, coupled with his own imagination, clinical expertise, and problem solving, to design a functional training program. The program should aim first at developing the most basic prerequisite skills and build to move advanced skills as the patient's abilities develop.

In most cases a patient will have many functional goals. The therapeutic program must progress him toward all of these goals. Fortunately there is much overlap of prerequisites between skills. Thus a person working on maintaining a balanced wheelie position is potentially progressing himself toward independence in negotiating ramps, curbs, stairs, and uneven terrain in a wheelie. Furthermore, work aimed at developing one ability can benefit other, seemingly unrelated, activities. For example, the strengthening and motor learning that result from practicing manual wheelchair propulsion are likely to help a patient's transfer abilities.

Example: Descend Ramp in a Wheelie. To learn to descend ramps in a wheelie, a cord-injured person needs adequate strength and range of motion in finger flexion, elbow flexion and extension, and shoulder and scapular motions. He also needs to be able to assume a wheelie position, maintain his balance point, glide forward, and control his wheelchair as it descends a slope in a wheelie.

The program design will depend on the individual's needs. If he has any deficits in prerequisite strength or range, the program should include exercises to address these deficits. This exercise program should occur concurrently with functional training.

The functional training program should also be tailored to the individual's needs, addressing areas of deficit in prerequisite skills. If the patient has none of the skill prerequisites, functional training should start with the most basic: assuming and maintaining a balanced wheelie position. When the patient is able to perform these maneuvers, he can practice gliding in a wheelie. After he has mastered that skill, he can work on descending ramps in a wheelie. By building his skill in this manner, the patient progresses to independence in descending ramps in a wheelie.

REFERENCES

Heinneman, A., Magiera-Planey, R., Schiro-Geist, C., & Gimines, G. (1987). Mobility for persons with spinal cord injury: An evaluation of two systems. *Archives of Physical Medicine and Rehabilitation, 68*, 90–93.

McClay, I. (1983). Electric wheelchair propulsion using a hand control in C4 quadriplegia. *Physical Therapy, 63*(2), 221–223.

O'Neil, L., & Seelye, R. (1990) Power wheelchair training for patients with marginal upper extremity function. *Neurology Report, 14*(3), 19–20.

Swarts, A., Krouskop, T., & Smith, D. (1988). Tissue pressure management in the vocational setting. *Ar-chives of Physical Medicine and Rehabilitation, 69*, 97–99.

Waters, R., & Lunsford, B. (1985). Energy costs of paraplegic locomotion. *Journal of Joint and Bone Surgery, 67-A*(8), 1245–1250.

14

Ambulation

Ambulation is a priority concern for many people following spinal cord injury. This is common knowledge among health professionals who work with cord-injured patients. Especially during the early weeks and months after injury, much of a patient's questioning often centers on his future capacity to walk.

The high priority of walking is understandable when one considers the value that our society places on standing and walking. Our attitudes about different postures are reflected in our language. Sitting down epitomizes passivity. ("I'm not going to take that sitting down.") In contrast, standing is seen as a measure of power, competence, and potency. ("Stand up and take it like a man.")

To Walk or Not to Walk?

Walking is clearly a priority for patients. However, it is an area of conflict for many health professionals. This is because research and experience have shown that people with spinal cord injuries are likely to abandon their ambulation skills after rehabilitation. Even those who have successfully learned to walk with orthoses and Lofstrand crutches are likely to opt for wheelchair mobility (Heinemann, Magiera-Planey, Schiro-Geist, & Gimines, 1987). Most find that wheelchairs are more practical than walking, enabling them to travel faster and with less energy expended. This is true even for people who can walk with two ankle-foot orthoses (AFOs) and assistive devices (Waters & Lunsford, 1985).

A reasonable question arises: If research and experience have shown that a cord-injured person is likely to abandon ambulation, why should the rehabilitation team spend time, money, and energy gait training? The answer is twofold.

First, though most patients give up ambulation following rehabilitation, some *don't*. Can we deny people the opportunity to walk because they *probably* will give it up? If we do, some would-be walkers will never get the chance. Second, a patient may receive psychological benefit from gait training even if he ultimately uses a wheelchair. Until he has had the opportunity to experience ambulation after his injury, he may not be able to accept wheelchair mobility. ("They wouldn't let me try. I know if I could just try . . .") Once he has tried walking with orthoses and assistive devices and has seen how difficult it is, he may be more ready to accept the alternative. Wheelchair mobility then becomes a matter of choice, representing independent and convenient mobility rather than symbolizing disability.

Ideally any cord-injured person who wishes to attempt ambulation should be given the opportunity to do so, as long as there is no medical contraindication. Even a patient who has a high lesion may benefit from the attempt.

Even if one agrees in theory that everyone should be given a chance to walk, the high cost of orthoses remains a barrier. It is hard to justify spending over a thousand dollars on a pair of orthoses for a person with a high cervical lesion, knowing that he is likely to give up ambulation after a few gait-training sessions.

Offering the opportunity for gait training to all cord injured patients will be more practical if the cost can be minimized. This can be done by postponing the purchase of orthoses until patients have demonstrated the potential for functional ambulation. If the physical therapy department has adjustable orthoses or a bank of donated orthoses, patients can begin gait training without purchasing orthoses. The equipment can then be purchased toward the end of gait training, after an individual has shown the ability and drive required to walk independently.

Although all patients should be provided with the opportunity to try walking, they should not be pressured into attempting ambulation if they are not interested. Unlike transfers, mat activities, and wheelchair skills, walking with orthoses is not a "survival" skill required for independent living (A patient who is not motivated to persue survival skills should not be forced to, but certainly a therapist should attempt to convince him of the need to learn these skills).

Likewise, gait training should not supersede functional training in survival skills. If a patient has limited funding for functional training, more practical skills should take precedence.

If functional ambulation is a goal in therapy, the program should address the following skills: balanced standing, ambulation over even surfaces and obstacles, rising from a wheelchair and sitting back down, falling safely and getting up from the floor, and donning and doffing the orthoses. This chapter presents a description of these ambulation skills,[1] as well as suggestions on how to teach them.

The descriptions of techniques and training presented in this chapter should be used as a guide, not as a set of hard and fast rules. The motions used to perform a given functional task vary between people. This variability is due to differences in body build, skill level, range of motion, muscle tone, and patterns of strength and weakness. During functional training the therapist and patient should work together to find the exact techniques that best suit that particular individual.

Functional Electrical Stimulation

No chapter on ambulation after spinal cord injury would be complete without a mention of functional electrical stimulation (FES).[2] Since the midseventies, research has been done on eliciting contractions in paralyzed musculature for ambulation. Using FES and assistive devices, people with complete spinal cord lesions have been able to walk over even surfaces, over mild inclines, and to ascend and descend stairs (Marsolias & Kobetic, 1987; Peckham, 1987). FES has also been used to augment ambulation with orthoses (McClelland, Andrews, Patrick, Freeman, & El Masri, 1987; Watkins, Edwards, & Patrick, 1987).

To date, ambulation using FES remains experimental and available to a limited number of people. A variety of problems remain to be solved, including safety, electrode failure, increased spasticity, miniaturization, standardization of electrode placement, convenience, patient compliance, affordability, and design for daily use in the community (Kralj, Bajd, & Turk, 1988; Marsolias & Kobetic, 1988; Peckham, 1987; Robinson, Kett, & Bolam, 1988; Thoma et al., 1987). Because FES is a recent development, long-term follow-up is lacking; the question remains as to whether people walking using

FES will ultimately find wheelchair mobility to be more practical.

It is hoped that functional electrical stimulation will make this chapter obsolete at some point in the future. However, much progress is needed before FES can be offered as a standard component of functional rehabilitation following spinal cord injury.

PRACTICE IN DEPARTMENT AND "REAL WORLD"

The physical therapy department in a rehabilitation center should be equipped with curbs of varying heights, stairs, and a ramp. This equipment is useful for initial practice of obstacle negotiation. However, practice should not end with mastery of these artificial obstacles. Many obstacles that a patient will encounter outside of the department will be more difficult to negotiate. For example, ascending a cement curb from a street is likely to be more difficult than ascending a wooden curb from a linoleum floor. The "real world" is full of uneven sidewalks, long and steep staircases, and uneven surfaces such as grass and sand. Functional training should include practicing ambulation skills outside of the department so that the patient will be better prepared to function in the "real world" following rehabilitation.

PHYSICAL AND SKILL PREREQUISITES

Each functional activity involves a particular set of skills. Each activity also has strength, joint range of motion, and muscle flexibility requirements. A deficiency in any of these skill or physical requirements will impair a person's performance of the activity.

The descriptions of functional techniques below are accompanied by charts that summarize the physical and skill prerequisites. Exact values for the physical prerequisites are not given because the requirements vary among individuals. For example, a person who is very skillful in coming to stand from the floor may require less hamstring flexibility for this activity than does someone who is less skillful.

AMBULATION SKILLS

Balanced Standing

Balanced standing is the most basic ambulation skill; before a person can walk, he must be able to remain upright in a standing position. With total pa-

---

[1] This chapter does not attempt to present all possible ambulation skills. An individual who is unable to master a skill described in this chapter may fare better with a variation of that technique or with an altogether different method.

[2] FES is also called FNS, or functional neuromuscular stimulation.

ralysis of the lower extremities, knee-ankle-foot orthoses (KAFOs) provide stability at the feet, ankles,
and knees. A cord-injured person with this level of
paralysis uses his arms, head, and upper trunk to
stabilize his hips.

In the absence of innervated lower extremities,
posture is the key to balanced standing. The position
of stability is illustrated in Figure 14–1A. In the balanced standing posture, the cord-injured person
stands with his pelvis forward so that his weight line
falls posterior to his hip joints. This position results
in an extension moment at the hips. Since hip extension is restricted by the Y ligaments, the hips are
stable in this posture.

In contrast to extension, hip flexion is not restricted by ligaments. In the absence of muscular
control, the hips will flex without restriction if a
flexion moment exists at the hips. Thus if a cord-
injured person standing with KAFOs changes his
posture so that his weight line falls anterior to his
hips, he will lose his stability at the hips. He will
"jacknife" as a result of this unrestricted hip flexion
(Fig. 14–1B).

Attaining and maintaining a balanced standing
posture is accomplished using the head-hips relationship. With his hands stabilized on parallel bars

or Lofstrand crutches, the cord-injured person can
push his pelvis forward by retracting his scapulae
and throwing his head back. Tucking the head forward and protracting the scapulae will move the pelvis posteriorly.

Functional ambulation requires the ability to
stand balanced without weight on both hands, at
least briefly. The functional ambulator must be able
to free at least one hand to move his crutches, to
open doors, and to reach for objects.

Ambulation Over Even Surfaces
This chapter will focus on ambulation with Lofstrand crutches and two KAFOs. Walking is most
feasible when the cord-injured person has fully intact upper extremities, although limited drag-to ambulation has been achieved by people with complete
cervical lesions. Walking is most readily achieved
and practical when abdominal musculature is innervated.

Charts 14–1 and 14–2 summarize the physical
and skill prerequisites for independent ambulation
over even surfaces.

Four-Point. When walking with a four-point gait, a
person moves one crutch or one foot at a time. This
gait pattern is slow but safe, since at least three

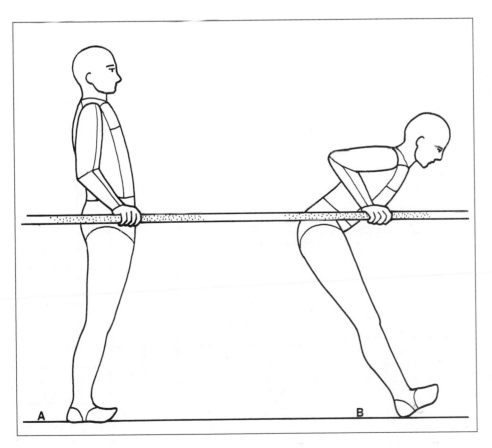

Figure 14–1. Balanced standing. **A.** Position of stability: pelvis forward with weight line posterior to hip joints. **B.**
"Jacknifing": stability lost if
weight line passes anterior to
hips.

Chart 14–1 Ambulation Over Even Surfaces—Physical Prerequisites

	Four-point gait	Swing-through gait	Swing-to gait	Drag-to gait	Stepping back or to the side
Strength					
Trapezius	√	√	√	√	√
Deltoids	√	☑	√	√	√
Biceps, brachialis, and/or brachioradialis	√	√	√	√	√
Serratus anterior	☑	☑	☑	☑	☑
Pectoralis major	☑	☑	☑	●	☑
Latissimus dorsi	☑	☑	☑	√	☑
Triceps	☑	☑	☑	●	☑
Wrist and hand musculature	●	√	√	●	●
Abdominals	●	●	●	●	●
Quadratus lumborum	●				●
Iliopsoas	●				
Range of Motion					
Scapular Elevation	√	√	√		
Depression	√	√	√	√	√
Abduction	√	√	√	√	√
Adduction	√	√	√	√	
Downward rotation	√	√			
Shoulder Flexion	√	√	√	√	√
Extension	√	√			
Elbow Extension	☑	☑	☑	√	√
Hip Extension	☑	☑	☑	☑	
Knee Extension	☑	☑	☑	☑	☑
Ankle Dorsiflexion	√	√	√	√	√

√ = Some strength is needed for this activity, or severe limitations in range will inhibit this activity.

☑ = A large amount of strength or normal or greater range is needed for this activity.

● = Not required, but helpful.

points (crutches and feet) remain in contact with the floor at all times. A four-point gait pattern also requires less energy expenditure than does a swing-through gait (Waters, Yakura, Adkins, & Barnes, 1989).

The cord-injured person preparing to walk should start in a balanced standing posture with his hips extended, pelvis forward, lumbar spine in lordosis, scapulae retracted, and head erect (Fig. 14–2**A**). From the starting position, he shifts his weight off one crutch. While balanced on his feet and one crutch, he lifts the unweighted crutch and moves it forward (Fig. 14–2**B**).

After moving the crutch, the person steps with his contralateral foot (For simplicity, the leg that is moving or about to be moved will be called the swing leg). To step, he shifts his weight off of the

Chart 14–2 Ambulation Over Even Surfaces—Skill Prerequisites

	Four-point gait	Swing-through gait	Swing-to gait	Drag-to gait	Stepping back or to the side
Control pelvis using head-hips relationship[a]	√	√	√	√	√
Balanced standing	√	√	√	√	√
Weight shift in standing	√	√	√	√	√
Lift and move one crutch	√			√	√
Step forward with one leg	√				
Step to side or back with one leg					√
Lift and move two crutches		√	√	(√)	
Swing-through step		√			
Swing-to step			√		
Drag-to step				√	
Distance/efficient ambulation	√	√	√	√	

[a] Refer to Chapter 11 for a description of this skill and therapeutic strategies.

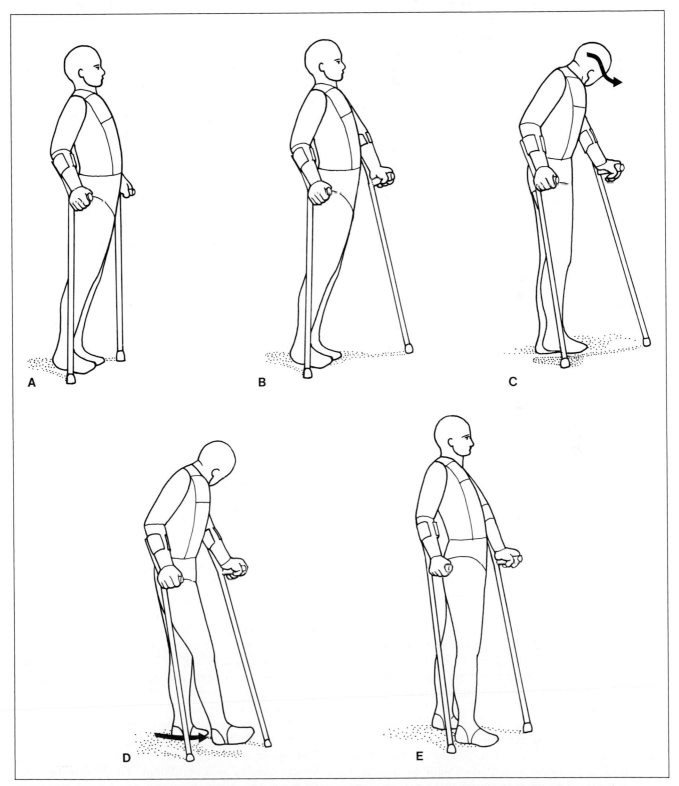

Figure 14–2. Four-point gait. **A.** Balanced standing posture. **B.** One crutch advanced. **C.** Lifting one leg by elevating pelvis on that side. Head tucked down and laterally away from swing leg. **D.** Once lifted, leg swings forward as a pendulum. **E.** Balanced standing posture with one leg advanced.

swing leg, presses down on the crutches, and elevates the swing side of his pelvis (Fig. 14–2C).

Elevation of the swing side of the pelvis can be accomplished using the latissimus dorsi, quadratus lumborum, or abdominal musculature if these muscles are innervated. The cord-injured person can supplement this muscular action with the head-hips relationship: while shifting his weight and pushing on his crutches, he tucks his head down and laterally away from the swing leg. At the same time he extends his elbow on the swing side, lifting that shoulder. As the torso pivots on the shoulders, the swing side of the pelvis lifts.

With one side of the pelvis lifted, the leg swings forward as a pendulum (Fig. 14–2D). If the individual's hip flexors are innervated, he can use them to step actively.

After stepping, the cord-injured person regains a balanced standing posture, pushing his pelvis forward by lifting his head and retracting his scapulae (Fig. 14–2E). From the balanced standing posture, he repeats the above-described process and steps with his other leg.

Swing-Through. A swing-through gait is faster than a four-point gait but requires more energy and entails a greater risk of falling.

A cord-injured person about to walk should start in a balanced standing posture with his hips extended, pelvis forward, lumbar spine in lordosis, scapulae retracted, and head erect (Fig. 14–3A). While in this posture he lifts his crutches and moves them forward (Fig. 14–3B).

To take a step, the person leans on his crutches and lifts his pelvis (and legs) by extending his elbows, depressing and protracting his scapulae, and tucking his head (Fig. 14–3C). Once the pelvis lifts enough for the feet to leave the ground, the torso and legs will swing forward as a pendulum (Fig. 14–3D).

When the person's heels strike (Fig. 14–3E), he should move quickly to stabilize himself. Pushing his pelvis forward using scapular retraction, throwing his head back, and pushing on the crutches, he returns to a stable standing posture (Fig. 14–3F). Once in this posture, he balances on his feet while he repositions his crutches forward. He is then in position to take another step.

Swing To. A swing-to gait is similar to a swing-through gait. The difference is that the person steps to, not past, his crutches. This gait pattern is slower than swing through, but it involves a smaller risk of falling.

The maneuvers used to perform a swing-to gait are the same as those used for a swing-through gait, except that the person drops his feet before they swing past his crutches (Fig. 14–4). At the end of the step, the feet and crutches are approximately colinear. This is an unstable position, as the base of support is shallow in the anteroposterior dimension. To maximize his stability while walking with a swing-to gait, the cord-injured person should quickly reposition his crutches anteriorly once he has completed a step and resumed a balanced standing posture.

Drag-To. Using a drag-to gait pattern, a person does not lift his trunk; his feet remain on the floor. The feet are dragged to, but not past, the crutches. This is a slow, energy-consuming gait. However, it requires less strength than the other gait patterns and thus may be the only option for someone with a very high lesion.

As is true with the other gait patterns, the person walking with a drag-to gait starts in the balanced standing posture and repositions his crutches anteriorly before taking a step. Depending on his stability in standing, he can reposition his crutches simultaneously or one at a time. To step, he leans on his crutches, extends his elbows, and depresses his scapulae enough to unweight his legs and drag his feet toward the crutches.

After moving his feet, the cord-injured person uses head and scapular motions to regain a balanced standing posture. As with a swing-to gait, he should quickly reposition his crutches at this point to increase his anteroposterior stability.

Stepping Backward or to the Side. This skill is used when walking sideways or backwards. It is also used to reposition a single foot when, for example, a person places his feet in preparation to sit down in a wheelchair.

To step backward or to the side, the cord-injured person lifts his leg using the same technique as is used in a four-point gait. He shifts his weight off one leg and lifts it using the latissimus dorsi, quadratus lumborum, abdominals, or motions of the head and upper trunk, or a combination thereof to lift that half of the pelvis.

With his leg lifted, the cord-injured person positions his foot by moving his pelvis. Using head and upper trunk motions to move his pelvis, he swings the leg as a pendulum. To step to the side, he moves his head and upper trunk back and forth laterally. To step backward, he moves his head up and down. In either direction he drops his pelvis (by lifting his head) to place his foot when it has swung to the desired position.

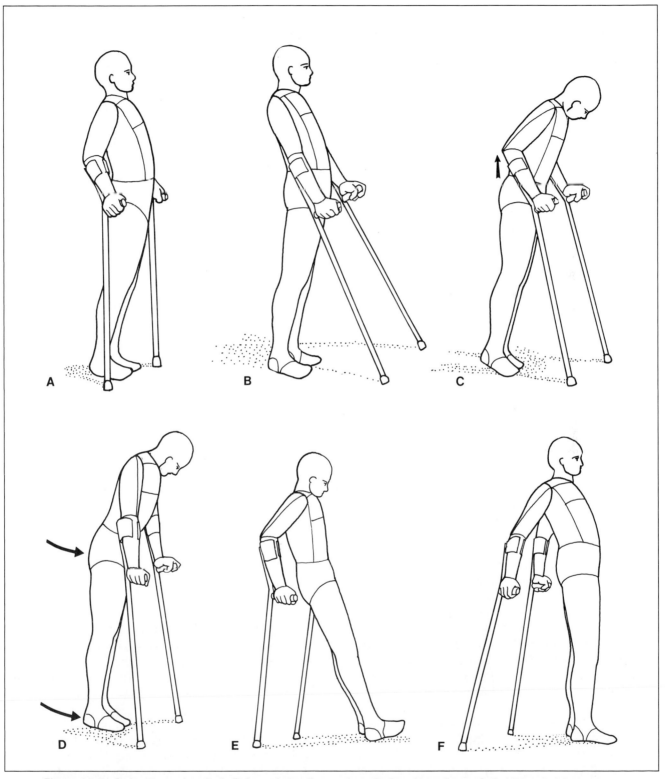

Figure 14–3. Swing-through gait. **A.** Balanced standing posture. **B.** Crutches advanced. **C.** Lifting pelvis and legs by extending elbows, depressing and protracting scapulae, and tucking head. **D.** Once lifted, torso and legs swing forward as a pendulum. **E.** Heels strike. **F.** Balanced standing posture regained by lifting head, retracting scapulae, and pushing on crutches to push pelvis forward.

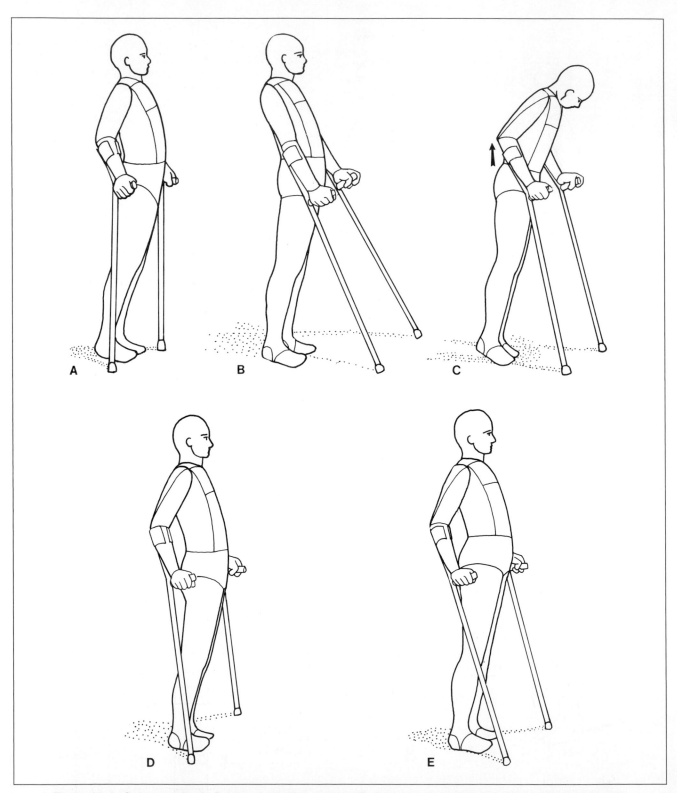

Figure 14–4. Swing-to gait. **A.** Balanced standing posture. **B.** Crutches advanced. **C.** Lifting pelvis and legs by extending elbows, depressing and protracting scapulae, and tucking head. **D.** Feet are advanced to, not past, crutches. Balanced standing posture resumed. **E.** Crutches quickly repositioned anteriorly for greater stability.

Chart 14—3 Ambulation Over Obstacles—Physical Prerequisites

	Ramps	Curbs	Stairs
Strength			
Trapezius	√	√	√
Deltoids	√	√	√
Biceps, brachialis, and/or brachioradialis	√	√	√
Serratus anterior	☑	☑	☑
Pectoralis major	☑	☑	☑
Latissimus dorsi	☑	☑	☑
Triceps	☑	☑	☑
Wrist and hand musculature	√	√	√
Abdominals	●	●	●
Quadratus lumborum	●	●	●
Iliopsoas	●	●	●
Range of Motion			
Scapular Elevation	√	√	√
Depression	√	√	√
Abduction	√	√	√
Adduction	√	√	√
Downward rotation	√	√	√
Shoulder Flexion	√	√	√
Extension	√	√	√
Elbow Extension	☑	☑	☑
Hip Extension	☑	☑	☑
Knee Extension	☑	☑	☑
Ankle Dorsiflexion	√	√	√

√ = Some strength is needed for this activity, or severe limitations in range will inhibit this activity.
☑ = A large amount of strength or normal or greater range is needed for this activity.
● = Not required, but helpful.

Negotiation of Obstacles

Independence in ambulation over even surfaces will enable a person to walk indoors within the confines of a single-level home or work environment. To walk in the community, obstacle negotiation skills are necessary. Techniques for negotiation of ramps, curbs, and stairs are presented below.

Charts 14–3 and 14–4 summarize the physical and skill prerequisites for independent ambulation over obstacles.

Ramps

The greatest challenge when walking up or down a ramp is avoiding being thrown down the slope. When a person wearing orthoses with immobile ankle joints stands on a slope, his orthoses, and therefore his hips, are thrown in the downhill direction.

Practice in ramp negotiation should not be lim-

Chart 14—4 Ambulation Over Obstacles—Skill Prerequisites

	Ascend ramps	Descend ramps	Ascend curbs	Descend curbs	Ascend stairs	Descend stairs
Swing-to ambulation over even surfaces	√					
Swing-to ambulation up a slope	√					
Swing-through ambulation over even surfaces		√	√	√	√	√
Swing-through ambulation down a slope		√				
Balanced standing	√	√	√	√	√	√
Reposition crutches while standing	√	√	√	√	√	√
Step up curb or step			√		√	
Step down from curb or step				√		√

ited to the gentle 1:12 grade of a standard public incline. Many, if not most, ramps in the community are far steeper than this. The patient who intends to walk in the community should develop the skills needed to ascend and descend ramps as steep as possible within his potential.

Ascend. When ascending a ramp, the cord-injured person should keep his crutches well in front of his feet. To maximize hip stability, he should keep his body angled up the hill, with his pelvis well forward. He should use a step-to (or step-toward) gait, not a swing-through pattern.

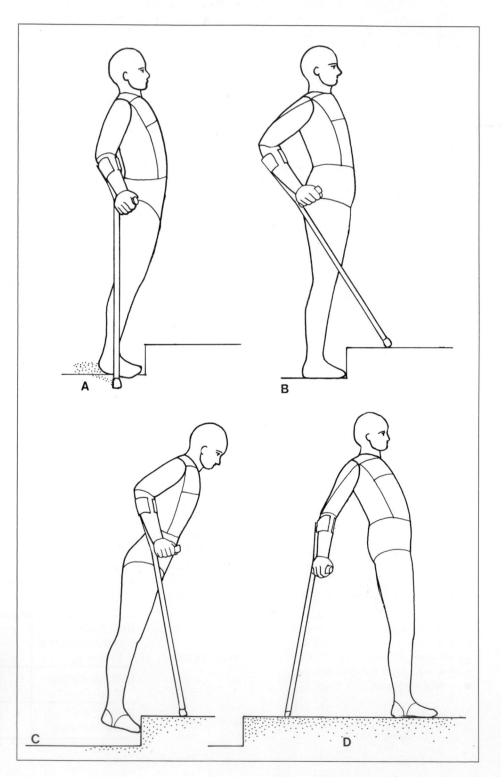

Figure 14–5. Ascending curb. **A.** Balanced standing posture with toes at edge of curb. **B.** Crutches onto curb. **C.** Lifting feet onto curb by leaning on crutches, extending elbows, and depressing scapulae. **D.** Pelvis pushed forward by throwing head back and retracting scapulae.

Descend. When descending a ramp, the slope tends to throw the hips toward a stable position. A swing-through gait pattern can be used.

Curbs

To be independent in ambulation in the community, curb negotiation skills are required. Although ramps have become common, they still are not universally present.

Ascend. To ascend a curb, the person approaches it face-on. He positions his feet with the toes at the edge of the curb (Fig. 14–5A), assumes a balanced standing posture, then places his crutch tips on the higher surface of the curb, a few inches from the edge (Fig. 14–5B).

From the starting position the person lifts his feet onto the curb. He does this by leaning forward on the crutches, tucking his head, extending his elbows, and depressing his scapulae (Fig. 14–5C). As his feet lift, the toes will drag up the vertical surface of the curb. When the toes lift past the curb, his torso and legs will swing forward as a pendulum.

The cord-injured person ascending a curb can step to or past his crutches. When his feet land, he throws his head back and retracts his scapulae to push his pelvis forward and regain a balanced standing posture (Fig. 14–5D).

Descend. When descending a curb, the person approaches it face-on. He assumes a balanced standing posture with his feet a few inches from the edge of the curb and places his crutch tips close to the edge of the curb (Fig. 14–6A).

From the starting position, the person steps off the curb. He does this by leaning on the crutches, tucking his head, extending his elbows, and depressing his scapulae. When the feet lift, his torso and legs will swing forward as a pendulum (Fig. 14–6B).

When the person's feet have swung past the edge of the curb, he drops them. (When "dropping" his legs he quickly lowers his torso/legs/feet with eccentrically controlled elbow and shoulder motions.) When his feet land, the cord-injured person regains a balanced standing posture, pushing his pelvis forward by throwing his head back and retracting his scapulae (Fig. 14–6C).

Stairs

If a cord-injured person walks in the community, he will inevitably comes across stairs. Many public and private buildings have stairs at their entrances. Within buildings, elevators are not always present and working.

In the stair negotiation techniques presented below, the person does not use a rail. The techniques are described in this way because rails are not always available in the community. The methods described can be adapted easily: when negotiating stairs using one crutch and one rail, the person holds the crutch not in use in the hand that holds the other crutch (Fig. 14–7).

Ascend. Ascending stairs is similar to ascending a series of curbs. The curb-negotiation techniques described above can be used to ascend stairs front-on (facing up the stairs).

In an alternative approach, the crutch walker can ascend stairs backwards. In the starting position for this technique, the person stands facing away from the stairs. He should stand in a balanced posture with his feet in front of the first stair and his crutches anterior to his feet (Fig. 14–8A).

From the starting position the person places his crutches on the lowest step (Fig. 14–8B). He then leans on the crutches, extends his elbows, and depresses his scapulae to lift his feet onto the step (Fig. 14–8C). When his feet lift past the step, his torso and legs will swing backward as a pendulum. When his feet land, he throws his head back and retracts his scapulae to push his pelvis forward and to regain a balanced standing posture (Fig. 14–8D).

Descend. Descending stairs is much like descending a series of curbs. A technique similar to the curb-negotiation method described above can be used to descend stairs. The cord-injured person places his crutches close to the edge of the step on which he stands, lifts his feet, and his torso and legs swing forward as a pendulum.

The difference between descending a step and a curb is that when descending a step in a stairway, the crutch walker has a limited area on which his feet can land safely. Thus when negotiating stairs, he must control the length of his step. If his feet land too far from their starting position, he will miss the next step.

While a cord-injured person descends a step, his feet may swing past the next step. To avoid missing the step, he should allow his feet to swing back over the step before he drops them.

Coming to Stand From a Wheelchair

Functional ambulation requires the ability to get into a standing position. The techniques described below center on rising from a wheelchair. They can be adapted to surfaces other than wheelchairs.[3]

---

[3] If an individual plans to ambulate in the community, during functional training he should practice getting up and down from other sitting surfaces such as toilets, cars, and standard chairs.

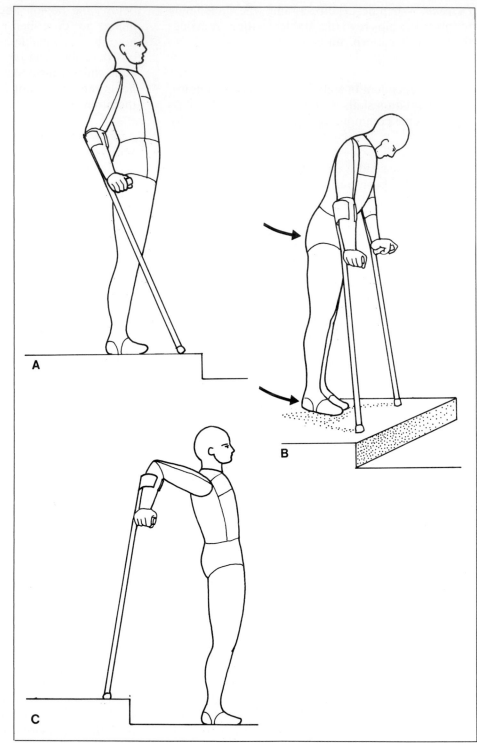

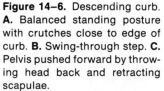

Figure 14–6. Descending curb. **A.** Balanced standing posture with crutches close to edge of curb. **B.** Swing-through step. **C.** Pelvis pushed forward by throwing head back and retracting scapulae.

Charts 14–5 and 14–6 summarize the physical and skill prerequisites for coming to stand from a wheelchair.

Both Hands on Armrests. This method for standing from a wheelchair is the most readily achievable method. Since the person gets onto his feet while both hands remain on the wheelchair, the method is easier, steadier, and requires less skill than the other techniques presented. However, rising from a wheelchair using this method takes longer, since more steps are involved.

To rise from his wheelchair using this method, the crutch walker first locks the chair's brakes and

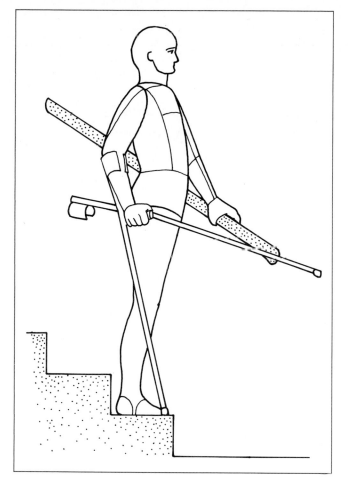

Figure 14–7. Descending stairs using a rail and one crutch, carrying second crutch.

Chart 14—5 Coming to Stand From Wheelchair—Physical Prerequisites

	Both hands on armrests	One hand on armrest and one on crutch	Both hands on crutches
Strength			
Trapezius	√	√	√
Deltoids	☑	√	√
Biceps, brachialis, and/or brachioradialis	√	√	√
Serratus anterior	☑	☑	☑
Pectoralis major	☑	☑	☑
Latissimus dorsi	√	☑	☑
Triceps	☑	☑	☑
Wrist and hand musculature	√	√	√
Abdominals	●	●	●
Range of Motion			
Scapular — Elevation	√	√	√
Scapular — Depression	√	√	√
Scapular — Abduction	√	√	√
Scapular — Adduction	√	√	√
Scapular — Upward rotation	√	√	√
Scapular — Downward rotation		√	√
Shoulder — Flexion	√	√	√
Shoulder — Extension	√	√	√
Shoulder — Internal rotation	√	☑	☑
Elbow — Flexion	√	√	√
Elbow — Extension	☑	☑	☑
Hip — Flexion	√	√	√
Hip — Extension	☑	☑	☑
Knee — Extension	☑	☑	☑
Ankle — Dorsiflexion	√	√	√
Combined hip flexion and knee extension	☑	☑	☑

√ = Some strength is needed for this activity, or severe limitations in range will inhibit this activity.

☑ = A large amount of strength or normal or greater range is needed for this activity.

● = Not required, but helpful.

places his crutches where he will be able to reach them once he is on his feet. He then positions his buttocks so that he is sitting at the front edge of his seat, resting on the side of his pelvis.

Once he is positioned appropriately in his seat, the person locks the orthotic knees and positions his legs in preparation to stand. The superior leg should rest on top of or slightly anterior to the other leg (Fig. 14–9**A**).

In the next step the person turns and places his hands on the armrests (Fig. 14–9**B**). He then gets onto his feet using the head-hips relationship: he presses down on the armrests, protracts his scapulae, and twists his head and upper trunk down and laterally. His lateral twist should be toward the side of the chair on which he sits (Fig. 14–9**C**). As he twists his head and upper trunk, his pelvis will lift up and over his feet. Once on his feet, the person uses the head-hips relationship to attain his balance point.

The crutch walker now stands with his hands on the wheelchair's armrests (Fig. 14–9**D**). His next

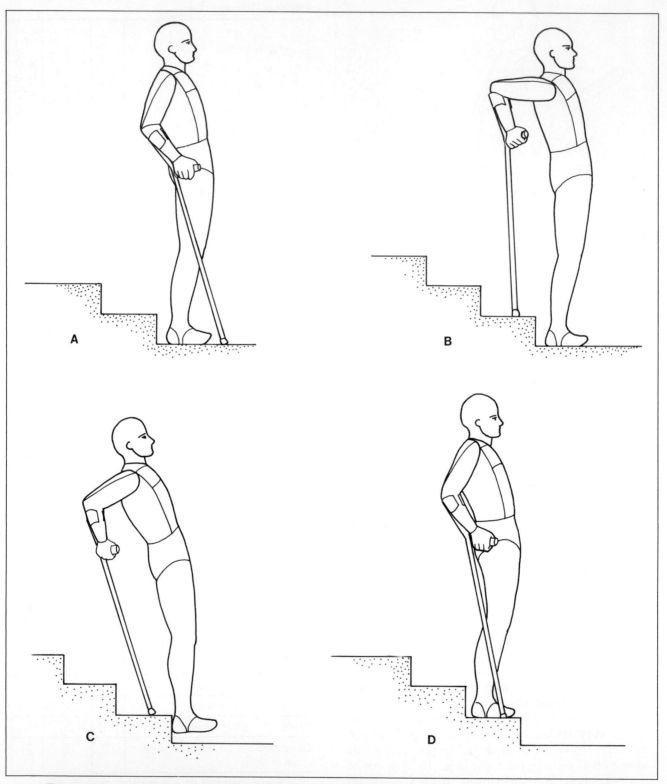

Figure 14–8. Ascending stairs backwards. **A.** Balanced standing posture with feet a few inches from lowest step. **B.** Crutches onto step. **C.** Lifting feet onto step by leaning on crutches, extending elbows, and depressing scapulae. **D.** Balanced standing posture regained.

Chart 14—6 Coming to Stand From Wheelchair—
Skill Prerequisites

	Both hands on armrests	One hand on armrest and one on crutch	Both hands on crutches
Move buttocks using head-hips relationship[a]	√	√	√
Position legs in preparation to stand	√	√	√
Hands on armrests, assume standing position from wheelchair	√		
Standing in front of wheelchair with hands on armrests, grasp crutch	√		
Standing with one hand on armrest and one on crutch, grasp second crutch	√	√	
Standing with crutches positioned forward, walk crutches back	√		
One hand on armrest and one on crutch, assume standing position from wheelchair		√	
Balanced standing	√	√	√
Both hands on crutches, assume standing position from wheelchair			√
While standing, lift and move both crutches			√

[a] Refer to Chapter 11 for a description of this skill and therapeutic strategies.

task is to substitute his crutches for the armrests. To grasp the first crutch, he shifts laterally to unweight one hand. While balancing on his feet and one hand, he grasps a crutch and positions it on his free arm (Fig. 14–9E). He then places the crutch tip on the floor, lateral to the wheelchair. Shifting his weight onto the crutch, the person unweights his other hand and grasps the remaining crutch. After positioning the second crutch on his arm, he places the crutch tip on the floor, lateral to the wheelchair. From this position he achieves an upright standing posture by walking his crutches back (Fig. 14–9F).

One Hand on Armrest, One on Crutch. When standing up from a wheelchair using this method, the crutch walker gets onto his feet with only one hand on the wheelchair. The other hand rests on a crutch, which provides a much less stable base of support. For this reason this method requires more skill than does coming to stand with both hands on a wheelchair. The advantage of the method presented here is that it is quicker than coming to stand with both hands remaining on the chair.

The person starts by locking the wheelchair's brakes and placing his crutches within easy reach. He then moves his buttocks to the front edge of the seat, locks the orthotic knees, and positions his legs and buttocks so that his legs extend diagonally from the seat.

After positioning his legs, the person grasps a crutch and positions it on his arm. The crutch should be held in the hand that is furthest from the chair. After grasping the crutch, the individual should place his free hand on the armrest that he faces (Fig. 14–10A).

The person now sits diagonally at the front of his seat, with one hand on an armrest and one on a crutch. From this position he pushes down with both hands, keeping his head tucked. If he performs the maneuver correctly, his pelvis will lift and his feet will drag toward the chair (Fig. 14–10B). When the legs reach a vertical or nearly vertical position, he pushes his pelvis forward to attain a balanced standing posture (Fig. 14–10C).

Once on his feet in a balanced posture, the person shifts his weight laterally onto the crutch. He then lifts his free hand, grasps the second crutch (Fig. 14–10D) and positions his arm in it, and places the crutch tip on the floor (Fig. 14–10E). After repositioning his crutches as necessary, he is ready to walk.

Both Hands on Crutches. This is the fastest method of rising to standing from a wheelchair. It also requires the most skill; rising from a chair while balancing on two crutches is a very challenging maneuver.

The person starts by locking his wheelchair's brakes, moving his buttocks to the front edge of the seat, locking his orthotic knees, and positioning his legs so that they extend straight forward from the seat. He then grasps both crutches, positions them on his arms, and places the crutch tips lateral to the wheelchair (Fig. 14–11A).

To stand from his chair, the crutch walker pushes down forcefully on the crutches. As he first lifts from the chair, he should keep his trunk flexed forward at the hips (Fig. 14–11B). As his legs move

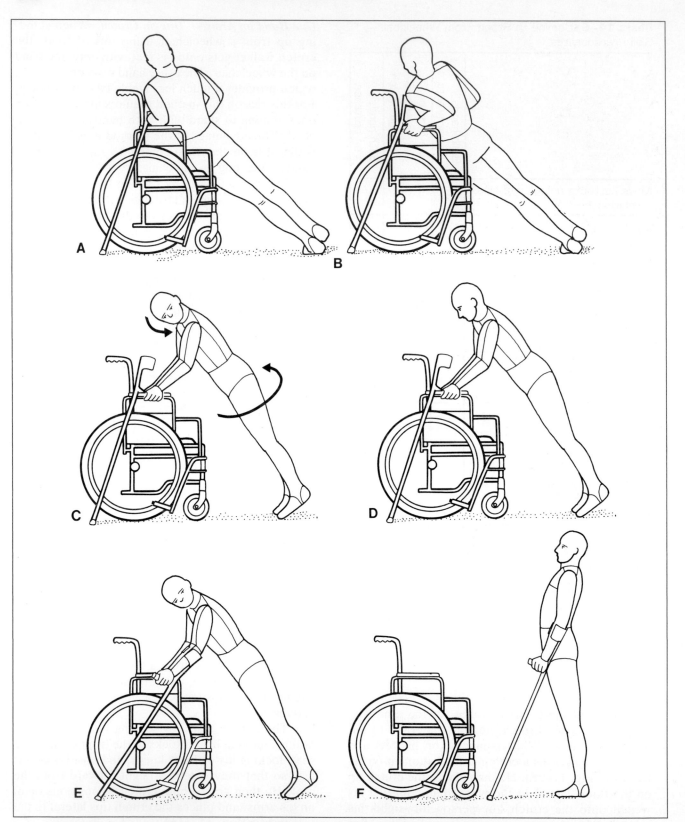

Figure 14–9. Coming to stand from a wheelchair, both hands on armrests. **A.** Sitting at front edge of seat, resting on side of pelvis. **B.** Hands on armrests. **C.** Onto feet using head-hips relationship. **D.** Standing with hands on armrests. **E.** Crutch positioned on arm. **F.** Upright standing.

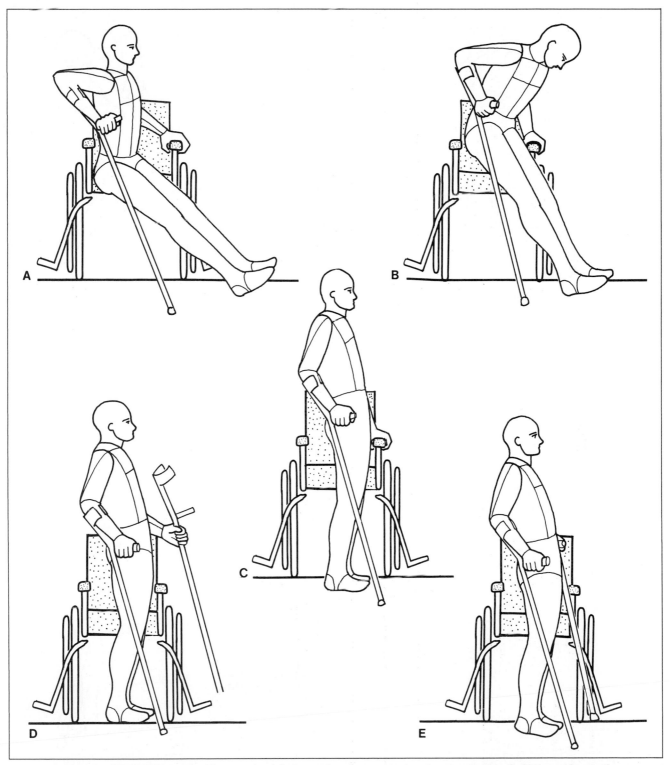

Figure 14–10. Coming to stand from a wheelchair, one hand on armrest and one on crutch. **A.** Sitting at front edge of seat with one hand on armrest and one on crutch. **B.** Lifting pelvis by tucking head while pushing on crutch and armrest. **C.** Balanced standing posture. **D.** Grasping second crutch. **E.** Second crutch placed on floor.

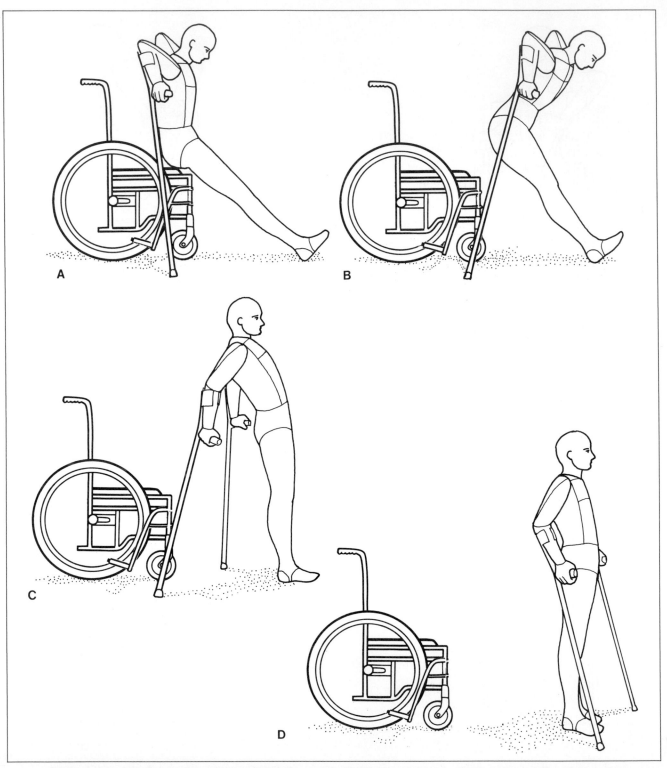

Figure 14–11. Coming to stand from a wheelchair, both hands on crutches. **A.** Sitting at front edge of seat with both hands on crutches. **B.** Rising from wheelchair. **C.** Scapular retraction and head-hips relationship used to push pelvis forward. **D.** Balanced standing posture with crutches repositioned anteriorly.

toward vertical, he extends his trunk toward and then past vertical by pushing on the crutches, lifting his head, and retracting his scapulae to push his pelvis forward (Fig. 14–11C). As he reaches a vertical standing position, he quickly repositions his crutches anteriorly. In this manner he assumes a balanced standing posture (Fig. 14–11D).

Sitting Down From a Standing Position

Functional ambulation requires the ability to sit down safely after walking. The techniques described below center on sitting on a wheelchair. They can be adapted to surfaces other than wheelchairs.

The challenge of rising from a chair is obvious: the cord-injured person must lift himself onto his feet, maintaining his balance throughout the maneuver. Returning to the chair has a less obvious challenge: the individual must lower himself into the chair without traumatizing his skin or tipping the chair. He avoids these problems by controlling his descent so that he lands squarely on the seat rather than on an armrest or on the backrest, and he lands without undue force.

Charts 14–7 and 14–8 summarize the physical and skill prerequisites for sitting down from a standing position.

Both Hands on Armrests. This maneuver is similar to coming to stand with both hands on the armrests, performed in reverse. While lowering himself to sitting, the cord-injured person supports himself with both hands on the wheelchair. Because the wheelchair provides such a steady base of support, this method of sitting from a standing position requires the least skill to perform safely.

In the starting position the individual stands facing the wheelchair with his feet in front of and slightly lateral to the casters (Fig. 14–12A). The appropriate foot position depends on the person's height. The feet should be placed so that when the crutch walker pivots on them, he will land squarely on the seat.

Standing in front of the wheelchair, the person shifts his weight onto one crutch and removes his unweighted hand and forearm from the other crutch. He then leans the unused crutch against the wheelchair and places his free hand on an armrest. Shifting his weight onto the armrest, he removes his other hand and forearm from its crutch, leans the crutch against the wheelchair, and places his hand on the armrest (Fig. 14–12B).

The person is now standing in front of the wheelchair supporting himself with a hand on each armrest. In the next step, he turns and lowers him-

Chart 14–7 Sitting Down From a Standing Position—Physical Prerequisites

		Both hands on armrests	Both hands on crutches
Strength			
Trapezius		√	√
Deltoids		√	√
Biceps, brachialis, and/or brachioradialis		√	√
Serratus anterior		☑	☑
Pectoralis major		☑	☑
Latissimus dorsi		√	☑
Triceps		☑	☑
Wrist and hand musculature		√	√
Abdominals		●	●
Range of Motion			
Scapular	Elevation	√	√
	Depression	√	√
	Abduction	√	√
	Adduction	√	√
	Upward rotation	√	√
	Downward rotation		√
Shoulder	Flexion	√	√
	Extension	√	√
	Internal rotation	√	☑
Elbow	Flexion	√	√
	Extension	☑	☑
Hip	Flexion	√	√
	Extension	☑	☑
Knee	Extension	☑	☑
Ankle	Dorsiflexion	√	√
Combined hip flexion and knee extension		☑	☑

√ = Some strength is needed for this activity, or severe limitations in range will inhibit this activity.

☑ = A large amount of strength or normal or greater range is needed for this activity.

● = Not required, but helpful.

Chart 14–8 Sitting Down From a Standing Position—Skill Prerequisites

	Both hands on armrests	Both hands on crutches
Position self in preparation to sit in wheelchair	√	√
Standing facing wheelchair, place hands on armrests	√	
Move pelvis using head-hips relationship[a]	√	√
Balanced standing	√	√
Facing wheelchair with hands on armrests, turn and lower self into chair	√	
Standing facing away from wheelchair, lower self into chair		√
While standing, lift and move both crutches	√	√
Step forward, back, and to the side	√	√
Weight shift in standing	√	

[a] Refer to Chapter 11 for a description of this skill and therapeutic strategies.

self into the chair. The direction of the turn is determined by the position of his feet in relation to the wheelchair. The turn should be toward the feet: if the feet are to the left of the chair, the head and upper trunk should turn toward the left. The person should twist his head and upper trunk with enough force to provide the momentum to turn his buttocks fully around toward the seat. As he turns, he releases one armrest. (If turning to the left, he releases the right armrest.) He can either throw his free arm in the direction of the turn (Fig. 14–12C) to add momentum to the turn or place his hand on the far rear corner of the seat. After landing, he unlocks the orthotic knees and repositions his buttocks on the seat as needed.

Both Hands on Crutches. Using this method to sit down from a standing position, a person supports himself on two crutches while lowering himself into a wheelchair. This maneuver requires more skill than is required if he supports himself on the armrests.

In the starting position for this maneuver, the crutch walker stands well in front of the wheelchair, facing away from it (Fig. 14–13A). The appropriate foot position depends on the individual's height. The person should place his feet so that when he pivots on them, he will land squarely on the seat. It is critical that he places his feet an appropriate distance from the chair. If he stands too far from the chair, he will miss the seat when he sits. If he stands too close to the chair, he will hit the backrest instead of the seat and may tip the chair over backwards.

Standing facing away from the wheelchair, the crutch walker balances on his feet and repositions his crutches posteriorly (Fig. 14–13B). The exact placement of the crutches will vary among individuals. The person should position the crutches so that he will be able to pivot on them and lower his buttocks onto the seat.

After positioning his crutches, the person lowers himself into the wheelchair. Supporting his weight on the crutches, he tucks his head forward. This causes his pelvis to move backward out of the position of stable standing, and he "jacknifes" at the hips (Fig. 14–13C). He then lowers himself onto the seat. After landing, he unlocks the orthotic knees and repositions his buttocks on the seat as needed.

Falling Safely

Ambulation involves a risk of falling. Anyone who walks, especially if he has impaired motor and sensory function, is likely to fall eventually. Anyone who learns to walk with orthoses and assistive devices should learn to fall in a way that will minimize the risk of injury.

When falling, there are two things that a crutch walker can do to minimize his risk of injury. First, he can move his crutches out of the way so that he does not injure himself by landing on a crutch or by having a crutch exert excessive force on his arm. While falling, the person throws his crutches laterally (or laterally and posteriorly) away from the path of fall. He should aim to get the crutch tips up off of the floor, so that the crutches do not act as fulcrums on his arms when he lands.

The second thing that a person can do when he falls is to break his fall with his arms. He should land on his palms and cushion the fall by allowing the elbows and shoulders to "give" when he lands. He must *not* hold his arms rigid as he falls onto them.

Charts 14–9 and 14–10 summarize the physical and skill prerequisites for falling safely and assuming a standing position from the floor.

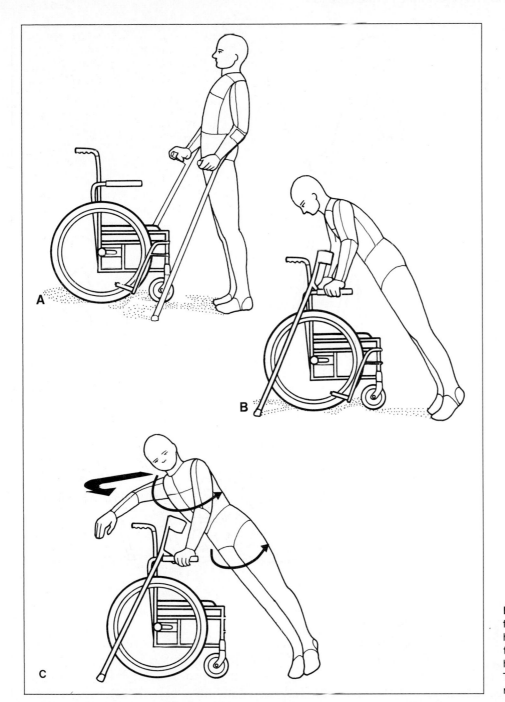

Figure 14–12. Sitting down from standing position, both hands on armrests. **A.** Standing facing wheelchair. **B.** Both hands placed on armrests. **C.** Turning toward hand on armrest.

Assume Standing Position From the Floor

After getting onto the floor, either by falling or by design, a person needs to be able to get back up. This task is challenging but feasible for people with intact upper-extremity function.

To prepare to rise from the floor, the person gets into a prone position with his hips adducted and externally rotated. He then places a crutch on either side of himself. The crutch tips should point away from his feet, and the grips should be at or caudal to the level of his greater trochanters. In this position the crutches will be within reach when he is ready to use them.

After positioning his crutches and legs, the person places his palms on the floor next to his shoulders (Fig. 14–14A). He then moves from prone to plantigrade by lifting his pelvis from the floor using the head-hips relationship, pushing down and for-

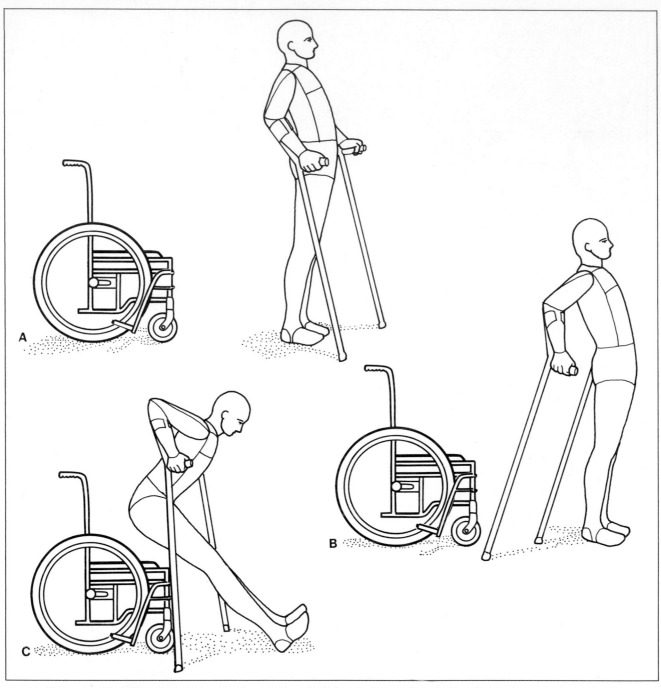

Figure 14–13. Sitting down from standing position, both hands on crutches. **A.** Standing facing away from wheel-chair. **B.** Crutches repositioned posteriorly. **C.** Lowering self onto wheelchair seat.

ward (away from his feet) while tucking his head (Fig. 14–14**B**). When he has lifted his pelvis as high as he can, he walks his hands toward his feet while keeping his head tucked. This maneuver will elevate the pelvis further (Fig. 14–14**C**).

As the person walks his hands toward his feet, his legs become more vertical. By walking his hands back, he moves his legs as far as he can toward (not

past) vertical. The remaining steps involved in coming to stand will be easier with more vertically oriented legs.

Once the individual has walked his hands back as far as he can, he shifts his weight and balances on one hand. He then grasps a crutch with his unweighted hand (Fig. 14–14**D**).

In the next step the person balances on one

Chart 14—9 Falling Safely and Standing From the Floor—Physical Prerequisites

	Fall safely	Stand from the floor
Strength		
Trapezius		√
Deltoids	√	√
Biceps, brachialis, and/or brachioradialis	√	√
Serratus anterior	☑	☑
Pectoralis major	☑	☑
Triceps	☑	☑
Wrist and hand musculature	√	√
Abdominals		●
Range of Motion		
Scapular Elevation		√
Abduction	√	√
Adduction	√	√
Upward rotation	√	☑
Downward rotation		√
Shoulder Flexion	√	☑
Extension		√
Internal rotation		√
Horizontal adduction		√
Horizontal abduction	√	☑
Elbow Flexion	√	√
Extension	√	☑
Hip Flexion		√
Extension		☑
Knee Extension		☑
Ankle Dorsiflexion		√
Combined hip flexion and knee extension		☑

√ = Some strength is needed for this activity, or severe limitations in range will inhibit this activity.
☑ = A large amount of strength or normal or greater range is needed for this activity.
● = Not required, but helpful.

Chart 14—10 Falling Safely and Standing From the Floor—Skill Prerequisites

	Fall safely	Stand from the floor
Throw crutches	√	
Catch self on hands	√	
Position self in prone[a]		√
Position crutches in preparation to stand		√
Assume plantigrade posture from prone		√
Dynamic balance in plantigrade and modified plantigrade		√
In plantigrade, walk hands toward feet		√
In plantigrade, grasp and position crutch		√
In modified plantigrade with one hand on crutch, grasp and position second crutch		√
From modified plantigrade supported on two crutches, push torso to upright		√
Standing with crutches positioned forward, walk crutches back		√

[a] Refer to Chapter 12 for a description of this skill and therapeutic strategies.

crutch while grasping the remaining crutch with his free hand (Fig. 14–14E). For many this is the most challenging part of coming to stand from the floor. Balancing on one crutch will be easiest if the crutch tip is aligned with the midline of the torso. Placement of the proximal aspect of the crutch varies between individuals. Three positions are illustrated in Figure 14–15.

While propping on one crutch, the person grasps the other crutch with his free hand and positions it on his forearm (Fig. 14–14F). He then shifts his weight onto this crutch. If the forearm cuff of the first crutch is not on his forearm, he can now balance on the other crutch while repositioning this cuff. Supporting himself on both crutches, he then pushes to a standing position: using the head-hips relationship, he pushes his pelvis forward (Fig. 14–14G). Once standing, he walks his crutches back until he is upright (Fig. 14–14**H**).

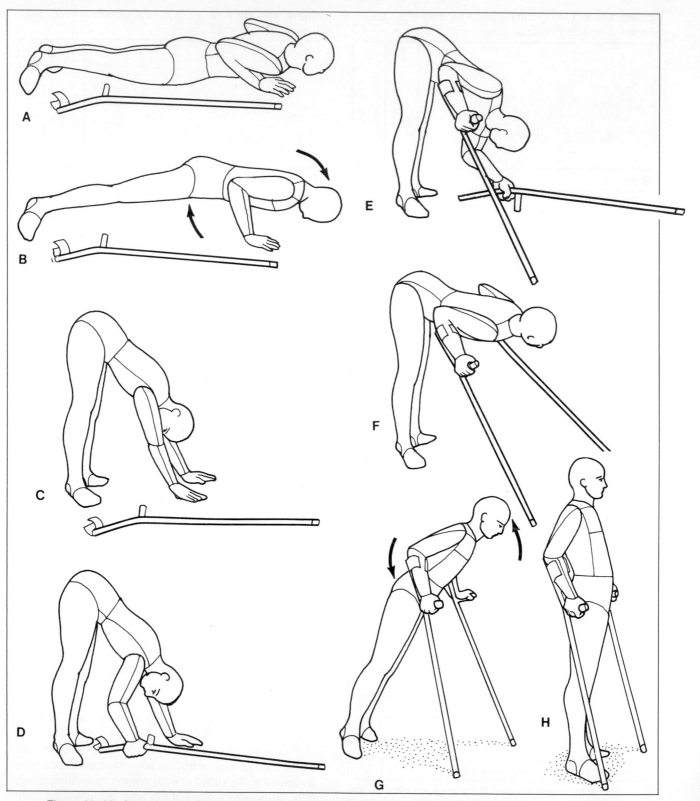

Figure 14–14. Assuming standing position from the floor. **A.** Starting position: prone with legs and crutches positioned appropriately, palms on floor. **B.** Lifting to plantigrade using head-hips relationship. **C.** Pelvis elevated fully. **D.** Grasping first crutch. **E.** Balancing on one crutch while grasping second crutch. **F.** Forearm cuffs positioned. **G.** Pushing trunk upright. **H.** Upright standing.

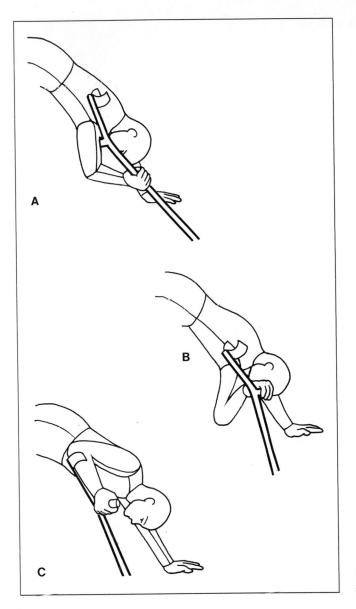

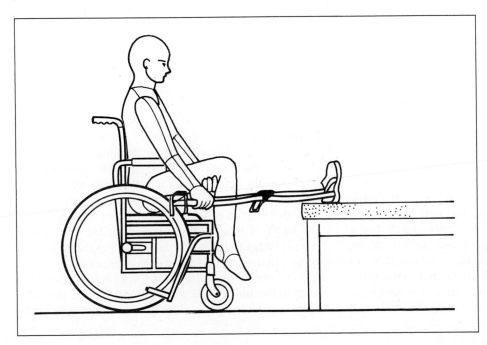

Figure 14–15. Three crutch position options for coming to stand from the floor.

Figure 14–16. Donning orthosis while sitting in wheelchair.

Don and Doff Orthoses

Independent functioning with orthoses requires the ability to put them on and take them off. For people with intact upper-extremity functioning, this is the easiest of the ambulatory skills to master.

A cord-injured person can put his orthoses on while sitting in bed or in his wheelchair. The technique is essentially the same in either location. When donning an orthosis while sitting in a wheelchair, the person props the orthosis on furniture to support it with the knee in extension (Fig. 14–16). Whether in bed or in a wheelchair, he first positions his orthosis and opens the shoe and all straps. He then lifts his leg and positions it over the orthosis, with his knee flexed. He slides his foot into the shoe, checks to make sure that his toes are positioned appropriately, then fastens the shoe and all straps.

Removing an orthosis is generally easiest if the individual remains seated in his wheelchair. This task simply involves opening all straps and the shoe and lifting the leg out of the orthosis.

THERAPEUTIC STRATEGIES

General Strategies

To accomplish a functional goal, the patient must acquire both the physical and skill prerequisites for that activity. For example, when working on ambulation with a swing-through gait, a cord-injured person must develop adequate strength and range in the extremities, as well as develop the ability to balance in standing, lift the trunk by pushing down on lofstrand crutches, and resume and maintain a balanced standing posture.

When developing skill prerequisites for a functional goal, the patient should start with the most basic prerequisite skills and progress toward more challenging activities. (A person had best develop the ability to maintain an upright standing posture before attempting to take a step.)

Before asking a patient to attempt a new skill, the therapist should explain and demonstrate the technique. The demonstration should provide a clear idea of the motions involved and the timing of these motions. The patient should also be shown how the new skill will be used functionally.

During functional training, the therapist should remember that every cord-injured person will perform a particular activity differently. Each has a unique combination of body build, coordination, strength, and flexibility, and these characteristics influence the manner in which he performs functional tasks. For example, each patient is unique in the exact motions that he uses and the timing of these motions as he stands up from the floor. What has worked for the last patient may be a total disaster for the next. The challenge of functional training is finding the timing and maneuvers that best suit the individual involved.

As a therapist and patient work together on a skill, they can learn from failed attempts by analyzing the problem. Is the patient strong enough to perform the maneuver? Is he flexible enough? Is he shifting his weight too far or not far enough? Are his crutches placed appropriately?

Strategies for addressing the various prerequisite skills are presented below.

Equipment. Before attempting any of these skills, the therapist should check the patient's equipment. The parallel bars or crutches should be adjusted to the appropriate height. The standard height for assistive devices is used: as the patient stands in a balanced posture with his shoulders relaxed and his hands on the parallel bars or on the crutches, his elbows should be in 20 to 30 degrees of flexion.

The therapist must evaluate the orthoses carefully to make sure that they fit and function well and are aligned appropriately. The ankles should be held in slight dorsiflexion, and the knees should lock securely in full extension. The orthoses must not exert excessive pressure on any area of skin. The therapist should check for potential sources of trauma to the skin, such as rough seams in leather components or nail points protruding from the soles of the shoes.

During gait training, the therapist and patient should check the patient's skin frequently for problems caused by abrasion or excessive pressure. The skin is at risk anywhere it comes in contact with the orthosis.

Parallel Bars. Any cord-injured person who lacks functioning hip extensors will be very unstable when he first gets onto his feet. For this reason the most sensible place to initiate gait training is in the parallel bars. This equipment provides stable support for early practice. However, parallel bars are a double-edged sword. The very stability that makes them a secure place to begin standing and walking can cause problems. Parallel bars will support a person's weight regardless of whether he pulls, pushes, or leans on them. No other assistive device can provide this degree of support. A patient who develops the habit of leaning laterally or pulling on parallel bars is likely to have difficulty making the transition to ambulation with Lofstrand crutches.

To prepare a patient for the eventual transition to ambulation outside of the parallel bars, the therapist should encourage him to avoid leaning laterally or pulling on the bars. This should be stressed from the beginning of gait training, to avoid the development of bad habits. When pressing on the bars, the patient should direct the force vertically downward. By maintaining his hands in an open position while standing and walking, he can avoid inadvertently pulling on the bars.

No matter how careful a patient and therapist have been to avoid developing bad habits in the parallel bars, the transition from bars to crutches is a challenging one because crutches provide a much less stable base of support than do parallel bars. Even someone who walks independently and skillfully in the parallel bars is likely to require close spotting, even significant assistance when he first ventures out of the bars. The therapist should keep the difficulty of this transition in mind. Deterioration in the patient's performance when he first practices with crutches is not necessarily an indication that he needs to return to the parallel bars for further preparatory practice.

Guarding. Guarding is required during much of gait training to ensure the patient's safety. The challenge of guarding well is to keep the crutch walker safe without interfering with his gait or motor learning.

Hands-on spotting while walking with a cord-injured person is best done from behind. A therapist who stands behind the patient is less likely to get in the way of his head and trunk motions and feet as he steps. When practicing stairs or curbs, the therapist is likely to find it easier to guard the patient when standing below him.

When a patient loses his balance while walking, the natural reaction for many therapists is to pull his pelvis (via a gait belt) up and toward the therapist. This guarding technique is not effective with cord-injured people, since a backward tug on a patient's pelvis will throw his hips into an unstable position. Uncontrolled forward flexion of the trunk on the hips ("jacknifing") is likely to result.

A therapist should guard in such a way that the patient's balance is restored, not hindered, when assistance is given. When a cord-injured person lacking innervated hip extensors loses his balance, the therapist should push his pelvis forward and pull his upper trunk back. This will return him to a balanced standing posture (Fig. 14–17).

When a therapist makes a postural correction for a patient or catches him when he starts to lose his balance, the patient should be made aware of this assistance. Especially if the therapist has a hand on an area with impaired sensation, the patient may not realize that the therapist has assisted him. As a

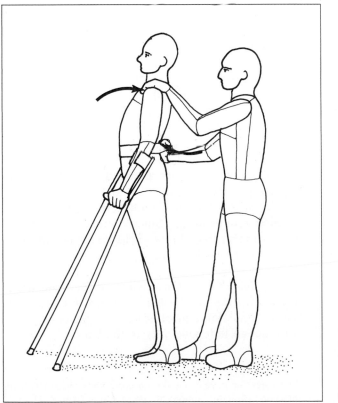

Figure 14–17. Forces applied when helping a patient maintain or return to a balanced standing posture.

result, he will not realize that he has made an error that needs to be corrected.

There are two ways in which a therapist can make a patient aware of his mistakes and of the assistance being given. First, the therapist can provide verbal feedback. ("I had to catch you just now. You were falling to the left.") Verbal feedback is especially important when a patient first attempts a skill. In the second strategy, the therapist guards in a way that enables the patient to feel his mistakes. Specifically, when he starts to "jacknife" or lose his balance to the side, the therapist does not catch him or correct his posture until he has fallen far enough that he can sense what has happened.[4] This strategy is not appropriate when the patient first attempts a skill. Standing for the first time, or walking outside of the parallel bars for the first time, can be frightening enough as it is. The therapist should begin allowing partial falls only after the patient has overcome his initial fear of the activity.

Close guarding is required during most of gait training. At some point, however, a person who plans to walk independently must practice walking without spotting. The transition from walking with guarding to walking alone can be a test of nerves for both the patient and the therapist. To ease this transition, and to maximize the patient's safety throughout the process, the shift should be gradual. As (and *only* as) an individual demonstrates that he can safely perform a skill unassisted, the therapist's guarding should be withdrawn. The patient and therapist first progress from walking with contact guarding to walking with the therapist's hands hovering inches away, ready to grab if needed. They then progress to walking with the therapist standing nearby, ready to dive and grab. When both parties are ready, the patient walks while the therapist watches from a distance[5] and prays, and finally just prays. In this manner the patient and (perhaps more so) the therapist can be weaned from guarding.

Specific Strategies

Balanced Standing. Training in balanced standing should include practice maintaining a balanced standing posture as well as practice moving in and out of that posture while standing upright. Before a patient begins practice in balanced standing, he

should have had prior practice using the head-hips relationship to control his pelvis.[6]

The therapist should demonstrate and explain the balanced standing posture, showing how head and shoulder motions can be used to move the pelvis and stabilize the hips. The patient should stand with his head erect, chest forward (scapulae retracted), and pelvis forward. His feet should be a few inches apart.

During early training, the patient gains an awareness of his pelvis' motions in standing and develops skill in controlling these motions. He should practice moving his pelvis using head and scapular motions. As he moves in and out of a balanced posture, he should attend to sensory cues that tell him of his pelvis' position. Practice should include experiencing how his hips "jacknife" when his weight line falls anterior to his hips.

During initial training, the therapist can assist the patient to a balanced standing posture in the parallel bars. The therapist can help him maintain the posture and give him feedback and suggestions. As the patient's skill develops, the therapist should reduce the assistance provided. Once the patient can balance well with both hands on the parallel bars, he can practice balancing with one hand, then both hands, lifted. If he has difficulty balancing, the alignment of the orthotic ankles may need to be adjusted.

When a cord-injured person walks, his feet do not always land where he wants them to. A patient will be better prepared for ambulation if he learns to balance, at least briefly, with his feet in less than optimal positions. Training in standing balance, then, should be done with the feet in various positions. The patient should start with his feet in the easiest position (close to parallel and a few inches apart) and progress to balancing with his feet in more challenging positions.

Initial practice of standing balance should take place in the parallel bars. Once the patient has progressed to walking in the bars and is ready to start working with lofstrand crutches, he should practice standing with crutches. Since crutches provide less stable support than do parallel bars, balancing with them is more challenging.

Independent Work: Once a patient has had initial practice in the parallel bars and has demonstrated that he can catch himself if he loses his balance, he can practice independently in the bars.

---

[4] This is not to say that the patient should be allowed to plummet halfway to the floor each time he starts to lose his balance. A few inches of free fall is generally enough to catch a person's attention.

[5] Before walking alone, the patient must be proficient in falling safely.

---

[6] Strategies for developing skill in controlling the pelvis using head and shoulder motions are presented in Chapter 11.

Weight Shift in Standing. Before practicing weight shifts in standing, the patient must be able to maintain a balanced standing posture. To practice shifting his weight while standing with a given assistive device (parallel bars or lofstrand crutches), the person should be adept in balanced standing using that assistive device.

The patient can begin weight shifting with lateral shifts, with his feet side by side a few inches apart. As his skill improves, he can progress to shifting his weight with his feet in other positions. If he is to walk with a four-point gait, the patient must develop the capacity to stand with one foot diagonally in front of the other and shift his weight onto the forward foot.

During early weight-shifting practice, the therapist can assist the patient into position in the parallel bars and guard him as he shifts his weight. The therapist can help him get a feel for the motion by placing a hand against his trunk or shoulder and having him push against the hand. As the patient's skill improves, the therapist can withdraw the resistance and the guarding. When gait training has progressed to the point where the patient is ready to start ambulation outside of the parallel bars, he should practice weight shifting with Lofstrand crutches.

Independent Work: Once an individual has had initial practice in the parallel bars and has demonstrated that he can catch himself if he loses his balance, he can practice weight shifting independently in the bars.

Lift and Move One Crutch. To lift a crutch while standing, a person must be able to maintain a balanced standing posture and weight shift with two crutches. He will be better prepared to practice moving a crutch if he has practiced lifting a hand while standing in the parallel bars.

The patient should practice lifting a crutch while the therapist guards and provides assistance as necessary. As his skill improves, the assistance can be withdrawn.

Step Forward With One Leg. Balanced standing and weight shifting are prerequisites for learning to step forward with one leg. To practice stepping using a given assistive device (parallel bars or Lofstrand crutches), the patient should be adept in standing and weight shifting using that assistive device. He should also be skillful in the use of the head-hips relationship before attempting to step with one leg.

Practice should start with the patient standing in the parallel bars with one hand in front of the other. (The hand opposite the stepping leg should be anterior.) From this position he practices shifting his weight off the leg and lifting his pelvis on the unweighted side. When his pelvis tilts enough to lift the foot off the ground, the leg swings forward as a pendulum or by muscle action, depending on whether the iliopsoas is innervated.

The patient elevates his pelvis using the quadratus lumborum, latissimus dorsi, abdominal musculature, or the head-hips relationship, or a combination thereof. Whichever method he uses, the therapist can help him learn the motion by demonstrating, assisting with the motion, and providing verbal and tactile feedback during practice.

A patient with innervated quadratus lumborum, latissimus dorsi, or abdominals may build the groundwork for stepping by practicing elevating his pelvis in side lying. Utilizing quick stretch and resistance, the therapist can facilitate motor learning and strengthening.[7]

If using the head-hips relationship to elevate his pelvis, the patient may use exaggerated motions when first practicing, tucking his head far down and to the side. As he develops a feel for the maneuver, he can reduce his head and upper trunk motions.

Practice stepping should begin in the parallel bars, with the therapist spotting and assisting as needed. As the patient's skill improves, the assistance should be withdrawn. Once proficient in the parallel bars, the patient should progress to working outside of the bars with crutches. Before attempting to step with crutches, he should have developed his dynamic balance skills in standing with these assistive devices.

Independent Work: Once a patient has had initial practice in the parallel bars and has demonstrated that he can catch himself if he loses his balance, he can practice stepping independently in the bars.

Step to the Side or Back With One Leg. The patient must be proficient in using the head-hips relationship, balanced standing, and weight shifting before attempting to step to the side or back. To practice stepping using a given assistive device (parallel bars or lofstrand crutches), the patient should be adept in standing and weight shifting using that assistive device. Prior practice in stepping forward should make learning to step back or to the side easier.

Practice should start with the patient standing

---

[7] For a more complete description of proprioceptive neuromuscular facilitation techniques, the reader should refer to the following references: Sullivan, Markos, & Minor, 1982; Sullivan & Markos, 1987.

in the parallel bars. From this position he practices shifting his weight off one leg and lifting his pelvis on the unweighted side. The techniques that he can use for elevating his pelvis and the therapeutic strategies for developing this skill are the same as described above for stepping forward with one leg.

With his leg lifted, the patient practices swinging it laterally or forward and back using head and upper trunk motions to move his pelvis. He may use exaggerated motions when first practicing. As he develops a feel for the maneuver, he can reduce his head and upper body motions.

Once he has learned to swing his leg, the patient can practice placing his foot by lowering his pelvis when his foot has swung to the desired position.

Practice should begin in the parallel bars, with the therapist spotting and assisting as needed. As the patient's skill improves, the assistance should be withdrawn. Once proficient in the parallel bars, the patient should progress to working outside of the bars with crutches. Before attempting to step with crutches, he should have developed his dynamic balance skills in standing with these assistive devices.

Independent Work: Once a patient has had initial practice in the parallel bars and has demonstrated that he can catch himself if he loses his balance, he can practice stepping to the side and back independently in the bars.

Lift And Move Two Crutches. Before attempting to lift and move two crutches at once, a patient must be proficient in balanced standing with crutches. He should also be able to lift both hands simultaneously while maintaining a balanced standing posture in the parallel bars. An individual who has acquired these skills should not have difficulty learning to lift and move both crutches with a brief period of practice.

Swing-Through Step. Before practicing this maneuver, a patient must be skillful in balanced standing, including moving in and out of the balanced posture. He should also be skillful in the use of the head-hips relationship. To practice stepping using a given assistive device (parallel bars or Lofstrand crutches), the individual should be adept in standing using that assistive device.

Practice should start with the patient standing in a balanced posture in the parallel bars with his hands anterior to his hips. From this position he should practice lifting his feet off the ground by leaning forward onto his arms while extending his elbows, depressing and protracting his scapulae, and tucking his head. When his feet leave the ground,

his trunk and legs will swing forward as a pendulum hanging from his shoulders. During gait training, the therapist should stress the passive nature of the feet's motion: the crutch walker's task is to lift his feet; gravity will provide the force to move them forward.

When the patient's heels strike, he should quickly regain the balanced standing posture. He does this by retracting his scapulae and throwing his head back, pushing his pelvis forward.

The therapist can help the patient learn the required motions by demonstrating, assisting with the motions, and providing verbal and tactile feedback during practice. The patient may use exaggerated motions when first practicing lifting his feet and regaining a balanced posture. As he develops a feel for the maneuver, he can reduce his head and upper body motions.

Practice should begin in the parallel bars, with the therapist spotting and assisting as needed. As the patient's skill improves, the assistance should be withdrawn. Once proficient in the parallel bars, the patient should progress to working outside of the bars with crutches. Before attempting to step with crutches, he should have developed his dynamic balance skills in standing with these assistive devices.

Independent Work: Once a patient has had initial practice in the parallel bars and has demonstrated that he can catch himself if he loses his balance, he can practice stepping independently in the bars.

Swing-To or Drag-To Step. To practice a swing-to or drag-to step, a patient must be skillful in balanced standing, able to move in and out of a balanced standing posture. He should also be skillful in the use of the head-hips relationship. To practice stepping using a given assistive device (parallel bars or Lofstrand crutches), the patient should be adept in standing using that assistive device.

A swing-to step is like a swing-through step, except that the feet land even with, not past, the crutches. In a drag-to step, the patient lifts his trunk only enough to drag his feet to or toward the level of his crutches. His feet do not leave the ground. Both gait patterns can be taught using the training strategies described for teaching a swing-through step.

Distance/Efficient Ambulation. Once a patient is able to walk with a given gait pattern using assistive devices, he will require practice to develop his endurance and perfect his skills. He should walk over increasing distances as his ability develops. He can also practice walking on uneven surfaces such as sidewalks and grass.

Independent Work: When a patient is able to walk safely and to fall without guarding, he can practice independently. When his distance capabilities have increased enough, he should be encouraged to walk to his various activities during the day and to walk during his free time in the evenings.

Ambulation Up and Down Slopes.
A person must be proficient in ambulation over even surfaces before beginning practice on ramps.

The patient is likely to be very unstable when first walking on ramps. This is especially true when ascending, since the inclined surface tends to throw the pelvis into an unstable position. The patient should be encouraged to keep his crutches well in front of his feet when ascending and to keep his body angled up the hill with his pelvis well forward. He should use a step-to (or step-toward) gait, not a swing-through pattern. When descending, he may step past his crutches.

Practice in ramp negotiation should start on gentle slopes. Once the patient masters a slope of a particular grade, he should progress to steeper inclines. Training in ramp negotiation can continue in this manner until the individual has reached his maximal potential.

Step Up and Down Curb/Step.
Before attempting ambulation over curbs or stairs, the patient must be proficient in ambulation over even surfaces.

During training, the therapist should emphasize maintaining control during ascent and descent and rapid resumption of a balanced standing posture once the feet have landed. Practice should start on small curbs. As the patient's skill increases, the curb height can be increased. Once the patient is skillful in negotiation of step-high curbs, he can progress to practicing on stairs.

Sitting in Wheelchair, Position Legs in Preparation to Stand.
To practice positioning his legs in preparation to stand, a patient must be skillful in stabilizing his trunk in a wheelchair.[8] Prior practice in leg management on a mat[9] will make practice in a wheelchair easier.

If an individual has the physical potential to come to standing from a wheelchair, he should be able to learn to position his legs without much dif-

ficulty. The therapist should demonstrate the maneuver and encourage the patient to practice.

Independent Work: After a brief period of supervised practice with feedback, the patient should be able to practice this skill independently.

With Hands on Armrests, Assume Standing Position from Wheelchair.
Before a patient begins working on this skill, he must be proficient in using the head-hips relationship to move his pelvis.

During initial practice, the therapist can demonstrate and assist the patient as he pushes himself into a standing position. The therapist should encourage him to use forceful and abrupt head and upper trunk motions to lift his pelvis. As the patient's skill develops, the therapist's assistance should be reduced.

This maneuver is most difficult at its beginning, when the person lifts himself from the seat. If an individual has difficulty lifting himself to a standing position from a wheelchair, he can work on the skill in reverse in the following manner. The therapist assists him to a standing position, facing the chair with one hand on each armrest. The patient's feet should be positioned in front of and slightly lateral to the casters. From this position he turns and lowers his buttocks slightly toward the seat and then pushes himself back to the starting position (Fig. 14-18). He should move over a small arc at first, lowering himself only as far as he can retain control of the motion and push back up. As his skill improves, he should increase the arc of motion. He should challenge his limits as he practices, working in a range in which he experiences difficulty but can maintain control. By pushing his limits in this manner, the patient gradually builds to the point where he can lower himself to the seat and push back up to standing.

Standing in Front of Wheelchair With Hands on Armrests, Grasp Crutch.
Anyone who has the physical potential to assume a standing position from a wheelchair should achieve this prerequisite skill without much difficulty. The patient can start by practicing weight shifting while standing in front of a wheelchair with his hands on the armrests. He can progress to lifting a hand, then grasping a crutch. The therapist can assist the patient into position and guard him as he practices.

Standing With One Hand on Wheelchair Armrest and One on Crutch, Grasp Second Crutch.
To practice this skill, a patient must be able to weight shift while standing with crutches and balance in standing with one hand lifted.

---

[8] This skill is addressed in Chapter 11.
[9] This skill is addressed in Chapter 12.

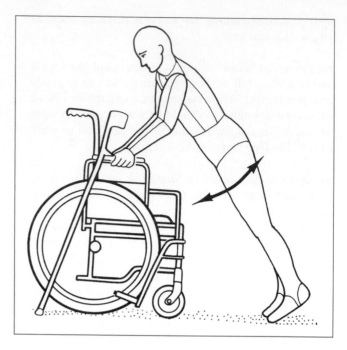

Figure 14–18. Practice lowering buttocks toward seat and returning to standing.

The patient stands in front of a wheelchair with one hand on an armrest and one on a crutch. He should face toward or sideways to the chair, depending on the method of coming to standing being practiced. From the starting position, the patient practices shifting his weight off the hand on the armrest. He can progress to lifting the unweighted hand, then grasping the second crutch. The therapist can assist the patient into position and guard him as he practices.

Standing With Crutches Positioned Forward, Walk Crutches Back. When performing this maneuver, a person starts in a position similar to that illustrated in Figure 14–14G. To attain an upright standing posture from this position, he shifts his weight from one side to the other and repositions each crutch as it is unweighted.

Before practicing this skill, a patient should be proficient in balanced upright standing and able to lift and reposition one crutch at a time while standing upright.

Walking the crutches back from a forward position is most difficult when the crutch tips are furthest from the feet. In this position the person is furthest from upright, and the greatest amount of weight is being borne through the crutches. As he walks his crutches toward his feet, he assumes a more upright posture. His weight is increasingly borne through his legs, and the task becomes easier.

Training in this skill will be easiest if the patient starts in the least challenging position and works toward the most difficult. He should start with his legs close to vertical, with the crutch tips a few inches in front of his feet. From this position he walks his crutches away from his feet and back again. Throughout these maneuvers, his pelvis remains anteriorly positioned to prevent "jacknifing." As his skill improves, he walks his crutches over greater distances, walking the crutch tips as far anteriorly as he can while maintaining control and retaining the ability to return to upright.

This skill can be practiced concurrently with the other prerequisite skills for coming to stand from a wheelchair or from the floor.

Independent Work: This skill is most readily practiced independently if the patient can get into position on his own. If he knows how to fall safely and has developed some skill in walking his crutches forward and back, he can practice independently over a floor mat. For added safety he can practice in front of a wall. When practicing in front of a wall, he should face away from the wall and position his feet far enough from the wall that he does not touch it while he practices but close enough that the wall will support him if he starts to fall backward.

With One Hand on Armrest and One on Crutch, Assume Standing Position From Wheelchair. Practice of this skill requires proficiency in using the head-hips relationship to move the pelvis. The patient must also be skillful in balanced standing with crutches, including moving in and out of a balanced standing posture.

During initial practice the therapist can demonstrate and assist the patient as he lifts himself into a standing position. The therapist should encourage him to use forceful and abrupt head and upper trunk motions to lift his pelvis. As the patient's skill develops, the assistance should be reduced.

With Both Hands on Crutches, Assume Standing Position From Wheelchair.

Before attempting this maneuver, the patient must be proficient in using the head-hips relationship to move his pelvis. He must also be skillful in balanced standing with crutches, including moving in and out of a balanced standing posture.

When teaching this skill, the therapist can demonstrate and then assist the patient as he lifts himself to standing. The therapist should encourage him to push forcefully and abruptly on his crutches and to keep his head tucked as his pelvis lifts. As the patient's legs move toward vertical, he must push his pelvis forward to attain a balanced standing posture. As his legs move past vertical, he must reposition his crutches anteriorly. During practice the patient can work on perfecting his motions and timing. As his skill develops, the therapist can reduce the assistance given.

Position Self in Preparation to Sit in Wheelchair.

When sitting down from a standing position, a cord-injured person wearing KAFOs pivots on his feet as he descends. Thus if he does not position his feet appropriately prior to sitting, he will not land correctly in the wheelchair. Instead of landing on the seat, his buttocks may hit the chair's backrest or armrest, or even miss the wheelchair altogether.

A patient should be able to step in all directions before practicing this skill. Training in foot placement for sitting is then a matter of finding the position that is best for that individual.

To find the optimal foot position, the therapist and patient can first make an educated guess, judging from the individual's leg length and predicting the path of his buttocks as he pivots on his feet. The patient can then position his feet and, with the therapist guarding closely, sit down in the chair. If he does not land appropriately on the seat, the patient and therapist should determine what was wrong with his initial foot position. (Were his feet too close to the chair? Too far away? Too far lateral to the chair's midline? Not lateral enough?) He can then try again with his feet in a different position. By this informed trial and error and by learning from their mistakes, the patient and therapist can find an appropriate foot position for sitting down in the chair.

This skill can be practiced concurrently with other skill prerequisites for getting in and out of a standing position from a wheelchair.

Standing Facing Wheelchair, Place Hands on Armrests.

To practice this skill, a patient must be proficient in the following balanced standing skills with Lofstrand crutches: moving in and out of a balanced standing posture, weight shifting, lifting a hand, and repositioning the crutches.

When working on this skill, the patient practices shifting his weight off of one crutch, leaning the crutch on the wheelchair, and placing his unweighted hand on an armrest. He then repeats these actions with his other hand.

During initial practice the therapist provides guarding and assistance as needed. As the patient's skill improves, the assistance can be reduced.

When practicing this skill, the patient should get into the habit of leaning his crutches against the wheelchair where he can reach them. When crutches are placed in this manner instead of being tossed aside, they are less likely to be damaged. In addition, the crutch that is placed within reach remains retrievable. Once a crutch is tossed, the patient loses the option to change his mind about sitting down.

Facing Wheelchair With Hands on Armrests, Turn and Lower Self into Chair.

Before practicing this maneuver, a patient should be proficient in using the head-hips relationship to move his pelvis.

In this maneuver the cord-injured person standing in front of his wheelchair turns approximately 180 degrees and drops into the chair. Since he releases an armrest while descending, the descent is not truly controlled: the person drops into the seat instead of lowering himself.

The therapist should encourage the patient to use head and upper trunk motions that are forceful and abrupt enough to generate the momentum required to turn his torso and land on his buttocks. The therapist should guard closely at first. As the patient's skill develops, the guarding can be withdrawn.

Standing Facing Away From Wheelchair, Lower Self into Chair.

Practice of this skill requires proficiency in using the head-hips relationship to move the pelvis and balanced standing skills with lofstrand crutches.

In this maneuver a crutch walker standing in front of a wheelchair flexes at the hips and lowers his buttocks into the chair. He should be able to control the descent to some degree, since both of his hands remain on his crutches while he descends.

Since the crutches do not provide a stable base of support, he is not likely to be in total control of the descent, able to stop or reverse his motion at will. However, he should have enough control to land without excessive force and with his buttocks squarely in the seat.

As the patient practices with guarding, the therapist should encourage him to control his motion as he "jacknifes" and lowers himself into the wheelchair. As his skill develops, the guarding can be withdrawn.

This skill can be practiced concurrently with other skill prerequisites for getting in and out of a standing position from a wheelchair.

When Falling, Throw Crutches and Catch Self on Hands.
The two components of this maneuver, throwing the crutches and landing on the hands, can first be practiced separately or in combination. Before training is complete, however, the patient must practice both together.

When throwing the crutches while falling, the aim is to position them so that they will not cause injury. The patient should be encouraged to throw his crutches laterally out of his path of fall. The crutch tips should swing upward so that they do not catch on the ground. The forearm cuffs may remain on the arms. To get a feel for the throw, the patient can practice throwing one crutch at a time while the therapist guards him. For added security while practicing throwing one crutch, the patient can stand outside of a set of parallel bars and hold the nearest bar.

When a patient practices falling and landing on his hands, the therapist should stress to the patient that he *must* allow his arms to "give" to absorb the shock. During initial practice the force of the fall should be minimized. The therapist can accomplish this by having the person fall over a short distance and by lowering him instead of allowing him to fall unrestrained. As the patient's skill develops, he can progress to falling unrestrained over a short distance and gradually build the distance over which he falls.

Lying on the Floor, Position Crutches in Preparation to Stand.
For a patient with the physical potential to get himself into a standing position from the floor, this prerequisite skill is not physically challenging. Training is simply a matter of determining the correct placement for the crutches.

When preparing to assume a standing position from the floor, the cord-injured person should position his crutches so that he will be able to reach them easily when the time comes. The appropriate

position will depend on how far back he walks his hands in plantigrade as he comes to stand. The crutches' hand grips are likely to be reached easily if they are positioned at or caudal to the level of the greater trochanters. The therapist and patient can determine the optimal crutch position through problem solving and trial and error, with the patient grasping the crutches in various positions while in plantigrade.

From Prone, Assume Plantigrade Posture.
To move from prone to plantigrade, a cord-injured person must be proficient in moving his pelvis using the head-hips relationship. Prior practice in using head and upper trunk motions to assume a quadruped position from prone will facilitate acquisition of this skill.

During early practice the therapist can assist the patient as he attempts to assume a plantigrade posture. The patient should be encouraged to push forcefully down and cephalad while tucking his head and upper torso to lift his pelvis. A strong and skillful individual may be able to move from prone to plantigrade with minimal practice. Others may require more training.

This maneuver is most difficult at its beginning, when the person lifts his pelvis from the floor. A patient who has difficulty assuming a plantigrade posture can work on the skill in reverse in the following manner. The therapist assists him into a plantigrade posture with his pelvis well off the ground. From this position the patient lowers himself slightly toward prone and pushes back to the starting position. He should move over a small arc of motion at first, lowering himself only as far as he can retain control of the motion and push back up. As his skill improves, he should increase the arc of motion. He should challenge his limits as he practices, working in a range in which he experiences difficulty but can maintain control. By pushing his limits in this manner, the patient gradually builds to the point where he can lower himself to prone and push back up to plantigrade.

Assuming a plantigrade posture can be practiced concurrently with other skill prerequisites used in coming to stand from the floor.

Independent Work: After a patient has developed some ability in this maneuver, he can work independently on a floor mat to increase his skill and the consistency of his performance. If he has difficulty lifting his pelvis, he can work with his feet stabilized by a wall. However, he must progress to pushing into plantigrade without his feet stabilized if he is to become independent in coming to stand from the floor without his feet stabilized on an object.

Dynamic Balance in Plantigrade and Modified Plantigrade. A patient need not be independent in attaining plantigrade or modified plantigrade postures to practice dynamic balance in these positions. To practice dynamic balance in a given posture, he should have well-developed dynamic balance skills in less advanced postures. Thus to practice in plantigrade, an individual should have good dynamic balance in quadruped.[10] Before beginning balance practice in modified plantigrade, he should have good dynamic balance in plantigrade.

In the plantigrade posture, a person is positioned with his feet and hands on the floor, his hips flexed, and his buttocks in the air (Fig. 14–19**A**). Modified plantigrade includes a variety of postures in which a person's feet are on the floor, his hips are flexed, and his hands are supported by a surface that is higher than the floor. The hand placement in the modified plantigrade postures involved in coming to stand from the floor include one hand on the floor and one on a crutch and both hands on crutches (Fig. 14–19**B** and **C**).

One task when practicing modified plantigrade with one hand on a crutch involves determining the crutch position that best suits the individual. Three crutch positions used in coming to stand from the floor are illustrated in Figure 14–15. While practicing balance in modified plantigrade, the patient can try the different crutch positions to see which one affords him the best control.

To develop dynamic balance in plantigrade or modified plantigrade, the patient can start with practice maintaining the posture. The therapist can assist him into position and have him attempt to maintain the posture using head, scapular, and upper trunk motions to control his pelvis. The therapist helps at first, reducing the assistance as the patient's skill improves. The patient can progress to maintaining the position while the therapist applies resistance in various directions.

Once an individual is able to stabilize himself in plantigrade or modified plantigrade, he can progress to shifting his weight in that posture, then weight shifting and lifting the unweighted hand, and finally maintaining his balance as he lifts a hand and reaches in different directions. All of these actions can be performed with and without resistance supplied by the therapist.

---

[10] Strategies for developing dynamic balance in quadruped are presented in Chapter 11.

Independent Work: If a patient can assume plantigrade or modified plantigrade without assistance, he can practice his dynamic balance on a floor mat independently.

In Plantigrade, Walk Hands Toward Feet. To practice walking his hands back while in a plantigrade posture, a patient should have well-developed dynamic balance skills in plantigrade. He does not have to be independent in assuming this posture.

An individual with good dynamic balance in plantigrade should be able to learn to walk his hands back with minimal practice. During early training, the therapist may help him control his pelvis as he attempts the maneuver. This assistance can be decreased as the patient's skill develops.

This skill can be practiced concurrently with other skill prerequisites used in coming to stand from the floor.

Independent Work: If a patient can assume a plantigrade posture without assistance, he can practice this skill independently on a floor mat. For added safety he can practice near a wall. When practicing near a wall, he should face away from the wall and position his feet far enough from the wall that he does not touch it while he practices but close enough that the wall will support him if he starts to fall backward.

In Plantigrade, Grasp and Position Crutch. In this maneuver the person moves from plantigrade to modified plantigrade. In the end posture he supports his weight with one hand on the floor and one on a crutch (Fig. 14–19**B**). A patient need not be independent in assuming a plantigrade posture to practice this skill, but he should have well-developed dynamic balance skills in plantigrade. The therapist can help the patient maintain his balance during early practice. As his skill builds, this assistance can be decreased.

This skill can be practiced concurrently with other skill prerequisites used in coming to stand from the floor.

Independent Work: If a patient can get into plantigrade and walk his hands toward his feet without assistance, he can practice grasping and positioning a crutch independently on a floor mat. For added safety he can practice near a wall. When practicing near a wall, he should position himself so that the wall is close enough to prevent a backward fall but does not support him as he practices.

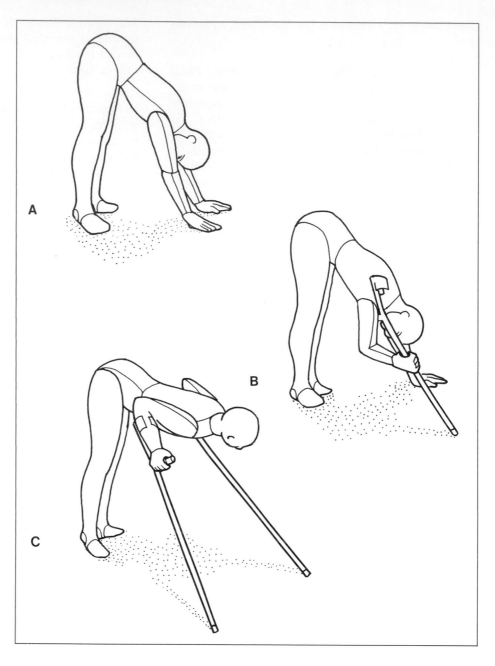

Figure 14–19. Plantigrade and modified plantigrade postures. **A.** Plantigrade. **B** and **C.** Modified plantigrade postures involved in coming to stand from the floor with KAFOs and Lofstrand crutches.

In Modified Plantigrade With One Hand on Crutch, Grasp and Position Second Crutch With Free Hand. In this maneuver the patient moves from one modified plantigrade posture to another. In the end posture he supports his trunk with two crutches (Fig. 14–19C). Before attempting this skill, he should have well-developed dynamic balance skills in modified plantigrade.

This skill is likely to require a moderate amount of practice, even for a skillful patient. The therapist and patient can use the strategies described above

for learning to move from plantigrade to one-crutch–supported modified plantigrade.

From Modified Plantigrade Supported on Two Crutches, Push Torso to Upright. The starting position for this maneuver is illustrated in Figure 14–19C. From this posture the cord-injured person lifts his trunk by pushing downward on the crutches. While raising his trunk, he pushes his buttocks forward by lifting his head.

During early practice the therapist can help the

patient stabilize his pelvis as he lifts his torso. This assistance can be removed as the patient's skill improves.

This skill can be practiced concurrently with other skill prerequisites used in coming to stand from the floor.

Independent Work: If a patient can get into two-crutch–supported modified plantigrade without assistance and if he is able to fall safely, he can practice pushing his torso to upright independently on a floor mat. For added safety, he can practice near a wall. When practicing near a wall, he should position himself so that the wall is close enough to prevent a backward fall but does not support him as he practices.

Donning and Doffing Orthoses. This skill should be readily achievable by anyone with the potential for independent ambulation. During early practice the therapist can provide suggestions and assist the patient as needed.

Independent Work: After a brief period of supervised practice with feedback, the patient should be able to practice this skill independently.

PROGRAM DESIGN

When using this text as a resource to assist in working toward a functional goal, the therapist should first read the text's description of that functional activity. Based on that description, the corresponding charts or both, the therapist can determine what physical and skill prerequisites are required to perform the skill. Taking into consideration the patient's evaluation results, the therapist can determine where the patient has deficits relevant to the functional goal. The program should then be designed to address these deficits, accomplishing the needed physical and skill prerequisites.

Many strategies are available for increasing strength and range of motion; the field of physical therapy has a variety of approaches for accomplishing these ends. The program may include any combination of the following: proprioceptive neuromuscular facilitation, progressive resistive exercises (concentric and eccentric), strengthening through functional tasks, isokinetic exercise, prolonged stretching, and electrical stimulation. Strengthening and stretching will also occur with increased activity. The patient can exercise independently, in groups, and one on one with the therapist.

This chapter presents functional training strategies for each prerequisite skill. The therapist can use these suggestions, coupled with his own imagination, clinical expertise, and problem solving, to design a functional training program. The program should aim first at developing the most basic prerequisite skills and build to more advanced skills as the patient's abilities develop.

In most cases a patient will have many functional goals. The therapeutic program must progress him toward all of these goals. Fortunately there is much overlap of prerequisites between skills. Thus a person working on weight shifting in standing is potentially progressing himself toward independence in ambulation over even surfaces and obstacles, getting in and out of a wheelchair, and coming to stand from the floor. Furthermore, work aimed at developing one ability can benefit other, seemingly unrelated, activities. For example, the strengthening and motor learning that result from practicing getting into plantigrade from prone may help a patient's uneven transfer abilities.

Example: Assume Standing Position From the Floor. To come to standing from the floor, a patient needs adequate strength in scapular protraction, shoulder flexion and horizontal adduction, and elbow extension. He must also have adequate joint range in these motions, as well as in shoulder extension and horizontal adduction, elbow flexion, and hip flexion. His hamstring flexibility should be greater than normal. In addition, he must be able to position himself in prone with his feet pointing outward, place his crutches, push himself into plantigrade, weight-shift and walk his hands toward his feet in plantigrade, grasp a crutch and balance on it, grasp the second crutch, push himself to standing, and walk his crutches back until he is upright.

The program design will depend on the individual's needs. If he has any deficits in prerequisite strength or range, the program should include exercises to address these deficits. Most patients will benefit from hamstring stretching and upper extremity strengthening.

If the patient has none of the skill prerequisites, functional training should start with the most basic: assuming, maintaining, and weight shifting in a plantigrade posture. When he is able to perform these maneuvers, the patient can practice grasping and positioning his crutches, pushing himself to standing, and walking his crutches back. By building his skill in this manner, he progresses to independence in getting to standing from the floor.

REFERENCES

Heinneman, A.; Magiera-Planey, R.; Schiro-Geist, C., & Gimines, G. (1987). Mobility for persons with spinal cord injury: An evaluation of two systems. *Archives of Physical Medicine and Rehabilitation, 68,* 90–93.

Kralj, A.; Bajd, T., & Turk, R. (1988). Enhancement of gait restoration in spinal injured patients by functional electrical stimulation. *Clinical Orthopaedics and Related Research, 233,* 34–43.

Marsolias, E., & Kobetic, R. (1987). Functional electrical stimulation for walking with paraplegia. *The Journal of Bone and Joint Surgery, 69-A(5),* 728–733.

Marsolias, E., & Kobetic, R. (1988). Development of a practical electrical stimulation system for restoring gait in the paralyzed patient. *Clinical Orthopaedics and Related Research, 233,* 64–74.

McClelland, M.; Andrews, B.; Patrick, J.; Freeman, P., & El Masri, W. (1987). Augmentation of the Owestry parawalker orthosis by means of surface electrical stimulation: Gait analysis of three patients. *Paraplegia, 25,* 32–38.

Peckham, P. (1987). Functional electrical stimulation: Current status and future prospects of applications to the neuromuscular system in spinal cord injury. *Paraplegia, 25,* 279–288.

Robinson, C.; Kett, N., & Bolam, J. (1988). Spasticity in spinal cord injured patients: 2. Initial measures and long-term effects of surface electrical stimulation. *Archives of Physical Medicine and Rehabilitation, 69,* 862–868.

Sullivan, P., & Markos, P. (1987). *Clinical procedures in therapeutic exercise.* Norwalk, CT: Appleton & Lange.

Sullivan, P.; Markos, P.; & Minor, M. (1982). *An integrated approach to therapeutic exercise: Theory and clinical application.* Reston, VA: Reston Publishing Company.

Thoma, H.; Frey, M.; Holle, J.; Kern, H.; Mayr, W.; Schwanda, G., & Stohr, H. (1987). State of the art of implanted multichannel devices to mobilize paraplegics. *International Journal of Rehabilitation Research, 10(4)* (Suppl. 5), 86–90.

Waters, R., & Lunsford, B. (1985). Energy costs of paraplegic locomotion. *Journal of Joint and Bone Surgery, 67-A(8),* 1245–1250.

Waters, R.; Yakura, J.; Adkins, R., & Barnes, G. (1989). Determinants of gait performance following spinal cord injury. *Archives of Physical Medicine and Rehabilitation, 70,* 811–818.

Watkins, E.; Edwards, D., & Patrick, J. (1987). ParaWalker paraplegic walking. *Physiotherapy, 73(2),* 99–100.

15

Incomplete Lesions

A spinal cord injury is classified as incomplete if any motor or sensory function is preserved more than three levels below the neurological level of injury (American Spinal Injury Association, 1989). People with incomplete lesions exhibit preserved neurological function below their lesions at the time of injury, varying degrees of neurological return as spinal shock resolves, or both. This sparing is the result of ascending or descending tracts or both that are left undamaged by the cord injury.

Approximately 54% of the spinal cord injuries sustained in the United States are incomplete. This amounts to approximately 4,200 incomplete spinal cord injuries sustained each year.[1] The proportion of cord lesions that are incomplete has risen sharply in the last few years, probably due to improvements in emergency management techniques (Kennedy, Stover, & Fine, 1986; National Spinal Cord Injury Association, 1988).

Neurological return following incomplete spinal cord injury can occur in a variety of patterns. The three major incomplete cord injury syndromes are Brown-Séquard, anterior cord, and central cord syndromes. Brown-Séquard syndrome is typified by paralysis and loss of proprioception on the side of the lesion and loss of sensitivity to pain and temperature contralaterally. In anterior cord syndrome, motor function and pain/temperature sensation are lost below the level of lesion, and proprioception is spared. With central cord syndrome, motor and sensory impairment are more severe in the upper extremities than in the lower extremities.[2] Clinical presentations often do not fit neatly into one of these syndromes. People may exhibit symptoms typical of a single syndrome or of two or more syndromes combined. In addition, the motor or sensory tracts

or both may be partially or completely disrupted in damaged portions of the cord.

Because of the varying degrees and patterns of neurological damage that can occur in an incomplete spinal cord injury, labeling by the level of neurological lesion alone has limited usefulness. For example, two people with incomplete C6 quadriplegia could have markedly different motor and sensory function preserved below their lesions. The Frankel scale, presented in Chart 15–1, is a functionally meaningful classification system for incomplete lesions.

Most neurological return following spinal cord injury occurs within the first postinjury year. However, motor or sensory return or both can occur for five or more years after injury (Piepmeier & Jenkins, 1988). The likelihood of experiencing significant return varies with the extent of neurological preservation evident at the time of initial admission (Chart 15–2).

Incomplete lesions tend to result in more spasticity than do complete lesions (Little, Micklesen, Umlauf, & Britell, 1989; Robinson, Kett & Bolam, 1988). Spasticity tends to be most severe among those with Frankel grade C lesions (Little, Micklesen, Umlauf, & Britell, 1989).

Psychosocial Considerations

Incomplete spinal cord injuries result in personal losses, regardless of the extent of neurological sparing. An individual who has significant return following spinal cord injury may learn to walk functionally but may exhibit an abnormal gait pattern. Or he may walk with a normal-appearing gait but be unable to play sports as skillfully as he did before his injury. He may be separated from loved ones during rehabilitation. His bowel, bladder, and genital functioning may not return to normal. His schooling may be delayed, or his vocational plans disrupted. He may sustain facial scarring from his halo orthosis. He may lose his illusions of immortality or invulnerability.

The losses caused by an incomplete spinal cord

---

[1] This estimation is probably inaccurate, due to underreporting of cases in which people either sustain minimal neurological damage or die soon after injury (Kennedy, Stover, & Fine, 1986).

[2] These syndromes are described in more detail in Chapter 2.

Chart 15—1 Frankel Classification of Degree of Incompleteness[a]

Frankel Grade	Description	Motor and Sensory Sparing Below the Zone of Partial Preservation	Muscle Grades Below the Zone of Partial Preservation
A	Complete	Absent	0/5
B	Incomplete, preserved sensation only	Sensation only	0/5
C	Incomplete, preserved motor nonfunctional	Minimal voluntary motor function	Majority of key muscles[b] less than 3/5
D	Incomplete, preserved motor functional	"Functionally useful" voluntary motor function	Majority of key muscles[b] at least 3/5
E	Complete return	Complete return of all motor and sensory function. (Reflexes may be abnormal.)	5/5

[a] (ASIA, 1989).
[b] Key muscles are identified in Chapter 2.

injury are real and painful. Yet it can be difficult for members of the rehabilitation team to recognize and respect feelings of loss among patients who have incomplete lesions. This is especially true when health professionals compare these patients to others who have more profound neurological impairments. Health professionals may see those with less severe functional losses as lucky. As a result they may overtly or covertly express to them that grief is not appropriate and even that they should be glad about their conditions.[3] In a like manner, people with extensive motor return may compare their losses with those of others and deny themselves permission to grieve. Thus the stage may be set for unresolved grief.

Learning to live with a disability involves more than the maximization of physical capacities and the acquisition of functional skills. It also involves psychological healing and social adaptation. For this reason psychosocial support is an important component of any rehabilitation program. During rehabilitation, health professionals support people as they mourn their losses and adjust to life following spinal cord injury.[4] This support should be provided regardless of the level or extent of the lesion.

---

[3] Many people with incomplete lesions may in fact come to see themselves as lucky and find comfort in the knowledge that their losses could have been worse. But this does not change the fact that losses have occurred and that these losses must be grieved.

[4] Chapter 4 presents a more complete description of the psychosocial sequelae of spinal cord injury and the process of adaptation after injury.

Education and Follow-Up

Education is an important component of any rehabilitation program. After spinal cord injury, people need to learn about the altered functioning of their bodies, the complications that can occur, and the avoidance and management of these complications. People with *incomplete* cord injuries must also learn about the significance of their lesions' incompleteness. They should be instructed about what to expect as time passes: the degree of motor and sensory return that is likely to occur and the probable timing of this return. Although definitive predictions are often not possible, patients can be apprised of the range of possibilities for neurological return and be informed about the rehabilitation team's best estimate of their ultimate outcomes. People with incomplete lesions should also be encouraged to monitor themselves for return and to inform the rehabilitation team when a significant change occurs.

Follow-up is another important component of health care following spinal cord injury. After dis-

Chart 15—2 Percent Who Progress to Higher Frankel Grade During Initial Hospitalization[a]

Frankel Grade On Admission	Percent Progressing To Higher[b] Grade
A	6.7
B	37.4
C	53.6
D	6.2

[a] (Kennedy, Stover, & Fine, 1986).
[b] Progress from A to B, C, or D; from B to C, D, or E; etc.

charge, periodic checkups make it possible to monitor and respond to changing physical and psychosocial needs, promote health, detect and treat complications early, and get feedback on the rehabilitation program. Follow-up has added significance for people with incomplete lesions. When neurological return occurs, further rehabilitation may be needed to maximize functional gains made possible by the return.

Rehabilitation professionals are contacted occasionally by people who state that they have suddenly experienced improved motor function after years of paralysis. Are these truly instances of sudden return out of the blue? Perhaps a more likely explanation is that these people have had a gradual return of neurological function that they did not notice. Impaired sensation and a lack of knowledge about the possibility of return may make it possible for motor return to go unnoticed. In these cases proper education and follow-up may have made it possible to detect and respond earlier to the changes in neurological status.

Functional Expectations

The functional potential of an individual with an incomplete lesion depends largely on the degree of motor return that he experiences. Muscle tone also affects function; severe spasticity can greatly impede progress. Sensation also impacts on function because somatosensory feedback is required for normal motor control.

With an incomplete spinal cord injury, the goals of treatment depend on the extent of return. When motor return is minimal, the functional potential is essentially the same as if the individual had a complete lesion at the same cord level. When significant motor return occurs in the trunk and extremities, a higher functional status can be achieved. In addition, the aim of treatment may go beyond mere function: more normal movement becomes a goal. Normalizing movement is an important aim because more normal motor patterns can result in higher functional status and greater social acceptability. For example, the therapist and patient may work to develop a normal gait pattern. Normalizing the gait can make it possible to walk for longer distances, since gait deviations reduce the efficiency of ambulation. A normal gait pattern will also facilitate reintegration into the community, as the individual will not appear "handicapped" when he walks.

Regardless of the extent of return that an individual experiences, he should learn to use any of his muscles that regain function. Return in even a single muscle may be exploited. For example, someone with isolated sparing in one iliopsoas may learn to use this muscle to assist in rolling or to lift his foot from the footplate of his wheelchair.

THERAPEUTIC STRATEGIES

Following *complete* spinal cord injury, a limited number of innervated muscles must be used to perform tasks that normally involve the muscles of the entire body. People with complete spinal cord lesions use muscle substitution, momentum, and the head-hips relationship to compensate for lost musculature. These abnormal motor patterns are taught during functional training; the emphasis of physical therapy treatment is on function rather than normalcy.

In contrast, people with *incomplete* spinal cord injuries may be capable of more normal movement patterns. Those who experience significant motor return may be able to function without abnormal use of muscle substitution, momentum, and the head-hips relationship. Yet coordinated motor function will not necessarily appear spontaneously as neurological return occurs. For this reason physical therapy should address normalcy of motion in addition to functional status in instances where significant return has occurred.

During normal functioning, the extremities do not act in isolation; muscles of the trunk, neck, and all extremities act in concert. Following incomplete spinal cord injury with significant motor return, this coordinated function of the entire body should be facilitated.

Proprioceptive Neuromuscular Facilitation

Proprioceptive neuromuscular facilitation (PNF) is ideally suited to the treatment of people with incomplete spinal cord injuries. This treatment approach places emphasis on normalizing movement of the entire body. PNF includes a variety of therapeutic activities, elements, and techniques that can be used to increase strength and range of motion, reduce spasticity, and develop coordinated motor control.[5]

PNF is a valuable treatment approach regardless of the extent of neurological return. Even if an individual does not experience sufficient motor return for ambulation, PNF can be used to enhance function and motor control. Coordinated movement of the trunk, neck, and extremities can be utilized in more basic activities such as rolling.

---

[5] For a more complete description of PNF, the reader should refer to the following references: Sullivan, Markos, & Minor, 1982; Sullivan & Markos, 1987.

Developmental Postures. Using PNF, motor control is developed in a variety of postures. Typically patients first work in basic postures such as side lying and supine. Coordinated movement is easier in these positions because of the low center of gravity and large base of support in these postures.

As a patient's ability to stabilize himself and move within a basic posture develops, he can work in progressively more challenging positions.[6] A more advanced posture is characterized by a higher center of gravity and a smaller base of support.

Stages of Motor Control. The PNF approach also involves progressing the patient from more basic to more advanced motor abilities. The four stages of motor control, progressing from most basic to most advanced, are mobility, stability, controlled mobility, and skill. Before one can exhibit a given level of motor control in a particular posture, one must be capable of the more basic levels of control in that posture. For example, walking (skill) requires the ability to weight shift (controlling mobility) in standing, which presuppposes the ability to maintain a standing posture (stability), which in turn requires adequate range of motion and ability to initiate motion (mobility). In therapy the patient develops basic motor abilities and then builds on them as his control improves.

Other Balance and Coordination Strategies

Exercises Based on Systems Model of Motor Control. The systems model of motor control emphasizes the interaction of the vestibular, visual, and somatosensory systems in postural control. Therapeutic strategies based on this approach address the development of motor capabilities under a variety of sensory conditions. Control is first developed in basic postures, with the patient performing simple activities such as small weight shifts. As the patient's motor control develops, he can work in more challenging postures and perform more complex activities. As the patient progresses, sensory conditions are also changed: the patient works on different supporting surfaces, and visual cues are altered. In addition, the therapist can disturb the patient's balance during the various activities, encouraging him to regain his balance[7] (Crutchfield, Shumway-Cook, & Horak, 1989).

---

[6] The selection of postures for treatment also involves consideration of postural influences on muscle tone.

[7] For a more complete description of the systems model and evaluation and treatment strategies based on this model, the reader should refer to the following reference: Crutchfield, Shumway-Cook, & Horak, 1989.

Therapeutic Ball Activities. A Swiss gymnastics ball can be used as an unstable supporting surface on which to sit. When a patient sits on a therapeutic ball, his balance and coordination are challenged as he works to control his and the ball's motions. By practicing stabilizing himself and moving on a ball, he can develop coordinated control of his trunk, neck, and extremities.[8]

Therapeutic ball activities are most appropriate for patients who have adequate trunk and lower extremity strength, range of motion, and coordination to stabilize themselves on balls with little or no assistance. To work on a therapeutic ball, the patient can be assisted into the position illustrated in Figure 15–1. Once on the ball, he can practice stabilizing himself there. After he has developed the capacity to maintain himself on the ball without assistance, he can practice shifting his weight in various directions, starting with small and progressing to larger movements. He can also practice rolling the ball slightly while sitting on it. While maintaining his balance, he should move the ball *a small distance* forward and back, side to side, diagonally, and in a circle. He should move only as far as he can while maintaining control over the motion. As his skill increases, he can increase the arc of motion. As an advanced activity, the patient can practice stabilizing and moving with one foot lifted from the floor.

Additional Treatment Strategies

In addition to developing coordination, the patient should work in physical therapy to maintain or increase his range of motion as needed and to strengthen weakened muscles. To accomplish these ends, the program may include any combination of the following: progressive resistive exercises (concentric and eccentric), strengthening through functional activities, isokinetic exercise, electrical stimulation, and prolonged stretching.

The physical therapy treatment program should also include functional training. The maneuvers that a given person uses to perform various activities will depend on his patterns of strength, range of motion, and muscle tone, as well as on his body build and level of skill. Because each individual with an incomplete spinal cord injury is so unique in his motor capabilities, functional training will involve a great deal of problem solving.

Following incomplete spinal cord injury, orthotics may be required to preserve structural integrity. Lower extremity orthotics in particular may

---

[8] Therapeutic ball techniques are not as comprehensive as PNF Work on an exercise ball should be used as an adjunct to, rather than a substitute for, a PNF treatment program.

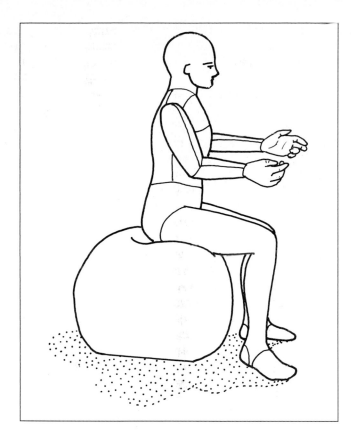

Figure 15–1. Starting position for therapeutic ball activities.

be needed during ambulation to protect the joints until muscular stability is adequate.

SUMMARY

Incomplete spinal cord injury can result in a wide variety of clinical presentations, ranging from minimal neurological sparing below the lesion to near-normal functioning. During rehabilitation, the patient should work to gain maximal use of and benefit from any musculature that retains or regains function. Rehabilitation should also include psychological support as the patient adapts to the injury's sequelae. Finally, education and follow-up are particularly important following incomplete spinal cord injury.

REFERENCES

American Spinal Injury Association. (1989). *Standards for neurological classification of spinal injury patients*. (Available from the American Spinal Injury Association, 2020 Peachtree Road NW, Atlanta, GA, 30309.)

Crutchfield, C.; Shumway-Cook, A., & Horak, F. (1989). Balance and coordination training. In R. Scully, & M. Barnes M. (Eds.), *Physical therapy* (pp. 825–843). Philadelphia: Lippincott.

Kennedy, E.; Stover, S., & Fine, P. (Eds.). (1986). *Spinal cord injury: The facts and figures*. Birmingham, AL: The University of Alabama Spinal Cord Injury Statistical Center.

Little, J.; Micklessen, P.; Umlauf, R., & Britell, C. (1989). Lower extremity manifestations of spasticity in chronic spinal cord injury. *American Journal of Physical Medicine and Rehabilitation, 68*(1), 32–36.

National Spinal Cord Injury Association. (1988). *Fact sheet #2: Spinal cord injury statistical information*. (Available from the National Spinal Cord Injury Association, 600 West Cummings Park, Suite 2000, Woburn, MA, 01801.)

Piepmeier, J., & Jenkins, N. (1988). Late neurological changes following traumatic spinal cord injury. *Journal of Neurosurgery, 69*(3), 399–402.

Robinson, C.; Kett, N., & Bolam, J. (1988). Spasticity in spinal cord injured patients: 2. Initial measures and long-term effects of surface electrical stimulation. *Archives of Physical Medicine and Rehabilitation, 69*(10), 862–868.

Sullivan, P., & Markos, P. (1987). *Clinical procedures in therapeutic exercise*. Norwalk, CT: Appleton & Lange.

Sullivan, P.; Markos, P., & Minor, M. (1982). *An integrated approach to therapeutic exercise: Theory and clinical application*. Reston, VA: Reston Publishing Company.

16

Sexuality and Sexual Functioning

Spinal cord injury impacts directly upon sexual behavior by altering genital functioning. In addition, the whole gamut of physical and social sequelae of spinal cord injury affect sexuality.

Sexuality

Sexuality is a central aspect of our lives. From birth on, our gender influences how we define ourselves and how we are seen by others. (Imagine a birth announcement that doesn't specify the infant's sex!) Because sexuality is such a basic component of our psychological makeup, it is an important ingredient of psychological health. Feelings of sexual inadequacy can impact strongly on a person's sense of identity and self-esteem (Boller & Frank, 1982).

> People treat you differently according to whether you're a boy or a girl; and from the way they react to you, you begin to build your image, your self-esteem. And if somebody or something takes away your sexuality, you don't know who you are or where you fit in.
> —Ellen Stohl (Kenney, 1987)

Sexuality is also important in our social relations. It is used to form and to maintain relationships, to wield power, to communicate with others (Romano, 1977), and to bolster self-esteem (Griffith et al., 1975). We express our sexuality not only, not even mostly, through sexual intercourse. Our attire, interactions with others, the images we present, our flirtations, smiles, and reactions to others are expressions of our sexuality. And yes, we express our sexuality in a wide variety of "sexual acts," ranging from holding hands to group sexual encounters.

Impact of Spinal Cord Injury. The essence of a person's sexual nature is in his or her mind. Spinal cord injury does not alter this. Following cord injury,

people continue to be sexual beings, with the same desires for sexual expression (Griffith, Tomko, & Timms, 1973; Halstead, 1984). Unfortunately, damage to the spinal cord brings on changes that can impede this expression.

Perhaps the most obvious way in which a spinal cord injury affects sexuality is in its affect on the person's physical capacity to perform sexual acts. Changes in genital functioning, motor abilities, sensation, range of motion, and muscle tone may interfere with a person's accustomed modes of sexual expression.

Spinal cord injury also brings logistical problems that can get in the way of sexual activity. Altered body language, the potential for bowel and bladder accidents, decreased spontaneity due to managing catheters, and the mechanics of undressing can complicate sexual encounters. In addition, a person with impaired mobility will face architectural and transportation barriers that will impede his or her ability to meet potential partners.

The social consequences of spinal cord injury add to the problem. Paralysis is a very visible disability; a person who uses a wheelchair or orthoses and assistive devices is readily identified as disabled. As a result, he or she is vulnerable to discrimination. People with disabilities are often viewed by others as sexless, devoid of sexual urges, and undeserving of sexual expression. In a society that places a high premium on physical appearance, disabled people are not seen as desirable partners. These societal attitudes can severely limit the opportunity for sexual expression (Brashear, 1978; Thornton, 1979; Cole & Cole, 1981; Kirk, 1977; Romano, 1977).

Attitudinal barriers to sexual expression also come from within. When a person sustains a spinal cord injury, his or her preexisting prejudices do not magically disappear. He or she is likely to see himself or herself, with a now "imperfect" body, as

275

undesirable, undeserving of sexual gratification, even neutered (Romano, 1977). A great deal of psychological discomfort is likely to result (Griffith et al., 1975).

The problems brought on by physical changes and internal and external attitudinal barriers are compounded by ignorance. People with spinal cord injuries often don't understand their own sexual potentials. Many find themselves totally in the dark regarding their sexual functioning and ways to go about finding sexual gratification (Romano, 1977).

In the past the focus of research and treatment in this area has been on the male, specifically on his genital functioning and fertility (Griffith et al., 1973). The freely expressed attitude was that the spinal cord-injured woman had an easier adjustment to make because the injury didn't impair her ability to perform in her accustomed role of passive participant in sexual activities (Cole, 1979; Bregman & Hadley, 1976).

This position, based on outdated notions of sex roles, is no longer defensible. Women now often take the initiative in sexual encounters, instead of waiting passively for men to approach them. And many women prefer positions other than the "missionary position" during intercourse. Like her male counterpart, a cord-injured woman may have difficulty with some of the positions and sexual activities to which she was accustomed prior to her injury. She will have the same potential for problems with bowel and bladder accidents interrupting intimate encounters and will be subject to society's discriminatory attitudes regarding sexuality and disability. She may feel unattractive as a result of her injury (Ray & West, 1984).

> I used to feel that I really couldn't have real relationships because I thought that, as a disabled woman, I wasn't as desirable. I figured that there was really no reason for anyone to be interested in me if he could have a woman who could walk, totally discounting my whole self and my uniqueness as a person. I didn't feel really good about myself until I started feeling sexually attractive, feeling that I could function, not competitively, but on an equal footing with any other woman.
>
> —Susan Schapiro (Corbet, 1980)

Some aspects of a woman's sexuality will not be as profoundly affected by cord injury as a man's. Her genital functioning will not be altered as much, and her fertility will not be affected. However, she may face more social difficulties, being more vul-

nerable than men to being perceived as unattractive and therefore unacceptable as a sexual partner (Bonwich, 1985). Health professionals should remember that spinal cord injury significantly affects sexuality whether the person is male or female.

Sexuality and the potential for sexual expression is a major concern for most people who sustain a spinal cord injury (Miller, Szasz, & Anderson, 1981). This concern often surfaces very soon after injury (Boller & Frank, 1982; Miller, Szasz, & Anderson, 1981). Faced with bodily changes and social stigma, a cord-injured person may feel less of a man or woman. Depression and lowered self-esteem can result (Cole & Stevens, 1975). Because of the psychological and social importance of sexuality, it is critical that this area is addressed during rehabilitation.

PHYSICAL ASPECTS OF SEXUAL FUNCTIONING

Although physical sexual responses are only a part of sexuality, they are certainly a significant part of it. Understandably, physical sexual responses are an area of great concern following spinal cord injury. Sooner or later after injury, people want to know about their capacity to perform various sexual acts, reach orgasm, and have children. Health professionals should be knowledgeable in this area, so that they can educate their patients appropriately.

Neurological Control of Genital Function

Male. The male's genital functions during sexual activity consist of erection, emission, and ejaculation.[1]

Erection is a vascular event, occurring when the erectile bodies of the penis (corpus cavernosa and corpus spongiosum) become distended with blood. It can be initiated by either parasympathetic or sympathetic stimulation. When this autonomic input causes the rate of flow of blood into the erectile bodies to exceed the rate of flow out, the penis becomes erect (Donovon, 1985; Gott, 1981; Weiss, 1978). Continuing autonomic stimulation is required to maintain the erection (Weiss, 1978).

Neurological control of erection involves the

---

[1] Some authors consider emission to be a part of ejaculation. In this chapter emission and ejaculation will be considered separate entities, as they represent two separate neurological events.

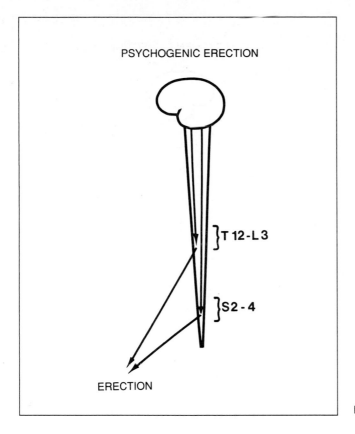

PSYCHOGENIC ERECTION

}T 12-L 3

}S 2 - 4

ERECTION

Figure 16–1. Neurological control of psychogenic erection.

thoracolumbar cord and the sacral cord, as well as higher centers. These higher centers include the cerebral cortex (Gott, 1981) and possibly the hypothalamus, putamen, septum, and reticular formation (Crenshaw, Martin, Warner, & Crenshaw, 1978; Fitzpatrick, 1974; Weiss, 1978). Efferent pathways from the cerebral cortex travel in the lateral columns near the pyramidal tracts. They synapse in the thoracolumbar (sympathetic) and sacral (parasympathetic) erection centers of the spinal cord. The input from higher centers provides both facilitation and inhibition of erection (Crenshaw, Martin, Warner, & Crenshaw, 1978).

Erection can be initiated from two different sources: psychological arousal or sensory stimulation in the genital area or pelvic viscera. Figures 16–1 and 16–2 illustrate the neurological control of the two types of erection. Psychogenic erections are brought on by psychological arousal. This arousal can be initiated by erotic thoughts or a variety of sensory experiences (smells, sounds, etc.). Erections brought on by sensory stimulation in the genital region or pelvic viscera are called reflex or reflexogenic erections. Normal functioning involves a combination of psychogenic and reflexogenic erection (Weiss, 1978). In fact, both are needed for an erection to be maintained (Geiger, 1979).

Reflex erections are mediated by the sacral cord. Parasympathetic efferents from S-2 through S-4 innervate the penile corporal arterioles, causing vasodilation when stimulated. Erection is initiated when sensory stimulation from the penis, perineal area, rectum, or bladder travels to S2-4. This stimulation causes firing of the parasympathetic efferents, resulting in erection (Gott, 1981; Geiger, 1979).

Psychogenic erections are mediated by the thoracolumbar and sacral cord. Sympathetic efferents from T-12 through L-3[2] (Gieger, 1979; Gott, 1981) are thought to innervate the arterioles of the penile corporal bodies with both vasodilator and vasoconstrictor fibers. A psychogenic erection occurs when impulses from higher centers cause the vasodilator sympathetic efferents to fire (Gott, 1981). Psychogenic erections may also be mediated in the sacral cord, occurring when facilitory impulses from the cerebral cortex cause the sacral efferents to fire (Weiss, 1978).

Emission is the process by which semen reaches the posterior urethra in preparation for eja-

[2] There is disagreement in the literature regarding the exact location of the thoracolumbar erection center. The center may extend from T-10 through L-2 (Boller & Frank, 1982) or from T-11 through L-2 (Donovon, 1985).

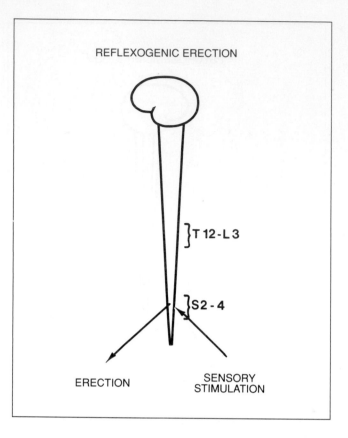

REFLEXOGENIC ERECTION

T 12 - L 3

S2 - 4

ERECTION

SENSORY
STIMULATION

Figure 16–2. Neurological control of reflexogenic erection.

culation. In emission, peristaltic contraction of the smooth muscle of the vas deferens causes sperm to be transported from the epididymus to the end of the vas deferens (ampulla; Gott, 1981). Secretions from the seminal vesicles and prostate are added to the sperm to form semen (Fitzpatrick, 1974). Contraction of the smooth muscle of the ampulla, seminal vesicles, and prostate (Geiger, 1979) and partial closure of the bladder neck causes the semen to enter the posterior urethra (Gott, 1981). Figure 16–3 illustrates the structures involved.

Neurological control of emission involves the cerebral cortex and both the sacral and thoracolumbar spinal cord (Fig. 16–4). Afferents from the genitals enter the second through fourth segments of the sacral cord. From there they ascend to the cerebral cortex. Efferents from the cerebral cortex travel via the anterolateral columns to the thoracolumbar cord, T-12 through L-3[3] (Fitzpatrick, 1974; Gott, 1981). Sympathetic efferents from the thoracolumbar cord innervate the vas deferens, seminal vesicles, prostate, and base of the bladder. The sympathetic outflow to these structures causes emission (Crenshaw, Martin, Warner, & Crenshaw,

1978; Gott, 1981). Emission can also occur as a result of direct input from the sacral cord to the thoracolumbar cord, without involvement of higher centers. Normally emission is stimulated by input from both sources (Crenshaw, Martin, Warner, & Crenshaw, 1978).

Ejaculation is the process by which semen is propelled from the posterior urethra. It involves contraction of striated musculature; the bulbocavernosus, ischiocavernosus, and other pelvic floor musculature (Geiger, 1979). The rhythmic contraction of these muscles, combined with closure of the bladder neck, propels the semen forward and out of the urethra[4] (Gott, 1981).

Ejaculation occurs as a result of a somatic sacral reflex (Fig. 16–5). Sensory afferents are activated when semen enters the posterior urethra as a result of emission. These afferents travel to S2-4, where they synapse with somatic efferents. Reflexive contraction of the bulbocavernosus and ischiocavernosus muscles results (Crenshaw, Martin, Warner & Crenshaw, 1978; Fitzpatrick, 1974; Gott, 1981), causing propulsion of the semen. The effer-

---

[3] There is disagreement in the literature regarding the area in the cord that controls emission. It may extend from T-10 through L-2 (Boller & Frank, 1982).

[4] Normal ejaculation, in which the semen is propelled forward, is called antegrade ejaculation. In retrograde ejaculation, semen is propelled back into the bladder. This occurs when the bladder neck fails to close during ejaculation or when the bladder neck has been resected surgically (Gieger, 1979).

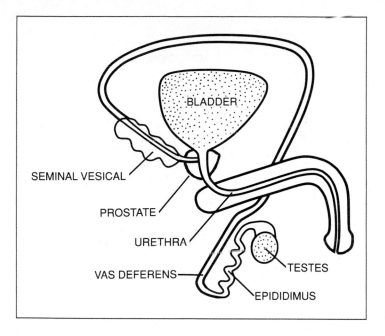

Figure 16–3. Structures involved in emission.

ents also stimulate reflexive contraction of the vesical sphincter, preventing retrograde ejaculation (Fitzpatrick, 1974). During ejaculation, the anal sphincter also contracts rhythmically (Geiger, 1979).

Female. The genital responses exhibited by women during sexual acts include vaginal lubrication; vascular engorgement of erectile tissue in the clitoris, the vagina, labia minora, and labia majora; contraction of the smooth muscle of the fallopian tubes;

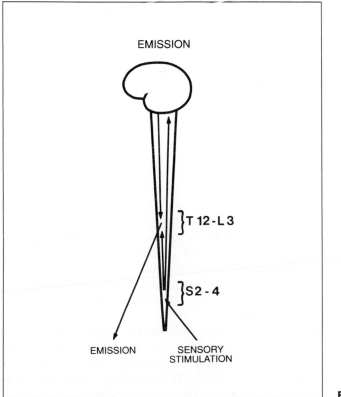

Figure 16–4. Neurological control of emission.

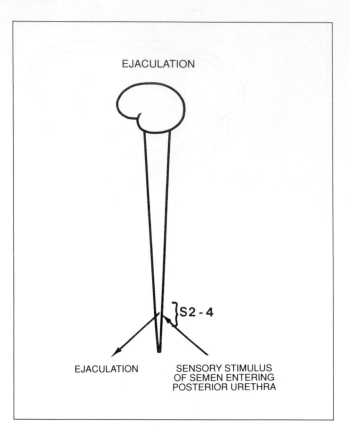

Figure 16–5. Neurological control of ejaculation.

and rhythmic contraction of the perineal musculature. The physical functioning of females during sexual activity has not been studied as extensively as the functioning of males.

Vaginal lubrication occurs as the result of secretion of mucus from Bartholin's glands into the vaginal opening. Mucus is also secreted by the vaginal epithelium. Lubrication occurs as a result of parasympathetic stimulation that arises from S2-4 (Boller & Frank, 1982; Griffith & Trieschmann, 1975; Guyton, 1987; Vick, 1984).

The engorgement of erectile tissue in the corpora cavernosa of the clitoris, vagina, labia minora, and labia majora that occurs during sexual activity is the result of vascular dilation. This dilation is the result of parasympathetic stimulation which arises from S2-4 (Boller & Frank, 1982; Guyton, 1987; Thews & Vaupel, 1985; Vick, 1984).

In the female equivalent of emission, the smooth musculature of the fallopian tubes, uterus, and paraurethral Skene glands contracts. The neurological control of these events is similar to the control of emission in the male (Fitzpatrick, 1974). These reactions are caused by sympathetic outflow from the thoracolumbar cord (Boller & Frank, 1982; Griffith & Treischmann, 1975).

As is true with ejaculation in males, the anal-

ogous female response involves striated musculature. It consists of rhythmic contraction of the bulbospongiosus (vaginal sphincter) and ischiocavernosus, pelvic floor (Boller & Frank, 1982), and anal sphincter. According to Fitzpatrick (1974), the neurological control of this response is similar to the control of ejaculation in the male. This muscular response is controlled by a somatic reflex involving S2-4 (Boller & Frank, 1982; Griffith & Treischmann, 1975).

Genital Function Following Injury

The impact that a spinal cord injury has on genital functioning is not completely understood. Much of our knowledge is based on studies that have been less than perfect. Most data have been gathered using retrospective surveys rather than observation. There has been inadequate control of variables such as marital status, time since injury, etiology, spasticity, and the influence of medication, surgery, and medical conditions (Griffith, Tomko, & Timms, 1973).

Despite these limitations, research has shown that the level and completeness of a lesion affect its impact on genital functioning. However, it is not possible to predict an individual's potential based on these factors. There are exceptions to any "rule

TABLE 16–1 STATISTICS ON MALE SEXUAL FUNCTIONING FOLLOWING SPINAL CORD INJURY

	UMN Lesions		LMN Lesions	
	Complete (%)	*Incomplete (%)*	*Complete (%)*	*Incomplete (%)*
Psychogenic erections	0	25	25–40	80–85
Reflexogenic erections	>90	95–100	0–25	90
Ejaculation[a]	¯1	¯25	14–35	≤70

[a] These statistics are based on studies that do not distinguish between emission and ejaculation and therefore are inflated.

of thumb" that one attempts to impose. It is important to keep this in mind when counseling patients.

Male. The preservation of erection, emission, and ejaculation capabilities after spinal cord injury varies with the level and completeness of lesion. Statistics on the sexual functioning of males following spinal cord injury are presented in Table 16–1.

In discussions of sexual functioning, cord lesions are often classified as upper motor neuron (UMN) or lower motor neuron (LMN) lesions. So-called UMN lesions leave the functioning of the sacral cord intact. People with these lesions display intact bulbocavernosus reflex[5] and anal sphincter tone. Most such lesions are above T12 (Gott, 1981).

So-called LMN lesions disrupt the functioning of the sacral cord. People with this level of lesion have a lax anal sphincter and absent bulbocavernosus reflex. Usually the lesion is below T12 in these cases (Gott, 1981).

Erection is the most likely of the genital functions to be preserved after spinal cord injury. This is due to the presence of erectile centers in two areas of the cord; a man with a spinal cord injury is likely to have either his thoracolumbar or sacral erection center functional.

The neurological basis of the erection capabilities of a person with a complete high lesion (UMN) are illustrated in Figure 16–6. With a lesion above T-12, the thoracolumbar erection center will no longer be in contact with the brain. As a result, psychogenic erections will not occur (Halstead, 1984). Although men with high lesions do not exhibit psychogenic erections, most retain the capacity for reflex erections. This capacity is due to the fact that the sacral segments of the cord remain functional: the intact sacral reflex arc makes reflex erections possible. Over 90% of men with complete UMN le-

sions have reflex erections (Geiger, 1979; Halstead, 1984; Weiss, 1978). The probability of both types of erection is increased if the lesion is incomplete. Of men with incomplete UMN lesions, 25% exhibit psychogenic erections, and 95% to 100% can have reflex erections (Halstead, 1984).

Lower lesions have a more detrimental effect on erections. Figure 16–7 illustrates the effect that a complete low lesion (LMN) will have on erections. A lesion below L-3 will leave all of the thoracolumbar erection center in communication with the brain. As a result, psychogenic erections will be possible. A lesion that falls within the thoracolumbar erection center (between T-12 and L-3) will lead to the inability to have psychogenic erections (Donovon, 1985). Of all men with complete LMN lesions, from 25% (Halstead, 1984; Weiss, 1978) to 40% (Gott, 1981) exhibit psychogenic erections. Reflex erections are less likely to be preserved, since low lesions are likely to disrupt the functioning of the sacral cord. Reports of the occurrence of reflex erections in men with complete LMN lesions range from 0% (Gott, 1981) to 25% (Halstead, 1984). Men with incomplete LMN lesions are more likely to retain the capacity to have erections. From 80% to 85% exhibit psychogenic erections, and 90% have reflex erections (Halstead, 1984).

In summary, many men with spinal cord injuries retain the capacity for penile erection. Men with high lesions are likely to exhibit reflex erections, and men with low lesions may have psychogenic or reflex erections. Incomplete lesions are most likely to result in sparing of erection.

Although most cord-injured men retain the capacity to have erections, many who have erections are unable to use them in coitus (Crenshaw, Martin, Warner, & Crenshaw, 1978; Fitzpatrick, 1974; Griffith, Tomko, & Timms, 1973). This makes sense when one recalls that the erections exhibited by neurologically intact men during sexual activity are sustained by input from both the thoracolumbar and sacral erection centers. Loss of input from either

---

[5] Contraction of the bulbocavernosus muscle upon percussion of the dorsum of the penis.

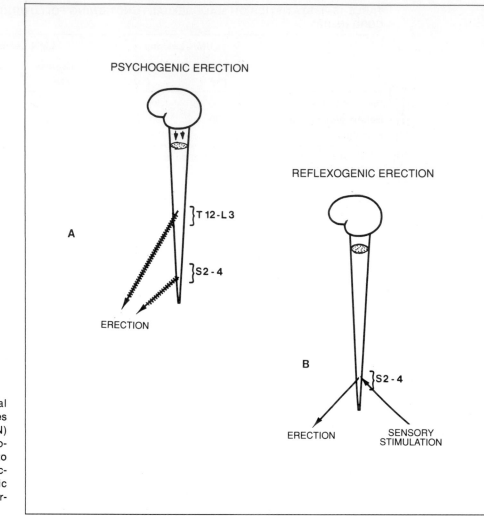

PSYCHOGENIC ERECTION

A

{T 12-L 3

{S2 - 4

ERECTION

REFLEXOGENIC ERECTION

B

{S2 - 4

ERECTION   SENSORY
STIMULATION

Figure 16–6. Neurological basis of erection capabilities after complete high (UMN) spinal-cord injury. **(A)** Psychogenic erection impaired due to loss of input from brain to erection centers. **(B)** Reflexogenic erection spared due to preservation of sacral reflex arc.

center may alter the quality of erection, the ability to sustain an erection, or both.

The data available on emission and ejaculation following cord injury are not as complete or accurate as that on erection. Many studies lump the two functions together, and data are lacking on emission itself. Donovon (1985) notes additional limitations of the studies done to date: data are gathered by survey, and there has been poor or no control of conditions that are common among cord-injured men and that are known to affect ejaculation (medication, bladder surgery, urinary tract infection).

Emission occurs as a result of sympathetic outflow from the thoracolumbar cord. Because this outflow is caused primarily by input from higher centers (Fitzpatrick, 1974; Gott, 1981), one would expect the effect of spinal cord injury on emission to be similar to its effect on psychogenic erection.

Figure 16–8 illustrates the neurological basis of the effect of a low cord injury (LMN) on emission.

If part or all of the T12 through L3 segments of the cord remain in contact with the brain, outflow from this area could cause emission. Higher lesions (UMN) that interrupt descending input to the thoracolumbar cord would be expected to impair emission (Fig. 16–9).

Ejaculation is the most neurologically vulnerable of the genital functions. This vulnerability is due to the fact that two separate spinal cord centers are involved. For ejaculation to occur, semen must be present in the posterior urethra; emission must occur. Emission is brought on by thoracolumbar outflow, in turn stimulated primarily by input from higher centers. An intact sacral arc is also required for true ejaculation, since ejaculation occurs as the result of a sacral reflex.

Figure 16–10 illustrates the effect of a complete low lesion (LMN) on ejaculation. A lesion that is low enough to preserve the thoracolumbar outflow required for emission is likely to interrupt the func-

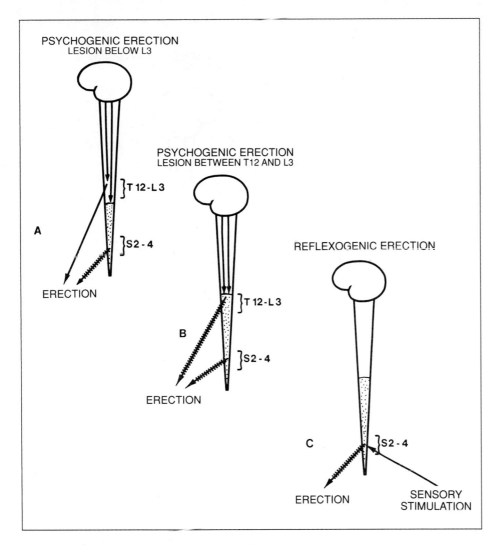

PSYCHOGENIC ERECTION
LESION BELOW L3

PSYCHOGENIC ERECTION
LESION BETWEEN T12 AND L3

A

}T 12-L3

}S2-4

ERECTION

B

REFLEXOGENIC ERECTION

}T 12-L3

}S2-4

ERECTION

C

}S2-4

ERECTION

SENSORY
STIMULATION

Figure 16–7. Neurological basis of erection capabilities after complete low (LMN) spinal cord injury. **(A)** With lesion below L3, psychogenic erection may be spared due to preserved input from brain to thoracolumbar erection center. **(B)** With lesion between T12 and L3, psychogenic erection impaired due to loss of input from brain to both sacral and thoracolumbar erection centers. **(C)** Reflexogenic erection impaired due to disruption of sacral reflex arc.

tioning of the sacral cord. Thus ejaculation is not likely to occur with a low lesion. Reports of the incidence of ejaculation among men with complete LMN lesions range from 14% to 35% (Gott, 1981). The incidence of ejaculation is greater with incomplete lesions. Up to 70% of men with incomplete LMN lesions ejaculate (Griffith, Tomko, & Timms, 1973). Since many studies do not distinguish between emission and true ejaculation, the figures on the incidence of ejaculation are inflated. In many instances, what is reported as ejaculation may actually be dribbling of semen due to emission.[6]

A complete lesion that is high enough to allow preservation of the sacral cord is likely to interrupt

the thoracolumbar cord's communication with higher centers. As a result, emission and therefore ejaculation are quite uncommon following complete UMN lesion, occurring in approximately 1% of these cases (Fig. 16–11). Approximately 25% of men with incomplete UMN lesions ejaculate (Fitzpatrick, 1974; Gott, 1981).

In summary, few spinal cord-injured men exhibit true ejaculation. For ejaculation to occur, emission must occur, and ejaculation and emission combined involve the cerebral cortex and both the thoracolumbar and sacral areas of the cord. Men with incomplete lesions are more likely to ejaculate than are those with complete lesions. In contrast to erectile capabilities, men with LMN lesions are more likely to ejaculate than are men with UMN lesions, and lower lesions result in more preservation of ejaculation than higher lesions (Gott, 1981). However, research flaws make the validity of the above trends questionable.

---

[6] For example, Geiger (1979) states that men with cauda equina lesions are more likely to ejaculate than men with higher lesions but that dribbling ejaculation is likely to be associated with flaccid pelvic floor musculature. This description is compatible with a complete LMN lesion and emission, not true ejaculation.

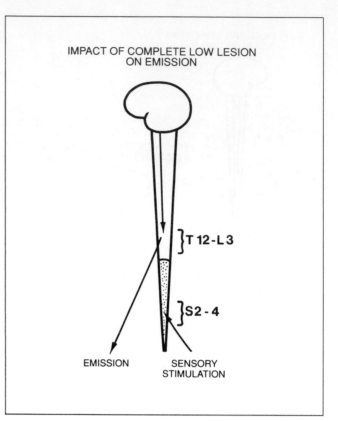

Figure 16–8. Neurological basis of impact of complete low (LMN) spinal cord injury on emission. Emission may be spared due to preserved input from brain to thoracolumbar cord.

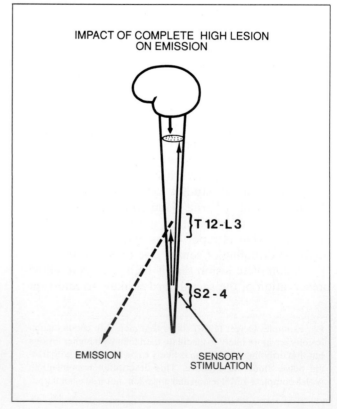

Figure 16–9. Neurological basis of impact of complete high (UMN) spinal cord injury on emission. Emission impaired due to loss of input from brain to thoracolumbar cord. A small minority may exhibit emission due to input from the sacral cord to the thoracolumbar cord.

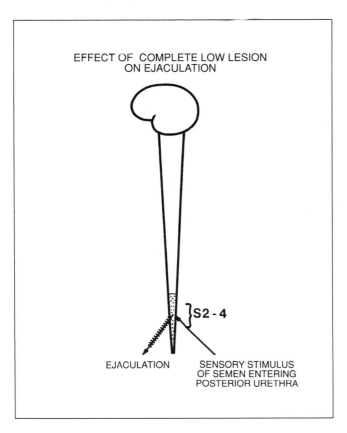

EFFECT OF COMPLETE LOW LESION
ON EJACULATION

}S2 - 4

EJACULATION   SENSORY STIMULUS
OF SEMEN ENTERING
POSTERIOR URETHRA

Figure 16–10. Neurological basis of impact of complete low (LMN) spinal cord injury on ejaculation. Ejaculation impaired due to disruption of sacral reflex arc.

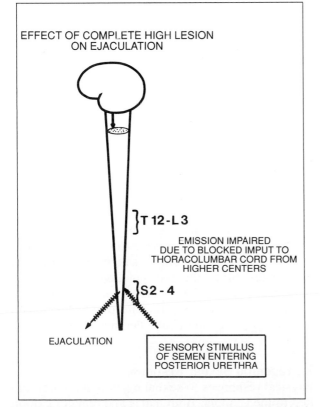

EFFECT OF COMPLETE HIGH LESION
ON EJACULATION

}T 12 - L 3

EMISSION IMPAIRED
DUE TO BLOCKED IMPUT TO
THORACOLUMBAR CORD FROM
HIGHER CENTERS

}S2 - 4

EJACULATION   SENSORY STIMULUS
OF SEMEN ENTERING
POSTERIOR URETHRA

Figure 16–11. Neurological basis of impact of complete high (UMN) spinal cord injury on ejaculation. Ejaculation impaired due to impaired emission, which results from loss of input from brain to thoracolumbar cord.

Female. Little is known about the genital functioning of women following spinal cord injury, as few studies have been done in this area. Clitoral and labial engorgement may occur (Donovon, 1985), and the vagina may moisten (Gatens, 1984). Other genital responses remain undocumented (Boller & Frank, 1982; Donovon, 1985).

Presumably, one can draw *tentative* conclusions regarding the genital responses of cord-injured women based on what is known about the functioning of their male counterparts. Clinical experience often supports this assumption (Geiger, 1979). Figures 16–12 and 16–13 illustrate the neurological basis of the (presumed) impact of complete spinal cord injury on the genital functioning of women.

The neurological control of vaginal lubrication and vascular engorgement of the genitalia is comparable to the control of penile erection in men. Based on what is known about the genital functioning of men after spinal cord injury, one would expect most cord-injured women to retain the capacity for vaginal lubrication and engorgement of the clitoris and labia. Following complete UMN lesion, most (over 90%) should exhibit these responses reflexively. They should not occur as a result of psychogenic excitation in these women. Following complete LMN lesion, few (0% to 25%) should exhibit vaginal lubrication and engorgement of the pelvic

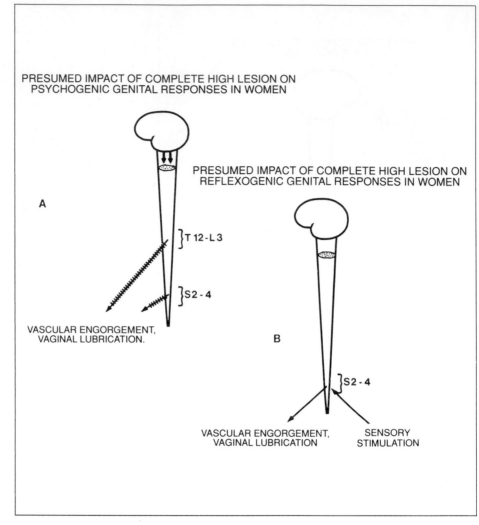

PRESUMED IMPACT OF COMPLETE HIGH LESION ON
PSYCHOGENIC GENITAL RESPONSES IN WOMEN

A

PRESUMED IMPACT OF COMPLETE HIGH LESION ON
REFLEXOGENIC GENITAL RESPONSES IN WOMEN

T 12 - L 3

S2 - 4

VASCULAR ENGORGEMENT,
VAGINAL LUBRICATION.

B

S2 - 4

VASCULAR ENGORGEMENT,
VAGINAL LUBRICATION

SENSORY
STIMULATION

Figure 16–12. Presumed impact of complete high (UMN) spinal cord injury on genital responses in women. **(A)** Psychogenic vascular engorgement and vaginal lubrication impaired due to loss of input from brain to thoracolumbar and sacral cord. **(B)** Reflexogenic vascular engorgement and vaginal lubrication spared due to preservation of sacral reflex arc.

structures reflexively. If women have a thoracolumbar center for these responses, some (25% to 40%) could be expected to exhibit these responses as a result of psychogenic stimuli.

Contraction of smooth musculature in the fallopian tubes, uterus, and paraurethral Skene glands is caused by outflow from the thoracolumbar cord, as is emission in men. Although data is lacking, one can draw *tentative* conclusions about the effects of cord injury based on neuroanatomy. A complete UMN lesion would be likely to disrupt these physical responses, and a LMN lesion should leave them intact in most instances.

Rhythmic contraction of striated pelvic musculature, the female analogue of ejaculation, is a sacral reflex. If the impact of spinal cord injury is equivalent in both sexes, one would expect few cord-injured women to exhibit this motor response. However, the statistics on ejaculation in males following cord injury are highly questionable, since

studies tend to report emission as ejaculation. Thus it is unknown how many cord-injured people exhibit the rhythmic contraction of striated pelvic musculature associated with ejaculation in men and its analogue in women.

Present knowledge of male genital responses after spinal cord injury remains imperfect, despite extensive research. The information available needs to be taken with a grain of salt when counseling individuals. Since the extrapolations about female responses presented above are presumptions based on imperfect knowledge, they need to be taken with an even larger grain of salt. Perhaps a whole shakerful.

Extragenital Sexual Responses

Physical responses to sexual excitation are not limited to the genitals. Both males and females exhibit nipple erection, engorgement of breast tissue, a light rash (''sex flush'') on the face and upper chest, pupil

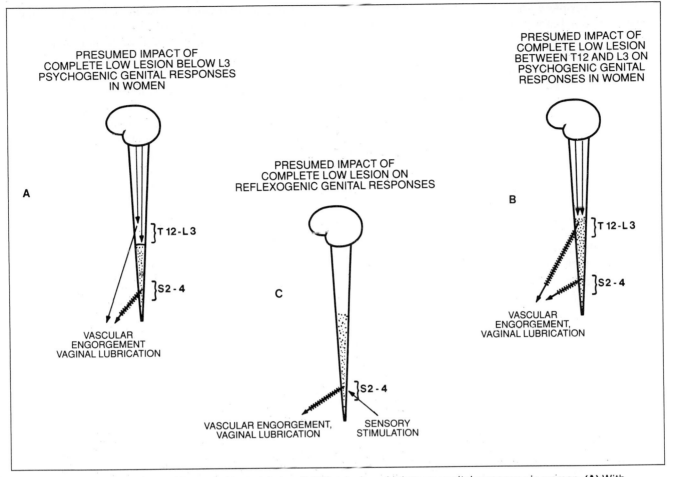

Figure 16–13. Presumed impact of complete low (LMN) spinal cord injury on genital responses in women. **(A)** With lesion below L3, psychogenic vascular engorgement and vaginal lubrication may be spared due to preserved input from brain to thoracolumbar cord. **(B)** With lesion between T12 and L3, psychogenic vascular engorgement and vaginal lubrication impaired due to loss of input from brain to sacral and thoracolumbar cord. **(C)** Reflexogenic vascular engorgement and vaginal lubrication impaired due to disruption of sacral reflex arc.

dilation, and increases in heart rate, respiration rate, and blood pressure (Geiger, 1979; Griffith, Trieschmann, Hohmann, Cole, Tobis, & Cummings, 1975; Thews & Vaupel, 1985). These responses are not affected by spinal cord injury, since they are mediated by higher centers.

Orgasm

Orgasm is an intensely pleasurable subjective experience. It is usually associated with ejaculation in the male and its physical equivalent in the female. However, orgasm does not have to be associated with these physical responses. It is "essentially a cerebral event" (Geiger, 1979).

Because orgasm is a mental event, it is not totally dependent upon genital sensation. Some men and women with complete spinal cord injuries still experience orgasm, even multiple orgasm (Cole, 1975). In the absence of pelvic innervation, fantasy and erotic imagery can be used to achieve orgasm (Cole, 1979). Some can achieve orgasm by concentrating on sensation from innervated areas and reassigning the sensation to their genitals (Cole, 1979; Griffith & Trieschmann, 1975). The orgasms experienced by people with spinal cord injuries are reported as satisfying, often followed by a resolution of sexual tension similar to that experienced by people without cord injuries (Cole, 1975; Cole, 1979).

The incidence of orgasm appears to vary with the level and completeness of lesion. It is rare among people with complete UMN lesions (Griffith, Tomko, & Timms, 1973; Halstead, 1984). It has been reported to occur occasionally (29%) in people with incomplete UMN lesions, less frequently (17%) among people with complete LMN lesions, and frequently (60%) following incomplete LMN lesion (Fitzpatrick, 1974).

A few people with UMN lesions report severe spasticity just before and during orgasm (Fitzpatrick, 1974). Following orgasm, some (both sexes) report that their spasticity is reduced or eliminated for a period of time (Griffith & Treischmann, 1975).

Fertility

Male. Few men with spinal cord injuries father children. Most estimates of the incidence of paternity following injury are 5% or lower (Donovon, 1985; Griffith, Tomko, & Timms, 1973; Gott, 1981).

Impaired erection and ejaculation are obvious sources of infertility after spinal cord injury. Techniques now exist that can be used to elicit ejaculation in otherwise anejaculatory cord-injured men, but these techniques remain experimental. One method of harvesting sperm, electroejaculation, involves electrically stimulating the seminal vesicles or obturator nerves (Brindley, 1980; Cole, 1979). Electroejaculation requires the presence of a functioning sacral cord. The success rate (percent of subjects yielding antegrade ejaculation) has ranged from 0% to 75% (Halstead, VerVoort, & Seager, 1987).

Unfortunately there is more to the problem of infertility than the inability to place semen in a partner's vagina. Even among men who are able to achieve ejaculation, "naturally" or through technological means, impregnation is unlikely. Men with spinal cord injuries tend to have testicular atrophy. They generally have low sperm counts, and the sperm tend to have low motility and an abnormally high incidence of malformation (Brindley, 1980; Cole, 1979; Donovon, 1985; Griffith, Tomko, & Timms, 1973; Halstead, VerVoort, & Seager, 1987). The cause of this impairment of spermatogenesis is unknown. Suggested reasons have included infection, impaired temperature regulation in the scrotum, nondrainage due to impaired ejaculation, and a lower state of overall health (Brindley, 1980; Boller & Frank, 1982; Fitzpatrick, 1974; Gott, 1981; Halstead, VerVoort, & Seager, 1987). With repeated ejaculations over time, testicular atrophy and the quality and quantity of sperm may improve (Griffith, Tomko, & Timms, 1973; Halstead et al., 1987; Siösteen, Forssman, Steen, Sullivan, & Wickström, 1990).

Female. Spinal cord injury does not change a woman's fertility (Boller & Frank, 1982; Donovon, 1985; Thornton, 1979). The menstrual cycle often stops at the time of injury, but it usually resumes within six months (Cole, 1979; Donovon, 1985; Fitzpatrick, 1974).

Cord-injured women can become pregnant and carry their babies to full term (Cole, 1979). The need for cesarean section (C-section) is not increased (Cole, 1975); most cord-injured women who become pregnant deliver healthy babies vaginally (Craig, 1990; Griffith, Tomko, & Timms, 1973; Verduyn, 1986).

Although a cord-injured woman remains fertile and can deliver normally, pregnancy has its risks. Most women with lesions above T7 exhibit autonomic dysreflexia during labor contractions (Verduyn, 1986; Wanner, Rageth, & Zach, 1987). With lesions above T6, the sensory level for the uterus, women may go into labor without realizing it[7] (Geiger, 1979; Thornton, 1979). Other hazards of pregnancy for cord-injured women include increased risk of anemia, urinary tract infections, decubiti, deep venous thrombosis, and rapid labor (Craig, 1990; Griffith, Tomko, & Timms, 1973; Thornton, 1979; Wanner, Rageth, & Zach, 1987). Premature labor is common (Verduyn, 1986).

Because of the complications of pregnancy unique to women with spinal cord injuries, it is advisable for their obstetricians to consult with rehabilitation specialists. With proper management, the increased risks of pregnancy should not pose a major threat to the health of the mother or child. Decubiti and urinary tract infections can be prevented with proper care. A physician aware of the risks of early and undetected labor can monitor the patient closely toward the end of pregnancy and take appropriate precautions when dilation begins. The symptoms of autonomic dysreflexia can be stopped or prevented with general anesthesia, epidural anesthesia, or various drugs[8] (Verduyn, 1986; Wanner, Rageth, & Zach, 1987).

Since women remain fertile following spinal cord injury, contraceptives are an important concern. The problems posed by the various contraceptive options are different after spinal cord injury. Oral contraceptives further increase a cord-injured woman's already elevated risk of deep venous thrombosis. An intrauterine device (IUD) can perforate the uterus, and the cord-injured woman may not detect the problem because of sensory deficits (Cole, 1979; Donovon, 1985; Thornton, 1979). A woman with impaired hand function would be likely to have difficulty inserting and removing a diaphragm or cervical cap. A diaphragm may be dislodged when a woman performs a Credé maneuver (a technique used for manual expression of urine

---

[7] Some report that this problem occurs in women with lesions above T10 (Cole, 1979; Wanner, Rageth, & Zach, 1987).

[8] Amyl nitrate, magnesium sulphate, demerol (Verduyn, 1986).

from bladder; See Chapter 17) to empty her bladder (Thornton, 1979). The combined use of condom and spermicidal foam is an effective method of birth control (Killien, 1984), but diminished hand function may complicate the insertion of foam. Assistive devices may make the task easier. Sterilization is an option for women who do not wish to bear children at any time in the future.

Because of the risks and logistical problems associated with the different methods of contraception, the choice may be difficult. The rehabilitation team should address the issue, assisting the patient in finding the solution that is most suitable for her.

THERAPEUTIC INTERVENTION

Spinal cord injury has a significant impact on sexuality. It can bring about profound changes in genital functioning, sensation, fertility, and the capacity for bodily movements used in sexual activity. Sexual encounters may be more difficult to orchestrate, and the prospect of incontinence at inopportune moments may be always lurking.

The alterations in physical sexual functioning and the inconvenience that they bring are only a part of the picture. Because a spinal cord injury changes a person from "normal" to "disabled," it places him or her at risk of being perceived as asexual, undesirable, and undeserving of sexual gratification, both by others and by himself or herself. Feelings of sexual inadequacy can undermine a person's self-worth and adaptation to the injury (Ray & West, 1984; Teal & Athelstan, 1975).

Despite the problems that spinal cord injury causes in the area of sexuality, people can adjust. No matter what the level of lesion, what motor abilities, what sensation or genital functioning, people can adapt. They can once again come to see themselves as sexual beings, forming and maintaining relationships, giving and receiving pleasure. But this will not happen automatically; time alone is not enough (Bregman & Hadley, 1976).

Goals of Intervention

The overall goals of the sexual component of a rehabilitation program after spinal cord injury should be for the person to become comfortable with himself or herself as a sexual being and to learn whatever is needed to make sexual fulfillment possible.

The rehabilitation team should affirm the cord-injured person's sexuality. The patient and family should receive the message that sexuality and sexual functioning are legitimate concerns and that a fulfilling sex life is a reasonable goal.

People with spinal cord injury also need to gain a basic understanding of how they can function sexually. This understanding should include physical sexual responses before and after injury, fertility, techniques for giving and receiving pleasure, and strategies for dealing with logistical problems such as spasticity or incontinence.

Knowledge in the area of sexuality and sexual functioning is important, but this information will be all but worthless to the person who does not feel worthy of sexual gratification. In a rehabilitation program, a patient should work to regain his or her sense of self-worth, sexuality, and attractiveness as a sexual partner (Ray & West, 1984).

Communication is a critical ingredient in all sexual encounters. Perhaps it becomes even more important following spinal cord injury. Patients may need to develop skills in meeting people, putting them at ease, dealing with misunderstandings or misgivings, initiating and refusing sexual activities, communicating likes and dislikes, and letting partners know what they can expect in a sexual encounter (Bregman & Hadley, 1976; Steger & Brockway, 1980; Thornton, 1979).

> I verbalized a lot of things: You know I'm paralyzed, you know I don't have much sensation, or if you don't know this, I'm gonna tell you. And I'm gonna show you. And I'm gonna reach out and touch you, and I'm gonna hold you because that's something I need to do and I want to do. And it's worked.
>
> —Mark Johnson (Corbet, 1980)

Knowledge, comfort with self, and communication skills are a good start. Ultimately the goal is for the cord-injured person to be able to put these things into practice. Patients should be encouraged to explore and experiment, learning how their bodies respond and what is now pleasurable. With their partners,[9] they can try different positions and sexual activities. The rehabilitation team can assist in this process by providing a private room for intimate encounters and providing support when needed.

Strategies

There are a variety of approaches to sexual rehabilitation following spinal cord injury. Several basic strategies are presented below. Most programs in-

---

[9] Not all patients have sexual partners available. Options in these cases include utilizing surrogates, encouraging patients to explore their bodies on their own, emphasizing strategies for finding sexual partners or any combination thereof.

corporate more than one of these strategies. Perhaps the perfect program would include elements of all of them.

Psychosexual and Physical Evaluation. In many centers sexual rehabilitation begins with an evaluation. One or more members of the rehabilitation team assess the patient's sexual functioning in much the same way that they evaluate other areas of function.

In taking a psychosexual history, a health professional investigates psychosocial issues that can impact on a cord-injured person's sexual adjustment. Areas of investigation can include the patient's past and present sexual attitudes and behavior, level of understanding of his or her sexual functioning, communication skills, present relationships, feelings about himself or herself as a sexual being, and present sexual desires and concerns (Boller & Frank, 1982; Miller, Szasz, & Anderson, 1981).

A sexual evaluation also includes a history of the patient's medical status. The health professional investigates the patient's history of urinary tract and bowel functioning and complications, genitourinary surgery, erection or menstruation and pregnancy, venereal disease, and contraception (Boller & Frank, 1982).

Finally, a thorough sexual evaluation includes an examination that investigates the patient's physical potential for sexual functioning. It can cover genital sensation and responses, a neurological evaluation, and rectal examination. The evaluation can include sperm count studies or pelvic examination, depending on the patient's sex (Boller & Frank, 1982; Eisenberg & Rustad, 1976; Miller, Szasz, Anderson, 1981). The evaluation can also include the patient's strength, range of motion, muscle tone, and functional status, as these areas are relevant to the individual's potential for participating in various sexual activities (Miller, Szasz, & Anderson, 1981).

An evaluation of psychosocial and physical sexual functioning and potential is a valuable part of a rehabilitation program. It provides the rehabilitation team and patient with an understanding of the patient's functioning and enables them to set goals and design a program accordingly. The evaluation itself can also be therapeutic, as it demonstrates to the cord-injured person that the rehabilitation team considers his or her sexuality and sexual functioning to be an important area of concern.

Education. In sexual rehabilitation, education is a must and a minimum. Patients should learn about their physical sexual responses and the responses of their partners: how the body responds to sexual stimuli, how and why a spinal cord injury impacts on this function, how these sexual responses can be elicited, and how they can be utilized in sexual encounters. People with spinal cord injuries need to know about their fertility and about contraceptive options if indicated. They should learn that sexual pleasure and even orgasm are still possible, whether or not the genitals remain innervated. And they should know how to deal with logistical problems such as urinary devices or altered genital functioning. Without this knowledge, a patient may be at a loss regarding how to go about pursuing sexual gratification. Worse, he or she may be unaware that sexual gratification is even possible.

The educational component of sexual rehabilitation can take many forms. The information can be presented in lectures, films, slides, group discussions, or question and answer sessions (Eisenberg & Rustad, 1976; Romano & Lassiter, 1972). Romano and Lassiter (1972) emphasize that education regarding sexuality should begin with instruction about the physical and emotional aspects of "normal" sexual functioning. The information can be presented as a "review." Like the general public, people with spinal cord injuries are likely to be ignorant in this area but reluctant to admit this ignorance.

Desensitization/Attitude. In our culture sexual activities are emotionally charged and value laden; sexual behavior is immersed in taboos, prescriptions, and proscriptions. People come to rehabilitation with compelling, deep-seated feelings about what they should and shouldn't do in a sexual encounter, what is desirable and what is wrong or disgusting. These preexisting attitudes can be a formidable barrier to sexual adjustment after spinal cord injury. They can prevent a person from experimenting comfortably with his or her sexual expression. Attitudes can even inhibit a person's ability to absorb the information presented in an educational program. To achieve sexual fulfillment following spinal cord injury, a person may need to reassess his or her attitudes regarding sexual behavior.

One strategy used to address attitude is the Sexual Attitude Reassessment (SAR) workshop. SARs are intensive, short-term workshops in which the participants are exposed to a variety of sexual behaviors among able-bodied as well as disabled people. The programs include lectures and audiovisual materials, small-group discussions, and panel discussions. The content becomes increasingly explicit as the program progresses. The aim of this approach is to desensitize the participants to sexual stimuli, enabling them to examine their sexual attitudes and to become more comfortable with their own sexuality, with sexuality among disabled people, and with the various ways in which sexuality can be expressed. Acceptance and a willingness to experiment with sexual expression are encouraged (Eisenberg & Rustad, 1976; Romano, 1977).

SARs have been shown to be effective in bringing about lasting attitude changes, with participants becoming more accepting of a variety of sexual behaviors (Halstead, 1978; Halstead, Halstead, Salhoot, Stock, & Sparks, 1977; Higgins, 1984). The SAR and adaptations of this approach are used widely throughout the country (Halstead, 1978; Halstead, Halstead, Salhoot, Stock, & Sparks, 1977).

Elements of desensitization and attitude change are incorporated in many sexual rehabilitation programs. Sexual issues can be addressed over time, with the presentations and discussions gradually becoming more explicit. Contact with cord-injured people who have adapted well sexually can assist with attitude change. In a program described by Steger and Brockway (1980), the process of desensitization is begun in a group setting with participants verbalizing common synonyms of sexual terms.

Behavioral Treatment.

Knowledge and attitude change can pave the way for sexual adjustment, but they may not be sufficient. Even armed with an understanding and acceptance of his or her potential for sexual functioning, a cord-injured person faces social barriers to sexual gratification. The injury may have brought about role changes, conflict, and communication difficulties in preexisting relationships. Meeting people and initiating sexual relations may be problematic; the cord-injured person is likely to have a strike or two against him or her by virtue of being disabled. Moreover, the person may find that he or she is no longer able to use some tried and true techniques for communicating desires and testing the waters. (The old knee press under the table, for example.)

A variety of communication skills may be helpful to the cord-injured person (or anyone) in developing and maintaining sexual relations. These skills include assertiveness, verbal and nonverbal expression of desires and needs, and techniques for meeting and seducing potential partners (Dunn, Lloyd, & Phelps, 1979; Romano & Lassiter, 1972). Someone who learns to project confidence in himself or herself as a sexual being and knows how to put a partner at ease is more likely to be successful sexually.

Various approaches can be used to develop communication skills for sexual encounters. Patients can role play, rehearse behaviors, and receive feedback on their communication. They can also practice expressing desires and giving feedback, both verbally and nonverbally (Romano & Lassiter, 1972; Steger & Brockway, 1980).

In addition to developing new communication skills, a cord-injured person needs to learn how his or her body now functions sexually. The partner must also learn and adapt if the relationship is to continue. The patient and partner need to be given the permission and opportunity to explore their bodies and relearn how to give and receive pleasure. To facilitate this exploration, patients can be instructed in sensory exercises and the use of fantasy. A couple[10] may be given "homework assignments" involving various sexual activities tailored to the couple's needs (Steger & Brockway, 1980; Thornton, 1979). For inpatients, private rooms can be made available to enable couples or individuals to explore and redevelop their sexual potentials (Miller, Szasz, & Anderson, 1981). These rooms may also be used to provide much-needed private time for couples and families (Cole & Cole, 1981).

Counseling.

Sexual adjustment following spinal cord injury requires some major adaptations. A patient may be faced with altered functioning and loss of sensation in the genitals, a body that no longer looks or works the same as it used to, urinary appliances and the threat of incontinence during sex, loss of fertility, and altered social relations with others. Counseling can help a person come to terms with these changes.

Group therapy can provide a nonthreatening atmosphere for discussing sexual concerns. Many find it helpful to get together with other cord-injured people to discuss their feelings and the problems that they anticipate or have already faced. Participants often find comfort in learning that others are facing problems similar to theirs (Eisenberg & Rustad, 1976; Romano & Lassiter, 1972). Group counseling sessions can also provide opportunities for problem solving and mutual support.

More individualized counseling can also be helpful in adjusting sexually after spinal cord injury. One approach involves seeing both the patient and partner, as both have adjustments to make. The two can be seen individually and as a couple. In joint sessions the couple can develop their communication skills and discuss their expectations and emo-

---

[10] If a partner is not available, the patient should be encouraged to experiment on his or her own.

tions with each other (Eisenberg & Rustad, 1976; Halstead, 1984).

Specific Suggestions. Specific suggestions can be an invaluable aid to sexual adjustment after spinal cord injury. A patient who is simply told to "experiment" and then turned loose to find his or her own way may have difficulty finding that way. He or she may be reluctant to experiment without at least some initial guidance. Unanswered questions such as "What do I do with this catheter?" or "How exactly can I have intercourse?" may leave the individual reluctant to try sexual activities. Specific suggestions about the logistics of sexual encounters can pave the way for more comfortable and confident exploration.

People with impaired genital sensation may benefit from suggestions for maximizing their pleasure during sexual encounters. They should be encouraged to explore their bodies and find what areas give pleasure when stimulated. People with spinal cord injuries often find that their lowest innervated dermatomes are more sensitive to touch. Many find stimulation of the earlobes, neck, and mouth to be extremely pleasurable. By concentrating on pleasurable sensations, using fantasy, and reassigning pleasurable sensations to the genitals, people with cord injuries can maximize their pleasure, even to the point of orgasm (Cole, 1979; Griffith & Trieschmann, 1975; Steger & Brockway, 1980; Thornton, 1979).

Suggestions regarding pleasuring techniques for the partner can also be helpful. Patients can be encouraged to try oral or manual stimulation of the partner's genitals. People with impaired hand sensation may find vibrators to be useful for stimulating their partners (Steger & Brockway, 1980; Thornton, 1979).

Another area to address is compensation for dysfunctional vaginal lubrication or penile erection during coitus. Women who do not have functioning sacral cords may not produce adequate vaginal lubrication for intercourse. In these cases a lubricant can be used. Women who have intact sacral reflex arcs may require manual stimulation to achieve adequate lubrication (Thornton, 1979). Erectile dysfunction in men is more problematic for those who wish to have intercourse. Men with intact sacral reflexes may be able to elicit or prolong erection by stimulating the penis, scrotum, inner thighs, pubic hair, anus, or lower abdomen. A vibrator or manual stimulation can be used (Gatens, 1984; Halstead, 1984). With or without a functioning sacral reflex arc, a man with erectile dysfunction can use the "stuffing" technique. In this technique the penis is manually "stuffed" into the vagina. This is most easily accomplished with the man on top and the partner's hips flexed (Szasz, 1987). If the woman has adequate voluntary control over her pubococcygeus muscle, she may be able to create a tourniquet effect and cause the penis to become partially erect (Cole, 1975). If the sacral reflex arc is intact, "stuffing" the penis may elicit a reflex erection (Halstead, 1984). Men with erectile dysfunction may also wish to consider penile prostheses or other physical aids designed to facilitate penile-vaginal intercourse. These physical aids are described in a separate section below.

Health professionals can also make suggestions regarding positions for intercourse. A cord-injured male may prefer the female-superior position, side-lying face to face with his partner or sitting in a chair or wheelchair with his partner in his lap, facing toward or away from him. A woman may prefer the male-superior position or side lying. If she has severe adductor spasticity, a rear approach may be best. A cord-injured woman may also have intercourse sitting in a wheelchair, sitting at the edge of the seat with her partner kneeling in front of her (Cole, 1975; Steger & Brockway, 1980; Szasz, 1987).

Understandably, patients are concerned about managing their indwelling catheters during intercourse. They may fear that they will injure themselves during intercourse or that the catheters will get in the way. Patients should be assured that they can remove catheters prior to sexual intercourse if they prefer, or they can safely leave them in place. A man can fold his urethral catheter back along the side of his penis, either cover it with a condom or leave it uncovered, and lubricate well (Cole, 1975; Cole, 1979). A woman who wishes to leave her urethral catheter in place should tape it to her thigh, out of the way (Cole, 1979). A suprapubic catheter should be taped to the abdomen, and an ileal conduit bag should be positioned out of the way (Cole, 1979; Romano & Lassiter, 1972).

People who manage their bladder incontinence without indwelling catheters may have urinary accidents during sexual activities. This is especially true for people who have reflexively functioning bladders; stimulation of the thighs, genitals, or other pelvic structures may initiate the voiding reflex. This risk can be reduced by voiding immediately prior to sexual activity (Thornton, 1979). In addition, individuals may wish to note which sexual stimuli tend to induce voiding and avoid these stimuli. It may also be wise to keep a towel handy and to inform partners of the possibility of bladder accidents (Cole, 1979; Romano & Lassiter, 1972).

These steps can reduce the embarrassment and inconvenience of any accidents that occur.

Bowel accidents during sexual activity are another area of concern. Patients should be reassured that a regular bowel program can minimize the possibility of having a bowel accident during sex (Thornton, 1979).

A common concern expressed by many patients is that the partner may contract a urinary tract infection during intercourse. Both parties should be assured that this is unlikely if standard hygiene practices are used (Cole, 1979). Patients may also be concerned about autonomic dysreflexia during sexual activity. This is more likely to occur but should not pose a major threat if handled correctly. Patients who are subject to autonomic dysreflexia (people with lesions above T6) should be told of the possibility. If a headache occurs during genital stimulation, the couple should stop the stimulation briefly. The headache should then resolve quickly. When it does, the couple can resume their sexual activity, avoiding the particular stimulation that appeared to bring on the headache (Cole, 1975).

People who require assistance in preparation for sexual activities (undressing, transfers, positioning, management of catheters) may find that having a sexual partner provide this assistance creates problems. Both parties may find it difficult to shift from nurse–patient to lover–lover roles. Moreover, the caretaker/lover may spend so much energy on the preparation that he or she has little left over for the sex. When problems such as these arise, an attendant can often be of help (Halstead, 1984).

In some sexual rehabilitation programs, patients are given suggestions for setting the mood in preparation for sexual activity. These suggestions include tips on creating a romantic environment (lighting, music) as well as getting both partners in the mood (massage, alcohol, fantasy, erotic films; Eisenberg & Rustad, 1976; Halstead, 1984; Steger & Brockway, 1980).

Suggestions on maximizing pleasure for both partners and on the mechanics and logistics of sexual activity can be of great assistance to a newly injured person. Ultimately, however, each person still must find his or her own way sexually. He or she will need to experiment, discovering what positions and activities yield the most pleasure and satisfaction.

Physical Aids. Various physical aids are available for men with erectile dysfunction who wish to include penetration in their sexual activity. Noninvasive options include the use of a firm casing that is worn over the penis or an artificial penis that can

either be strapped above the anatomical penis or held in the hand (Eisenberg & Rustad, 1976; Hale, 1979; Szasz, 1987). One option for men who have reflex erections is a constricting band that is placed around the base of the erect penis to trap blood within the erectile bodies and prolong the erection. Alternatively a vacuum pump may be used to achieve an erection, which is then maintained with a constricting band at the base of the penis (Zasler & Katz, 1989).

A man who wishes to have an anatomical erection can undergo surgical implantation of a prosthesis into the erectile tissue of his penis. There are two classes of penile prostheses: inflatable and rod type. Inflatable prosthesis include a pump and reservoir and can be inflated or deflated as needed (Szasz, 1987). Rod-type prostheses provide a permanent erection. In addition to providing erection for intercourse, penile prostheses can aid in intermittent catheterization (Iwatsubo, Tanaka, Takahashi, Akatsu, 1986) or in fit of condom catheters (Szasz, 1987).

Penile prostheses have their problems. These include mechanical failure, decubiti, infection, and scarring (Collins & Hackler, 1988; Donovon, 1985; Szasz, 1987). Rod-type prostheses appear to involve less of a risk, with a success rate of over 94%. In contrast, inflatable prostheses have a 48% rate of mechanical failure over time (Wyndaele, deMeyer, deSy, & Claessens, 1986). With either type of prosthesis, people who have unrealistic expectations will be dissatisfied. In view of the physical risks and possibility of dissatisfaction, patients should be selected carefully. Appropriate candidates are those who have realistic expectations, are motivated in their self-care, and have been through a period of adjustment following injury (Green & Sloan, 1986).

As an alternative to penile prostheses, men can achieve erection by injecting vasoactive drugs into their corpus cavernosum. Erection occurs within a few minutes of injection and lasts for 1 to 6 hours (Wyndaele, deMayer, deSy, & Claessens, 1986). Complications include priapism and scarring of the corpora cavernosa with resulting reduction of erectile capabilities (Zasler & Katz, 1989).

A variety of options are available for achieving erections. However, the rehabilitation team should keep in mind that erection and vaginal penetration are not prerequisites for a satisfying sex life.

(There's a prevalent belief that) if your neurology is such that you do not get an erection physiologically, then you must have an erection prosthetically. I have no objection to this procedure, but I do object to the procedure being offered to newly injured people who have not had an adequate trial at living an integrated life as a para or a quad, who have not learned to *like* themselves again, who still see themselves as some kind of abomination, who think the big thing in sex is genital activity.

—George Hohmann (Corbet, 1980)

Sexuality as a Part of the Overall Rehabilitation Program

Coming to terms with one's sexuality and sexual functioning is an important component of adjustment after spinal cord injury. Seen in this light, sexual rehabilitation is clearly a key ingredient of rehabilitation after cord injury.

Unfortunately sexuality is often neglected by the rehabilitation team. Because of poorly defined roles and discomfort with sexuality, each team member may avoid the topic, hoping that other team members will deal with it. The team may limit their intervention to discussion of fertility or avoid the issue altogether (Cole, 1975; Conine, 1984). Under these circumstances, patients are often reluctant to bring up the topic (Boller & Frank, 1982). They may find the subject too embarrassing or may perceive the team's silence as an indication that sex is no longer an appropriate area of concern for them (Cole & Cole, 1978). Even when patients take the initiative to bring up the topic, health professionals may dodge questions and avoid discussions on sexual functioning. This behavior is likely to increase patients' anxiety about their sexuality and sexual functioning (Griffith, Trieschmann, Hohmann, Cole, Tobis, & Cummings, 1975).

To ensure that sexuality is addressed adequately with every patient, sexual rehabilitation (with defined roles and goals) should be an official component of the program. It should not be left to chance, with each team member hoping or assuming that someone else is taking care of it.

Sexuality should be addressed with all cord-injured patients, regardless of whether they are male or female, old or young (Larsen & Hegaard, 1984), heterosexual or homosexual, involved in an intimate relationship or unattached. Sexual rehabilitation should be comprehensive, should begin early (Cole, 1975), and should be tailored to the needs of each individual. If a patient has a sexual partner, that person should be involved in the process, since he or she will also have adjustments to make (Griffith, Trieschmann, Hohmann, Cole, Tobis, & Cummings, 1975).

Team Approach. Successful sexual rehabilitation requires a team approach. The various members of the rehabilitation team should be comfortable affirming patients' sexuality, answering questions about sexual concerns, and supporting the sexual component of the rehabilitation program (Eisenberg & Rustad, 1976). Patients will then be able to discuss sexual concerns with whomever they feel the most comfortable.

Being an effective team member requires more than knowledge in the area of sexual functioning. Values and attitudes are also important. A health professional who is uncomfortable discussing sexual issues, who sees disabled people as sexless, or who is repulsed by the sexual options open to cord-injured people will not be an effective participant in sexual rehabilitation. In fact, he or she is likely to have a detrimental effect on patients. Overtly or covertly, the health professional may convey negative attitudes that undermine the patient's progress (Cole & Stevens, 1975; Griffith, Trieschmann, Hohmann, Cole, Tobis, & Cummings, 1975).

All members of the rehabilitation team should have the knowledge and attitudes needed to support patients in their sexual rehabilitation. Specialized training may be required to prepare team members for their roles in sexual rehabilitation. SAR workshops can be valuable experiences for health professionals, increasing their comfort with sexual issues and making them more likely to address these issues with their patients (Cole & Cole, 1981).

PLISSIT Model. Although the entire rehabilitation team should be able to support the sexual component of the program, not all health professionals must (or even can) provide intensive sexual therapy to their cord-injured patients. Different professionals will provide different input, depending on their comfort, experience, interest, and expertise. According to his or her strengths and inclinations, each individual will have his or her own level of involvement in the sexual aspect of rehabilitation.

The PLISSIT model of intervention[11] can be useful for the team approach to sexual rehabilitation. "PLISSIT" is an acronym representing the levels of intervention described in the approach: *P*ermission, *L*imited *I*nformation, *S*pecific *S*uggestions, and *I*ntensive *T*herapy. Using this model, health professionals can supply varying levels of intervention. The level that a given person provides can be determined by both the patient's need and the professional's expertise and comfort.

Permission giving is the most basic level of in-

---

[11] Developed By J. S. Annon.

tervention in the PLISSIT model. At this level the health professional gives the patient "permission" to be sexual; through verbal or nonverbal behavior, the health professional affirms the patient's sexuality and encourages him or her to explore its expression (Brashear, 1978; Higgins, 1984). This is the minimal level of intervention, which all members of the team should be able to provide. The "permission" from various health professionals will provide much-needed support to the patient.

At the next level of intervention, the health professional provides limited information: the patient is educated about his or her sexual functioning (Brashear, 1978; Halstead, 1984; Higgins, 1984). For cord-injured patients, the education can cover anatomy and physiology, genital functioning following injury, fertility, and birth control.

At the third level of intervention, the health professional provides the patient with specific suggestions (Brashear, 1978). Suggestions can cover the logistics and mechanics of sexual acts, meeting and seducing people, and giving and receiving pleasure. A variety of health professionals may provide this level of intervention, addressing issues most pertinent to their fields. For example, a nurse may discuss options for managing a catheter during sexual encounters, and a physical therapist may make suggestions regarding positioning during intercourse.

Intensive therapy is the highest level of intervention, provided by health professionals with specialized training (Brashear, 1978). Counseling, behavioral treatment, and attitude reassessment fall into this category of intervention.

SUMMARY

Spinal cord injury has profound effects on sexuality and sexual functioning. Changes in genital functioning, sensation, and musculoskeletal functioning may make a person's accustomed modes of sexual expression difficult or impossible. In addition, the physical and social sequelae of a cord injury are likely to disrupt a person's sense of self, including his or her sense of self as a sexual being. Logistical problems such as incontinence or difficulty in meeting people can further complicate the picture.

Sexual rehabilitation is an important component of rehabilitation after spinal cord injury. Different rehabilitation centers take a variety of approaches in addressing sexuality. Some or all of the following elements can be included in a sexual rehabilitation program: psychosexual and physical evaluation, education, desensitization, attitude reassessment, counseling, and specific suggestions.

REFERENCES

Boller, F., & Frank, E. (1982). *Sexual dysfunction in neurological disorders: Diagnosis, management, and rehabilitation.* New York: Raven Press.

Bonwich, E. (1985). Sex role attitudes and role reorganization in spinal cord injured women. In Deegan M. J., Brooks N. A. (Eds.), *Women and disability: The double handicap* (pp. 56–67). New Brunswick, NJ: Transaction Books.

Brashear, D. B. (1978). Integrating human sexuality into rehabilitation practice. *Sexuality and Disability*, *1*(3), 190–199.

Bregman, S., & Hadley, R. G. (1976). Sexual adjustment and feminine attractiveness among spinal cord injured women. *Archives of Physical Medicine and Rehabilitation*, *57*, 448–450.

Brindley, G. S. (1980). Electroejaculation and the fertility of paraplegic men. *Sexuality and Disability*, *3*(3), 223–229.

Cole, T. M. (1979). Sexuality and the spinal cord injured. In Green R. (Ed.), *Human sexuality: A health practitioner's text* (pp. 243–263). Baltimore: Williams & Wilkins.

Cole, T. M. (1975). Sexuality and physical disabilities. *Archives of Sexual Behavior*, *4*(4), 389–403.

Cole, T. M., & Cole, S. S. (1981). Sexual attitude reassessment programs for spinal cord injured adults, their partners and health care professionals. In Sha'ked A. (Ed.), *Human sexuality and rehabilitation medicine* (pp. 80–90). Baltimore: Williams & Wilkins.

Cole, T. M., & Cole, S. S. (1978). The handicapped and sexual health. In Comfort A. (Ed.), *Sexual consequences of disability* (pp. 37–43). Philadelphia: George F. Stickley Company.

Cole, T. M., & Stevens, M. R. (1975). Rehabilitation professionals and sexual counseling for spinal cord injured adults. *Archives of Sexual Behavior*, *4*(6) 631–638.

Collins, K., & Hackler, R. (1988). Complications of penile prostheses in the spinal cord injury population. *The Journal of Urology*, *140*, 984–985.

Conine, T. (1984). Sexual rehabilitation: Roles of allied health professional. In Krueger D. (Ed.), *Rehabilitation psychology: A comprehensive textbook* (pp. 81–87). Rockville, MD: Aspen Publishers.

Corbet, B. (1980). *Options: Spinal cord injury and the future.* Denver, CO: A. B. Hirschfeld Press.

Craig, D. (1990). The adaptation to pregnancy of spinal cord injured women. *Rehabilitation Nursing*, *15*(1), 6–9.

Crenshaw, R. T.; Martin, D. E.; Warner, H., & Crenshaw, T. L., (1978). Organic impotence. In Comfort A. (Ed.), *Sexual consequences of disability* (pp. 25–35). Philadelphia: George F. Stickley Company.

Donovon, W. H. (1985). Sexuality and sexual function. In Bedbrook G. M. (Ed.), *Lifetime care of the paraplegic patient* (pp. 149–161). New York: Churchill Livingstone.

Dunn, M.; Lloyd, E. E., & Phelps, G. H. (1979). Sexual assertiveness in spinal cord injury. *Sexuality & Disability, 2*(4), 293–300.

Eisenberg, M. G., & Rustad, L. C. (1976). Sex education and counseling program on a spinal cord injury service. *Archives of Physical Medicine and Rehabilitation, 57,* 135–140.

Fitzpatrick, W. F. (1974). Sexual function in the paraplegic patient. *Archives of Physical Medicine and Rehabilitation, 55,* 221–227.

Gatens, C. (1984). Sexuality and disability. In Woods N. F. (Ed.), *Human sexuality in health and illness* (3rd ed., pp. 370–398). St. Louis: C. V. Mosby.

Geiger, R. C. (1979). Neurophysiology of sexual response in spinal cord injury. *Sexuality & Disability, 2*(4), 257–266.

Gott, L. J. (1981). Anatomy and physiology of male sexual response and fertility as related to spinal cord injury. In Sha'ked A. (Ed.), *Human sexuality and rehabilitation medicine* (pp. 67–73). Baltimore: Williams & Wilkins.

Green, B. G., & Sloan, S. L. (1986). Penile prostheses in spinal cord injured patients: Combined psychosexual counseling and surgical regimen. *Paraplegia, 24,* 167–172.

Griffith, E. R.; Tomko, M. A.; and Timms, R. J. (1973). Sexual function is spinal cord-injured patients: A review. *Archives of Physical Medicine and Rehabilitation, 54,* 539–543.

Griffith, E. R., & Trieschmann, R. B. (1975). Sexual functioning in women with spinal cord injury. *Archives of Physical Medicine and Rehabilitation, 56,* 18–21.

Griffith, E. R., Trieschmann, R. B., Hohmann, G. W., Cole, T. M., Tobis, J. S., & Cummings, V. (1975). Sexual dysfunctions associated with physical disabilities. *Archives of Physical Medicine and Rehabilitation, 56,* 8–13.

Guyton, A. C. (1987). *Human physiology and mechanisms of disease* (4th ed.). Philadelphia: W. B. Saunders Company.

Hale, G. (Ed.). (1979). *The source book for the disabled: An illustrated guide to easier more independent living for physically disabled people, their families and friends.* New York: Paddington Press.

Halstead, L. S. (1984). Sexuality and disability. In Krueger D. W. (Ed.), *Emotional rehabilitation of physical trauma and disability* (pp. 235–252). New York: Spectrum Publications.

Halstead, L. S. (1978). Sexual attitude reassessment programs, rehabilitation professionals and the physically disabled. In Comfort A. (Ed.), *Sexual consequences of disability* (pp. 255–274). Philadelphia: George F. Stickley Company.

Halstead, L. S.; Halstead, M. M.; Salhoot, J. T.; Stock, D. D., & Sparks, R. W. (1977). A hospital-based program in human sexuality. *Archives of Physical Medicine and Rehabilitation, 58,* 409–412.

Halstead, L. S.; VerVoort, S., & Seager, S. W. J. (1987). Rectal probe electrostimulation in the treatment of anejaculatory spinal cord injured men. *Paraplegia, 25,* 120–129.

Higgins, G. E. (1984). Sexuality and the spinal cord injured: treatment approaches. In Krueger D. W. (Ed.), *Emotional rehabilitation of physical trauma and disability* (pp. 253–265). New York: Spectrum Publications.

Iwatsubo, E.; Tanaka, M.; Takahashi, K., & Akatsu, T. (1986). Non-inflatable penile prosthesis for the management of urinary incontinence and sexual disability of patients with spinal cord injury. *Paraplegia, 24,* 307–310.

Kenney, L. (1987). Meet Ellen Stohl. *Playboy, 34*(7), 68–75.

Killien, M. (1984). Sexuality and contraception. In Woods N. F. (Ed.), *Human sexuality in sex and illness* (3rd ed., pp. 204–221). St. Louis: C. V. Mosby Company.

Kirk, S. A. (1977). Society and sexual deviance. In Gochros H. L., & Gochros J. S. (Eds.), *The sexually oppressed* (pp. 28–37). New York: Association Press.

Larsen, E. & Hejgaard, N. (1984). Sexual dysfunction after spinal cord or cauda equina lesions. *Paraplegia, 22,* 66–74.

Miller, S.; Szasz, G., & Anderson, L. (1981). Sexual health care clinician in an acute spinal cord injury unit. *Archives of Physical Medicine and Rehabilitation, 62,* 315–320.

Ray, C., & West, J. (1984). Social, sexual, and personal implications of paraplegia. *Paraplegia, 22,* 75–86.

Romano, M. D. (1977). The physically handicapped. In Gochros H. L., & Gochros J. S. (Eds.), *The sexually oppressed* (pp. 257–267). New York: Association Press.

Romano, M. D., & Lassiter, R. E. (1972). Sexual counseling with the spinal-cord injured. *Archives of Physical Medicine and Rehabilitation, 53,* 568–572.

Siösteen, A.; Forssman, L.; Steen, Y.; Sullivan, L., & Wickström, I. (1990). Quality of semen after repeated ejaculation treatment in spinal cord injury men. *Paraplegia, 28,* 96–104.

Steger, J. C., & Brockway, J. (1980). Sexual enhancement in spinal cord injured patients: behavioral group treatment. *Sexuality and Disability, 3*(2), 84–96.

Szasz, G. (1987). Sexual management. In Ford J., & Duckworth B. (Eds.), *Physical management for the quadriplegic patient* (2nd ed., pp. 377–396). Philadelphia: F. A. Davis Company.

Teal, J. C., & Athelstan, G. T. (1975). Sexuality and spinal cord injury: some psychosocial considerations. *Archives of Physical Medicine & Rehabilitation, 56,* 264–268.

Thews, G., & Vaupel, P. (1985). *Autonomic functions in human physiology.* New York: Springer-Verlag.

Thornton, C. E. (1979). Sexuality counseling of women with spinal cord injuries. *Sexuality & Disability, 2*(4), 267–277.

Verduyn, W. H. (1986). Spinal cord injured women, pregnancy and delivery. *Paraplegia, 24,* 231–220.

Vick, R. L. (1984). *Contemporary medical physiology.* Reading, MA: Addison-Wesley Publishing.

Wanner, M. B.; Rageth, C. J., & Zach, G. A. (1987). Pregnancy and autonomic hyperreflexia in patients with spinal cord lesions. *Paraplegia, 25,* 482–490.

Weiss, H. D. (1978). The physiology of human penile erection. In Comfort A. (Ed.), *Sexual consequences of disability* (pp. 11–24). Philadelphia: George F. Stickley.

Wyndaele, J. J.; de Mayer, J. M.; de Sy, W. A., & Claessens, H. (1986). Intracavernous injection of vasoactive drugs, an alternative for treating impotence in spinal cord injury patients. *Paraplegia, 24,* 271–275.

Zasler, N., & Katz, G. (1989). Synergist erection system in the management of impotence secondary to spinal cord injury. *Archives of Physical Medicine and Rehabilitation, 70,* 712–716.

17

Bowel and Bladder Management

Most people with spinal cord injuries are incontinent; since the bowel and bladder are innervated by sacral cord segments, any complete lesion will result in fecal and urinary incontinence. Because of the profound impact that incontinence can have upon a person's health and lifestyle, bowel and bladder management are major concerns following spinal cord injury.

Effects of Incontinence

Incontinence is far more than an inconvenience. It is a serious medical problem that can have life-threatening results if not managed appropriately.

Kidney damage is one complication of urinary incontinence. It can result from an atonic bladder's inability to void when filled with urine. When a bladder does not empty itself, enough pressure can build to cause urine to reflux into the ureters. Hydronephrosis and eventual renal failure can result.

Kidney function is also threatened by urinary tract infection, a common sequela of urinary incontinence. When cord injury leads to incomplete bladder emptying, bacteria flourish in the stagnant urine that remains. Infections in the bladder can ascend to the kidneys, especially when urinary reflux occurs.

Incontinence can pose a more immediate threat to people with cervical or high thoracic lesions. Bladder distension or fecal impaction can trigger autonomic dysreflexia, a heightened autonomic response that can progress rapidly to death. Autonomic dysreflexia is discussed in more detail in Chapter 2.

Bowel or bladder incontinence can also cause decubiti. Feces or urine that remains in contact with the skin for prolonged periods can damage the skin. Once breakdown occurs, the person may have to restrict his activities while his skin heals, and the healed area will remain vulnerable to subsequent decubiti. The person may face prolonged hospitalization, sepsis, amputations, and even death.

In addition to its impact on physical health, incontinence can have profound psychosocial consequences. Our society places great importance on continence. We associate bowel and bladder accidents with infancy, insanity, and physical infirmity; incontinence is strongly devalued. As a result, bowel and bladder accidents can be a source of acute embarrassment and social isolation, as well as of serious problems with self-image.

BLADDER FUNCTION

To understand the ways in which a bladder can function after spinal cord injury, one must understand normal bladder functioning. Figure 17–1 illustrates the urinary tract and musculature involved in bladder control.

Normal Bladder Function

Urine flows from the kidneys to the bladder through the ureters. It exits through the urethra. In normal functioning urine can voluntarily be stored in the bladder or voided.

Several muscles are involved in bladder control. The wall of the fundus, or body, of the bladder contains the detrusor, which loops around the point of juncture of the urethra with the bladder (Feneley, 1986). The external urethral sphincter and the periurethral skeletal muscles of the pelvic floor surround the urethra distal to this point.

Normal bladder function depends upon the neurological control of the detrusor, external sphincter, and periurethral pelvic floor muscles. This control involves both autonomic and somatic innervation (Fig. 17–2).

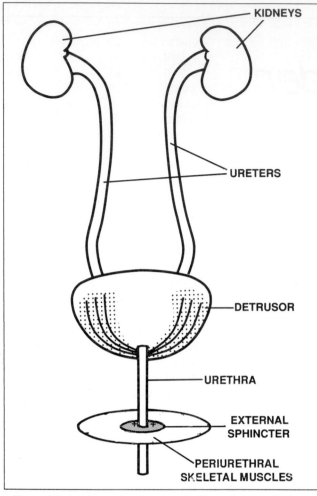

Figure 17–1. Urinary tract and musculature involved in bladder control.

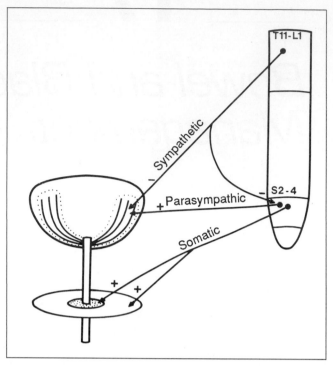

Figure 17–2. Motor innervation of the detrusor, external sphincter, and periurethral pelvic floor musculature.

Autonomic System. The detrusor, a smooth muscle, receives both parasympathetic and sympathetic innervation. The parasympathetic innervation arises from cell bodies in sacral cord segments 2, 3, and 4. Parasympathetic stimulation results in contraction of the detrusor. The bladder's sympathetic innervation arises from the 11th thoracic through the 1st lumbar segments of the cord (Feneley, 1986). The postganglionic fibers innervate the detrusor and have inhibitory synapses with the parasympathetic postganglionic fibers. Sympathetic stimulation causes relaxation of the detrusor.

Somatic System. The external urethral sphincter and the periurethral pelvic floor musculature are composed of striated muscle fibers. They receive somatic innervation from sacral cord segments 2 through 4.[1]

---

[1] Some research has suggested that the external urethral sphincter receives parasympathetic innervation (Feneley, 1986).

Reflexes Involved in Urination. Sympathetic tone dominates as the bladder fills. The resulting relaxation of the detrusor allows the pressure of urine in the bladder to remain low (Somjen, 1983).

Once the bladder reaches a critical volume (approximately 400 to 450 milliliters in most people), the autonomic input to the bladder changes. Sympathetic inhibition stops, and parasympathetic input to the detrusor causes an increase in tone. As a result, the pressure within the bladder increases (Somjen, 1983).

Increasing intravesical pressure activates stretch receptors within the bladder wall, eliciting the micturition reflex. In this reflex, parasympathetic input causes contraction of the detrusor (Fig. 17–3). Detrusor contraction increases the activation of the bladder's stretch receptors, which further stimulates the micturition reflex. This reflex soon fatigues, and the bladder returns to its former relaxed state. As time passes and further filling occurs, the reflex is stimulated again. This cycle of excitation and cessation of the micturition reflex repeats itself as the bladder continues to fill, becoming stronger as the pressure increases (Guyton, 1987).

When the volume of urine in the bladder and the strength of the micturition reflex raise the pressure in the bladder enough, the bladder neck is forced open. This activates stretch receptors in this

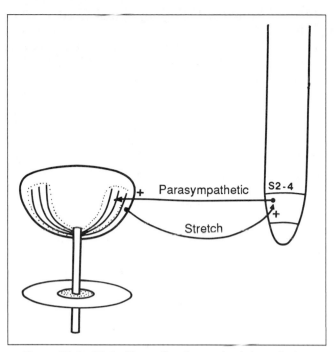

Figure 17–3. Micturition reflex. Increasing intravesical pressure elicits detrusor contraction.

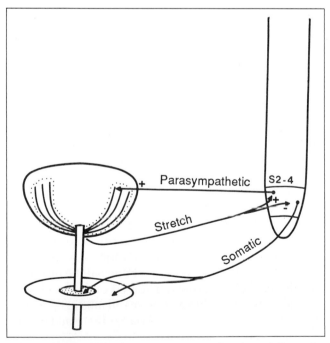

Figure 17–4. Reflexive response to urine forced through bladder neck: facilitation of micturition reflex and relaxation of external sphincter.

region, causing an increase in the strength of the micturition reflex and reflexive relaxation of the external sphincter (Guyton, 1987; Fig. 17–4).

Continence and Urination. Continence is maintained in part by the structure of the urethra and bladder. The bladder wall is folded over the urethra where these two structures join. Because of this fold, pressure in the bladder compresses the proximal portion of the urethra, blocking the flow of urine (Somjen, 1983). Elastic tissue in the proximal urethra adds to this functional sphincter (Feneley, 1986). These mechanisms for preventing the exit of urine from the bladder are adequate only with relatively low pressures. When the pressure becomes high enough to overcome the functional sphincter, the external sphincter and the periurethral pelvic floor muscles are needed to block the flow of urine.

The external sphincter and pelvic floor musculature are under both reflexive and voluntary control. The reflexive control makes continence possible without continual conscious vigilance against voiding. As the bladder fills, the pelvic floor musculature contracts reflexively. This muscle action compresses the urethra (Feneley, 1986).

Normal voluntary control over urination depends upon sensory input. Sensation from the bladder enters the sacral cord and ascends via the posterior columns and the lateral spinothalamic tracts to the medulla, thalamus, and on to the cerebral cortex (Feneley, 1986). The brain's control over urination originates in the cerebral cortex and brain stem (Guyton, 1987) and descends to the second through fourth segments of the sacral cord via the corticospinal and reticulospinal tracts (Feneley, 1986).

Urination at unwanted times is prevented voluntarily by inhibition of the micturition reflex and contraction of the external sphincter and the pelvic floor musculature (Fig. 17–5).

When the time and place are right for urination, descending input from the cerebral cortex facilitates the micturition reflex by direct action on the sacral reflex arc (Guyton, 1987). The resulting detrusor contraction increases the pressure within the bladder and pulls on the fold in the bladder where it joins the urethra. The urethra is opened, and urine passes into the urethra (Somjen, 1983). Cortical centers also inhibit the external sphincter and pelvic floor musculature, allowing urine to pass (Fig. 17–6).

Urination is also helped when voluntary relaxation of pelvic floor musculature allows the pelvic floor to drop. This drop allows urine to pass into the bladder neck, causing a reflexive increase of the micturition reflex (Guyton, 1987). The abdominal musculature can be used to assist voiding by exerting pressure on the bladder.

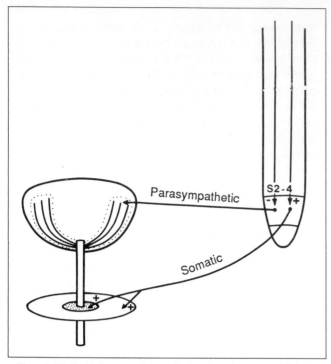

Figure 17–5. Voluntary delay of urination through inhibition of the micturition reflex and contraction of the external sphincter and pelvic floor musculature.

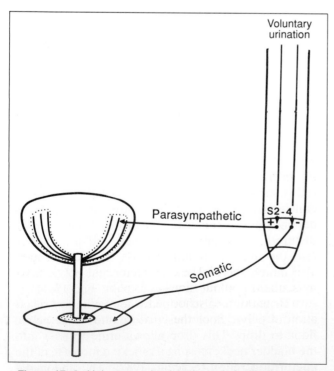

Figure 17–6. Voluntary urination through facilitation of the micturition reflex and relaxation of the external sphincter and pelvic floor musculature.

Bladder Function Following Spinal Cord Injury

Complete spinal cord injury results in the loss of voluntary bladder control and can disrupt reflexive control. The key factor determining bladder function after complete injury is whether or not the sacral reflex arc remains intact. With a high lesion, the sacral cord continues to function; the sacral reflex arc remains intact. Thus people with thoracic and cervical lesions tend to have reflexively functioning bladders. Lower lesions disrupt the functioning of the sacral cord, disrupting the sacral reflex arc. People with lumbar lesions tend to have bladders that reflexively empty only partially, if at all. With sacral cord (or cauda equina) lesions, reflexive emptying does not occur (Ruge, 1969).

It is important to note that the integrity of the sacral reflex arc, not the level of lesion, is the determining factor in bladder control following complete spinal cord injury. Lumbar and even high thoracic lesions can result in permanent loss of sacral reflexes (Comarr, 1977).

Areflexive Bladder. During spinal shock the bladder remains flaccid, with no reflex activity. It usually remains flaccid for 3 to 6 weeks after injury (Kraft, 1987).

The bladder remains areflexive permanently if the sacral reflex arc is disrupted. This occurs either when a cord lesion disrupts the functioning of the second through fourth segments of the sacral cord or when the cauda equina is injured.

Without input from the sacral cord, the bladder does not receive parasympathetic stimulation. As a result, the detrusor remains flaccid,[2] and the fold in the bladder wall over the urethra's point of entry obstructs the flow of urine. This blockage, combined with the absence of sacral voiding reflexes, results in urinary retention (Fig. 17–7).

The incontinence that occurs in an areflexive bladder is called overflow, or dribbling, incontinence. When enough pressure builds in the bladder, small amounts of urine are forced out through the urethra. A large volume of urine remains in the bladder. If it is not drained artificially, the bladder can become severely distended.

Reflexive Bladder. A reflexive bladder requires the presence of an intact reflex arc. Reflexive bladders are found in spinal cord-injured people who have

---

[2] The detrusor regains some automatic contractility after its innervation is lost, but this muscular function is "rarely satisfactory" (Somjen, 1983).

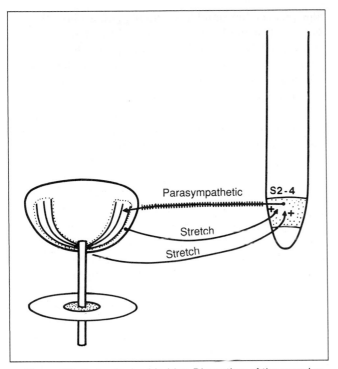

Figure 17–7. Areflexive bladder. Disruption of the sacral reflex arc causes loss of parasympathetic input to the bladder, leading to urinary retention.

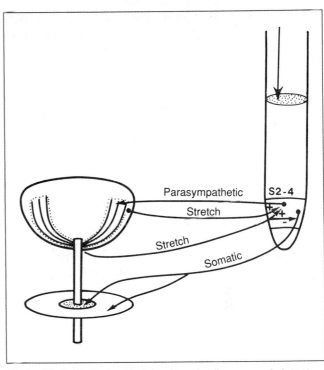

Figure 17–8. Reflexive bladder. Sacral reflexes remain intact but descending input is lost. Voluntary control is lost; bladder empties reflexively when full.

intact functioning in the S2-4 cord segments but whose descending input to these segments has been disrupted. When these conditions exist, the bladder empties reflexively once filling causes sufficient stretch of its wall (Fig. 17–8). Reflexive emptying can also be triggered by stimulating (stroking, pressing, hitting) the abdomen above the symphysis pubis, stroking the inner thigh, or pulling the pubic hair (Kraft, 1987; Rudy, 1984).

Sacral Sparing. Occasionally a person has a clinical picture of what appears to be a complete cord lesion, with the exception that he retains control of his bladder and bowels. This is called "sacral sparing" and is caused when a central cord lesion destroys all but the most peripheral fiber tracts.

Management of Urinary Incontinence
One goal of urinary management following cord injury is ensuring full emptying of the bladder. This artificial emptying is particularly important when the cord-injured person has an areflexive bladder. In these cases proper management is required to prevent the buildup of excessive pressure.

Whether the bladder functions reflexively or areflexively, it may not empty itself completely. A bladder that does not empty completely is vulnerable to urinary tract infections, as bacteria flourish in the stagnant urine. A urinary management program after cord injury ensures that the bladder is emptied periodically, eliminating stagnant urine and reducing the risk of infection.

Urinary tract infections do not result solely from stagnant urine. They can also result from the bladder management practices themselves. Appropriate attention must be paid to hygiene as catheters are applied, so that bacteria are not introduced into the urinary tract.

In addition to protecting the bladder, a urinary management program preserves the integrity of the patient's skin. Failure to maintain dry skin is likely to result in decubiti.

Finally, proper urinary management will prevent "accidents." The cord-injured person is likely to feel better about himself and find it easier to return to social life, school, and work if he is able to avoid soaking his clothes with urine at inopportune times.

Early Management. Since the bladder will not empty itself during spinal shock, it must be emptied artificially to prevent distention and its sequelae. Overdistention will damage the bladder wall, leaving it more vulnerable to infection and inhibiting its functioning following the passage of spinal shock (Pallett & O'Brien, 1985).

During spinal shock the patient is catheterized, either intermittently or using an indwelling catheter. Whichever method is chosen, sterile technique is required to prevent the introduction of bacteria into the bladder.

Intermittent catheterization requires more work for the nursing staff but has several advantages over the use of an indwelling catheter. If sterile procedure is used, the risk of infection is reduced by the use of intermittent catheters (Pallett & O'Brien, 1985; Rudy, 1984). Intermittent catheterization also allows a mild buildup of pressure in the bladder, facilitating a return of bladder tone as spinal shock resolves and sacral function returns. Acute management using intermittent catheterization increases the likelihood of success of bladder retraining (Pallett & O'Brien, 1985). Finally, indwelling catheters can cause ischemia of the urethral walls due to the constant pressure that they exert (Bromley, 1981).

Postacute Management: Bladder Retraining. As the acute phase following injury passes, the patient and health care team establish a more permanent program for managing bladder incontinence. The program of choice at this point often involves intermittent catheterization used in conjunction with other means of emptying the bladder.

The bladder retraining program is similar whether the patient's bladder is reflexive or areflexive. At the outset of the program, the patient empties his bladder on a regular basis and catheterizes himself after each voiding.[3] Regular emptying of the bladder and restriction of fluid intake prevent bladder overdistention.

The techniques used to induce voiding depend upon the manner in which the individual's bladder functions. If the bladder is reflexive, the person stimulates reflex emptying by tapping his abdomen above the pubis, stroking his inner thigh, or pulling his pubic hair (Kraft, 1987; Rudy, 1984). If his bladder is areflexive, he can express urine from his bladder manually, using the Credé maneuver (Pallett & O'Brien, 1985; Rudy, 1984). The Credé maneuver involves applying pressure to the abdomen, starting at the umbilicus and pressing downward. As the per-

son pushes his hand toward his pubis, he forces urine out of the bladder. This procedure may have to be repeated several times to get maximal emptying (Kraft, 1987). Alternatively, an individual with intact abdominal musculature may be able to empty his bladder by straining (Matthews, 1987; Rudy, 1984).

During bladder retraining, the patient catheterizes himself immediately after he has finished voiding. He then measures both the voided (expressed) and residual urine. (The urine that is removed by catheterization is called residual urine.)

Catheterization during a bladder retraining program serves two purposes. First, it ensures that the bladder periodically is emptied completely. In addition, catheterization makes it possible to measure the urine left in the bladder following expression, enabling the patient and health care team to determine how effectively he is able to empty his bladder. A large residual volume indicates that a large amount of stagnant urine remains in the bladder after expression. Because of the problems associated with residual urine, a major focus of an intermittent catheterization program is keeping this volume to an acceptably low level.

During the initial period of bladder retraining, the patient empties his bladder every four hours[4] using the methods described above, inducing voiding and then catheterizing (Kraft, 1987). As the patient becomes consistently more successful at expressing his urine, the intervals between catheterizations can be increased. An improved ability to express urine is evidenced by an increase in the volume of expressed urine and a decrease in the volume of residual urine. The time between catheterizations can be increased gradually to twice a day, daily, and once a week. Some people progress to the point where they catheterize every three weeks (Pallett & O'Brien, 1985) or even discontinue catheterization altogether (Kraft, 1987; Rudy, 1984). Of course, the cord-injured person continues to empty his bladder regularly between catheterizations.

A rise in residual volumes or a cessation of voiding between catheterizations indicates that a problem has developed. The person may have developed a urinary tract infection, or his urethra may be blocked. Whatever the cause, he must return to a more frequent catheterization schedule. Once the underlying problem has been resolved, he can once again gradually increase the intervals between catheterizations.

---

[3] Throughout this chapter the descriptions of bowel and bladder management techniques are phrased in terms of independent function. If a patient is unable to perform the techniques, the procedures are done by others.

---

[4] In some centers the bladder is emptied every six hours initially (Pallett & O'Brien, 1985).

It is generally accepted that residual volumes must be low for the frequency of intermittent catheterization to be decreased. However, different medical centers disagree as to what volume of residual urine can be considered to be acceptably low. Many agree that 100 milliliters is the maximal acceptable volume, but some centers have lower ceilings.

If urination occurs between planned voidings, measures need to be taken to keep the skin dry and to prevent embarrassing "accidents." For males, these goals are accomplished using an external catheter, attached via tubing to a collecting bag. During the day the urine can be collected in a leg bag, which is easily concealed under clothing. The problem of maintaining dry skin is more difficult for females, as they lack a point of attachment for an external catheter. To date, no satisfactory external catheter has been developed for females (Rudy, 1984; Shepherd & Blannin, 1986). Women who are unable to remain dry between planned voidings can use incontinence pads or indwelling catheters.

Alternative Postacute Management Programs. Most cord-injured people are able to empty their bladders well enough that they can wean themselves from an intermittent catheterization program. An estimated 10% to 30% are unable to do so (Pallett & O'Brien, 1985). These people may continue indefinitely to catheterize themselves periodically, usually every 4 to 6 hours (Matthews, 1987).

Alternatives to long-term intermittent catheterization include urethral or suprapubic indwelling catheters. Indwelling catheters are often used by individuals who have medical conditions that make fluid restriction unwise. Indwelling catheters can also be advantageous for people who are neither able to catheterize themselves nor to obtain reliable attendant care. Indwelling catheters can be left in place for up to 30 days (Kraft, 1987). Daily care simply involves keeping the perineal area and drainage bags clean, so care is less time consuming and requires less skill. Unless the catheter becomes blocked, bladder drainage is guaranteed. As a result there is a lower risk of autonomic dysreflexia or reflux (Matthews, 1987).

Unfortunately the long-term use of indwelling catheters also has significant disadvantages. Chronic urinary tract infection is almost assured[5] (Shepherd & Blannin, 1986), and the risk of kidney

and bladder stones is increased (Hall, Hackler, Zampieri & Zampieri, 1989). People with indwelling catheters must drink 3 to 4 liters of fluid daily (Kraft, 1987) to reduce the risk of bladder calculi. Males with indwelling *urethral* catheters can develop periurethral abscesses, urethrocutaneous fistulas, urethral diverticula, prostatitis, and epididymitis (Kiser & Herman, 1985). Females can develop urethral erosion (McGuire & Savastano, 1986). The insertion of a *suprapubic* catheter creates a new orifice, which may be experienced as mutilating (Matthews, 1987).

Sacral anterior root stimulators are a final option for bladder incontinence management. These stimulators are surgically implanted and allow the user to control voiding through electrical stimulation (Brindley, Polkey, Rushton, & Cardozo, 1986). This device remains experimental.

BOWEL FUNCTION

To understand the nature of bowel function after spinal cord injury, one must understand normal bowel functioning. Figure 17–9 illustrates the large intestine, rectum, internal and external anal sphincters, and puborectalis.

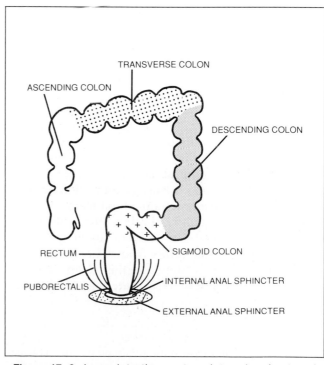

Figure 17–9. Large intestine, rectum, internal and external sphincters, and puborectalis.

---

[5] The incidence of bacteria with fever is greater, however, among people who depend on others for intermittent catheterization after discharge from the rehabilitation center (Cardenas & Mayo, 1987).

Normal Bowel Function

A normally functioning bowel can store or expel feces, depending on whether social circumstances are appropriate for defecation. Normal bowel function involves the control of the smooth muscle of the intestinal wall, the internal and external anal sphincters, and the pelvic floor musculature. This control comes from four separate sources: the autorhythmicity of the intestinal smooth muscle and the intrinsic, autonomic, and somatic nervous systems.

Autorhythmicity. Intestinal smooth muscle contracts rhythmically without any nervous input. Oscillations in the membrane potentials of the muscle fibers trigger action potentials that are conducted to nearby fibers. However, because the intestines are long and the conduction velocity of smooth muscle is slow, nervous input is required for the coordination of intestinal action (Somjen, 1983).

Intrinsic System. The gastrointestinal (GI) tract has its own intrinsic nervous system.[6] It extends from the esophagus to the anus and is responsible for coordinating the GI tract's actions. Of the three sources of neurological control of the gut, the intrinsic system is the most basic. In fact, even if all central nervous system (CNS) input is eliminated, the intrinsic system enables the intestinal tract to continue its usual functions of digestion, absorption, and propulsion of the food mass (Somjen, 1983).

The intrinsic system contains two nerve plexuses.[7] The submucosal plexus (of Meissner) is primarily sensory (Somjen, 1983) but is also involved in the control of secretion, and blood flow (Guyton, 1987). The myenteric plexus (of Auerbach) is primarily responsible for processing sensory information received from the submucosal plexus and coordinating the gut's movements (Somjen, 1983).

Peristaltic contractions are initiated and maintained by reflexes of the intrinsic system. Distention of a section of the intestine initiates reflexive contraction of the smooth muscle, propelling the food mass toward the anus. As the food mass is propelled, the next section of the intestine is distended and the peristaltic reflex is again stimulated.

The gastrocolic reflex is also mediated by the intrinsic nervous system. In this reflex, food or warm fluid (Hickey, 1986) entering the stomach causes reflexive evacuation of the colon (Guyton, 1987). This response is strongest following the first meal of the day (Matthews, 1987).

Autonomic System. The autonomic system coordinates the GI tract's actions with the rest of the body; sympathetic and parasympathetic input alters GI function in response to emotions and exercise. This control is achieved primarily through the autonomic system's influence on the intrinsic nervous system.

Sympathetic innervation of the GI tract arises from the T8 through L2 segments of the spinal cord (Guyton, 1987). Sympathetic input has a dampening effect on digestive functions. In general, it inhibits peristalsis, increases sphincter tone, reduces the secretion of digestive juices, and causes vasoconstriction.

Both the cranial and sacral divisions of the parasympathetic system innervate the GI tract. The cephalad portions of the digestive tract, from the esophagus through the transverse colon, receive innervation from the hypothalamus via the vagus nerve. The descending colon, sigmoid, and rectum receive parasympathetic innervation from sacral cord segments 2 through 4. In general, parasympathetic input has an excitatory effect on the intestines, resulting in an increase in peristaltic movements, secretion of intestinal juices, and relaxation of sphincters.

Somatic System. The external anal sphincter and pelvic floor muscles are composed of striated muscle fibers. They receive somatic innervation from sacral cord segments 2 through 4.

Reflexes Involved in Defecation. The intrinsic defecation reflex, mediated by the intrinsic system, is an important component of defecation. This reflex, elicited when feces enter the rectum, causes relaxation of the internal sphincter and peristalsis in the descending colon, sigmoid, and rectum (Fig. 17–10). However, the intrinsic defecation reflex is not usually strong enough to cause defecation (Guyton, 1987).

Normal defecation requires the parasympathetic defecation reflex. This is a sacral spinal reflex that is stimulated by filling of the rectum. The parasympathetic defecation reflex causes relaxation of the internal anal sphincter and an intensification of peristalsis in the descending colon, sigmoid, and rectum (Guyton, 1987; Fig. 17–11).

Continence and Defecation. The external anal sphincter and other muscles of the pelvic floor play

---

[6] Also called the enteric nervous system.

[7] Lundgren and Jodal (1983) list a third plexus, the subserous plexus.

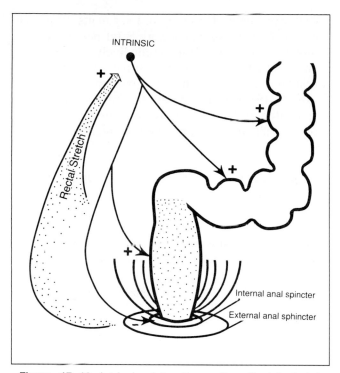

Figure 17–10. Intrinsic defecation reflex. Rectal stretch causes peristalsis and relaxation of the internal anal sphincter.

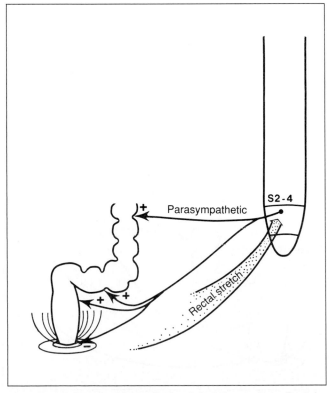

Figure 17–11. Parasympathetic defecation reflex. Rectal stretch causes intensification of peristalsis and relaxation of the internal anal sphincter.

a key role in continence. This musculature, though striated, remains active even at rest or during sleep (Devroede, 1983). The puborectalis is particularly important in maintaining continence. This striated muscle forms a sling around the rectoanal junction. Tonic contraction of the puborectalis creates a sharp angle between the rectum and the anal canal, preventing the passage of feces (Parks, 1986; Smout, 1987).

When feces enter the rectum and the internal sphincter relaxes, simultaneous contraction of the external anal sphincter prevents unwanted defecation. This contraction, caused by a sacral cord reflex (Devroede, 1983), is brief. Descending input determines whether the external sphincter's initial contraction continues (Guyton, 1987).

The descending input controlling defecation reflects the person's decision regarding whether or not he wants to defecate at that particular time. This voluntary control is dependent upon sensory input. The awareness of the need to defecate originates from stimulation of stretch receptors when feces move into the rectum. Receptors in the proximal anal canal distinguish between solid, liquid, and gas (Smout, 1987). The sensory input enters the spinal cord in sacral levels 2 through 4. It is not known where the ascending or descending pathways controlling defecation are located (Swash, 1987).

The brain's control over defecation originates in the cerebral cortex and descends to the second through fourth segments of the sacral cord. Voluntary control involves facilitation or inhibition of the external sphincter and pelvic floor musculature.

Defecation at unwanted times is prevented by maintained contraction of the external anal sphincter and pelvic floor musculature (Parks, 1986; Smout, 1987; Fig. 17–12). When defecation is prevented in this manner, the defecation reflexes subside after a few minutes. After several hours have passed or when additional feces enter the rectum, the reflexes are activated again (Guyton, 1987).

If feces enter the rectum at a time when defecation is possible, voluntary control involves inhibition of the external anal sphincter and pelvic floor musculature. With relaxation of the puborectalis, the rectoanal angle straightens and feces can pass into the anal canal (Smout, 1987). External sphincter relaxation allows the feces to exit the anus.

Defecation can be initiated voluntarily by closing the glottis and contracting the abdominals. When this straining is combined with relaxation of the puborectalis (Devroede, 1983), the resulting increase in intraabdominal pressure forces feces into the rectum, stimulating the defecation reflexes.

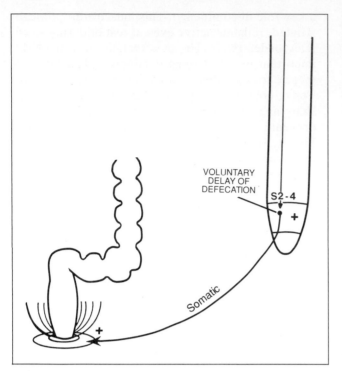

Figure 17–12. Voluntary delay of defecation through contraction of external anal sphincter and pelvic floor musculature.

Reflexive Bowel. If sacral cord segments 2 through 4 and the corresponding peripheral nerves remain intact, the bowel functions reflexively. The internal anal sphincter maintains its normal resting tone and relaxes reflexively when the rectum is distended (Miner, 1987). Because both the intrinsic and parasympathetic defecation reflexes remain functional, reflex defecation occurs when the rectum fills (Fig. 17–13).

Areflexive Bowel. The bowel functions differently in cases where the sacral reflex arc is interrupted, either from spinal cord or peripheral nerve damage. The intrinsic defecation reflex remains intact, but the stronger parasympathetic defecation reflex is lost. Without the parasympathetic defecation reflex, the bowel will not empty reflexively (Fig. 17–14). The internal anal sphincter remains active, although the tone is often low (Miner, 1987). As a result of this internal sphincter activity, coupled with an absent parasympathetic defecation reflex, feces can become impacted in the rectum (Pallett & O'Brien, 1985). Because the external anal sphincter (Rudy, 1984) and pelvic floor musculature (Parks, 1986) remain flaccid, some people with areflexive bowels

Bowel Function Following Spinal Cord Injury

Immediately after spinal cord injury, many patients exhibit paralytic ileus. This condition is characterized by atonia and an absence of peristalsis in the intestines. It usually appears within 24 hours of the injury and lasts about a week (Kraft, 1987). The cause of paralytic ileus is not known, but it may be due to the abrupt loss of parasympathetic input (Rudy, 1984).

Intestinal function returns spontaneously. Peristalsis resumes, pushing the products of digestion through the intestines, and the gastrocolic reflex returns. This resumption of intestinal function is possible because the intrinsic system remains intact following spinal cord lesions.

Although the intrinsic system remains intact, spinal cord injury disrupts the autonomic and somatic input to the GI tract. As a result, the portions of the intestines that are innervated below the level of the lesion will no longer alter their functions with emotions and exercise. Voluntary control of defecation will be lost, and reflexive defecation may also be lost. Following complete spinal cord injury, the process of defecation is comparable to bladder function after injury. The key factor is the integrity of the sacral reflex arc, not the level of the lesion.

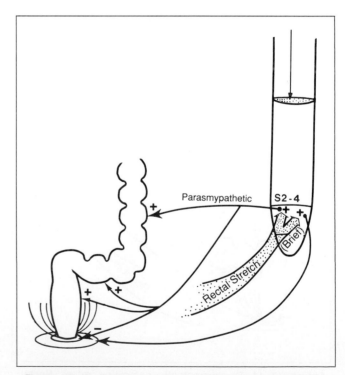

Figure 17–13. Reflexive bowel. Sacral reflexes remain intact, but descending input is lost. Reflexive defecation occurs when the rectum fills.

exhibit incontinence when stool passes unhindered from the rectum (Rudy, 1984).

An individual's sensory capacity following complete cord injury will also depend on the level of lesion. People with sacral lesions may experience a vague feeling of abdominal discomfort when the rectum fills. This sensation, absent in those with higher lesions, is carried by the sympathetic afferents (Devroede, 1983).

Management of Bowel Incontinence

After spinal cord injury, a bowel program is required to induce bowel movements at regularly scheduled intervals. Periodic emptying of stool will help prevent constipation and impaction, thus helping to prevent autonomic dysreflexia.

Bowel programs are also aimed at minimizing the occurrence of bowel movements at inconvenient or socially unacceptable times. This goal can be achieved by evacuating the bowels regularly. Prevention of bowel accidents is particularly important if the person is to return to a normal social life and work environment.

Reducing the occurrence of bowel accidents

has the added benefit of making it easier to keep the skin clean. (If someone has a bowel movement at the wrong time or place, it may be impossible to clean the skin immediately.) The result will be a reduced risk of decubiti.

Early Management. In the acute period following injury, the patient is monitored for paralytic ileus. If this condition develops, the loss of peristalsis can result in abdominal distention. Severe distention can cause vomiting, dehydration, and electrolyte imbalance. It can interfere with respiration by impeding the diaphragm's motions (Rudy, 1984). Distention can also damage the walls of the bowel, impairing future functioning.

If paralytic ileus develops, measures are taken to prevent distention. The gastric contents are aspirated, and the patient is not allowed to take any solids or liquids by mouth until his bowel sounds resume (Kraft, 1987).

Postacute Management: Bowel Retraining. After paralytic ileus resolves, a bowel training program can be initiated. The general pattern of a bowel training program is the same regardless of the level of lesion: the bowel is conditioned to empty at scheduled intervals.

At the outset of a bowel training program, a bowel movement is elicited at the same time every day.[8] This can be done in the morning or evening, depending on the patient's preferences. Since a bowel program can be a time-consuming process, the patient needs to decide whether a morning or evening schedule will be most suitable to his lifestyle.

Although the general pattern of a bowel training program is the same regardless of the person's level of lesion, the techniques employed to elicit a bowel movement vary. If the individual has a reflexively functioning bowel, a bowel movement is elicited by stimulation of reflexive defecation. After manually removing hard stool from his rectum (Kraft, 1987), the patient stimulates the parasympathetic defecation reflex. The reflex can be elicited using a suppository followed by digital stimulation of the rectum. The patient may need to relax his anal sphincter using digital stimulation (Boyink & Strawn, 1981) or by gently stretching the sphincter

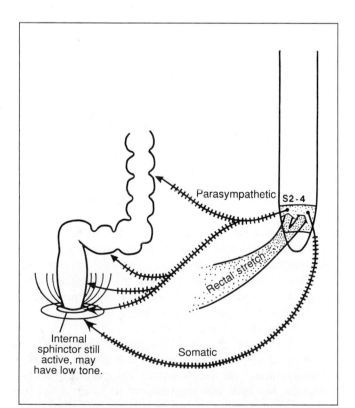

Figure 17–14. Areflexive bowel. Disruption of the sacral reflex arc causes loss of parasympathetic defecation reflex. Internal anal sphincter remains active; external sphincter is flaccid.

---

[8] There is disagreement in the literature regarding the frequency with which bowel movements should be elicited initially. Kiser and Herman (1985) suggest an every-other-day schedule. Kraft (1987) suggests that the bowel program should be performed daily for patients with flaccid bowels and every other day for those with spastic bowels.

(Pallett & O'Brien, 1985). Abdominal massage can promote the movement of feces toward the rectum. The pressure of the massage strokes should follow the pattern of the large intestine, moving from right to left (Pallett & O'Brien, 1985). The patient can also enhance the movement of feces into his rectum by contracting his abdominal musculature if it is innervated (Pallett & O'Brien, 1985).

A cord-injured person who does not have an intact sacral arc will have a flaccid bowel. Since the parasympathetic defecation reflex is absent, reflex emptying cannot generally be induced (Miner, 1987). The rectum is emptied by manual removal of the stool. Inserting a suppository several minutes before the manual evacuation can facilitate the process (Kraft, 1987). Contraction of the abdominal musculature can help move feces into the rectum (Pallett & O'Brien, 1985).

Several factors can be exploited to aid a bowel program. If the program follows a large meal, strong peristalsis elicited by the gastrocolic reflex will promote a bowel movement. Gravity can also be used to assist the program. Performing the bowel program while sitting upright will position the rectum and descending colon so that gravity assists in the movement of feces. If the bowel program is performed in bed, the person should lie on his left side. (Bedpans should *not* be used, as they are likely to cause decubiti.)

A bowel program can also be enhanced by ensuring that the stools are of a good consistency, formed but not hard. Cord-injured people can achieve this consistency by drinking adequate amounts of fluid and consuming a diet high in fiber. Stool softeners, laxatives, and medications that increase peristalsis are also employed by some.

During bowel training, the nursing staff keeps records of bowel movements. If the bowels do not move, or if constipation, diarrhea, fecal impaction, or unscheduled bowel movements occur, the problem needs to be addressed.

With consistent management, the bowel should begin to empty on schedule and not between times. When a patient experiences this success for 1 to 2 weeks (Matthews, 1987), he is ready to progress. Progress can take the form of a reduction of medications or suppositories or an increase in the time between defecations. The program should be progressed in only one area at a time (Matthews, 1987). For example, the suppository should not be eliminated at the same time that the interval between bowel programs is increased.

Ideally the patient works toward regulation of his bowels without suppositories or medication,

avoids accidents between scheduled bowel programs, and builds the time between programs. Some can gradually build up to three days between bowel movements (Boyink & Strawn, 1981).

INCONTINENCE MANAGEMENT TRAINING PROGRAM

During rehabilitation after spinal injury, the patient and health care team work together to establish bowel and bladder management programs. The techniques used to manage incontinence, described above, constitute only a portion of the training program. The health care team must do more than retrain the bladder and bowel. They must also teach the patient.

In an incontinence management training program, the cord-injured person should gain the knowledge required for him to carry out or direct the program on his own. He should acquire an understanding of the functioning of his bladder and bowels, the management techniques that he must use, the physical consequences of improper management, as well as complications to look out for, how to avoid them, and what to do if they develop.

It is not enough for the patient to understand his management program. He must also value it, or he is not likely to carry it out consistently.

During rehabilitation, the patient should also learn the physical skills involved in carrying out his bladder and bowel programs. Independence is possible even without innervation of the hand musculature. Self-catheterization and application of urinary collecting devices can be performed using either natural tenodesis or a tenodesis splint. Rectal stimulation can be performed using adaptive equipment.

If possible, the patient should become independent in his bowel and bladder programs. An individual who is unable to do so should develop the ability to instruct others in the management techniques. This ability will free him from dependence on family members or attendants who have been trained by the hospital staff.

During rehabilitation, the patient should be encouraged to participate in his bowel and bladder management. As he practices the physical techniques, his skill will improve. If he is involved in decision making and problem solving, he will be better prepared to direct his program after discharge. As an active participant, he may also come to value the program more.

Implications for Therapy

The nursing staff is responsible for the bulk of a patient's incontinence management training program: education and establishing bowel and bladder management programs. Physical and occupational therapy work with the patient to select equipment and to develop the necessary physical skills. These skills include gross activities such as sitting upright, toilet transfers, leg management, and maintaining an upright sitting position while reaching around to the anus. In therapy, the patient also acquires the manipulation skills used in self-catheterization, the application and removal of urinary collecting devices, dressing and undressing, and hygiene.

Understandably, incontinence can be an emotionally charged issue. Accidents that occur in therapy need to be handled in a matter-of-fact, tactful manner. The therapist should model comfort with the issue.

If a bowel or bladder accident occurs in therapy, it must be dealt with quickly. This expeditious management serves two purposes. First, it ensures that the individual's skin does not remain in contact with urine or feces for a prolonged period of time. As importantly, it helps to develop the habit of cleaning quickly following an accident. A therapist who ignores accidents that occur at inconvenient times (such as during group classes) models a lack of concern for hygiene. This can undermine the health care team's efforts to teach the patient to maintain clean, dry skin.

SUMMARY

Any spinal cord injury that disrupts the functioning of the sacral cord or interrupts its communication with the brain will result in incontinence. The manner in which the bowel and bladder will function depends upon the status of the sacral reflex arc.

During rehabilitation, the health care team and the patient work together to establish a satisfactory program for managing incontinence. This program provides a means of emptying the bowel and bladder and maintaining dry skin between planned emptyings, thus helping to prevent the serious physical and psychosocial problems that can result from incontinence.

REFERENCES

Boyink, M. A., & Strawn, S. M. (1981). Spinal cord injury: Postacurate phase. In Martin N., Holt N., &

Hicks D. (Ed.), *Comprehensive rehabilitation* (pp. 449–491). New York: McGraw-Hill Book Company.

Brindley, G.; Polkey, C.; Rushton, D., & Cardozo, L. (1986). Sacral anterior root stimulators for bladder control in paraplegia: the first 50 cases. *Journal of Neurology, Neurosurgery, and Psychiatry, 49*, 1104–1114.

Bromley, I. (1981). *Tetraplegia and paraplegia: A guide for physiotherapists* (2nd ed.). New York: Churchill Livingstone.

Cardenas, D., & Mayo, M. (1987). Bacteriuria with fever after spina cord injury. *Archives of Physical Medicine and Rehabilitation, 68*, 291–239.

Comarr, A. E. (1977). The neurogenic bladder. In Pierce D. S., & Nickel V. H. (Ed..), *The total care of spinal cord injuries* (pp. 165–169). Boston: Little, Brown & Company.

Devroede, G. (1983). Storage and propulsion along the large intestine. In Bustos-Fernandez L. (Ed.), *Colon: structure and function* (pp. 121–139). New York: Plenum Medical Book Company.

Feneley, R. C. L. (1986). Normal micturition and its control. In Mandelstam D. (Ed.), *Incontinence and its management* (2nd ed., pp. 16–34). Dover, NH: Croom Helm.

Gordon, D. L., & Stevens, M. M. (1981). Spinal cord injury: Acute phase. In Martin N., Holt N., & Hicks D. (Ed.), *Comprehensive rehabilitation nursing* (pp. 418–448). New York: McGraw-Hill Book Company.

Guyton, A. C. (1987). *Basic neurosocience: Anatomy and physiology*, Philadelphia: W. B. Saunders Company.

Hall, M., Hackler, T., Zampierri, T., & Zampieri, J. (1989). Renal calculi in spinal cord-injured patient: Association with reflux, bladder stones, and Foley catheter drainage. *Urology, 34*(3), 126–128.

Hickey, J. V. (1986). *The clinical practice of neurological and neurosurgical nursing* (2nd ed.). Philadelphia: J. B. Lippincott.

Kiser, C., & Herman, C. (1985). Nursing considerations: Skin care, bowel and bladder training, autonomic dysreflexia. In Adkins H. (Ed.), *Clinics in physical therapy: Vol. 6. Spinal cord injury*. New York: Churchill Livingstone.

Kraft, C. (1987). Bladder and bowel management. In Buchanan L. E., & Nawoczenski D. A. (Ed.), *Spinal cord injury: Concepts and management approaches* (pp. 81–98). Baltimore, Williams & Wilkins.

Lundgren, O., & Jodal, M. (1983). Nerves of the colon. In Bustos-Fernandez L. (Ed.), *Colon: Structure and function* (pp. 187–209). New York: Plenum Medical Book Company.

Matthews, P. (1987). Elimination. In P. J. Matthews, & C. E. Carlson (Ed.), *Spinal cord injury: A guide to rehabilitation nursing* (pp. 97–119). Rockville, MD: Aspen.

McGuire, E., & Savastano, J. (1986). Comparative urological outcome in women with spinal cord injury. *Journal of Urology, 135*, 730–731.

Miner, Ph. B. (1987). In Gooszen H. G., Ten Cate Hoedemaker H. O., Weterman I. T., & Keighley M. R. B. (Eds.), *Disordered defaecation: Current opinion on diagnosis and treatment* (pp. 145–152). Boston: Martinus Nijhoff Publishers.

Pallett, P. J., & O'Brien, M. T. (1985). *Textbook of neurological nursing*. Boston: Little, Brown & Company.

Parks, A. G. (1986). Faecal incontinence. In Mandelstam D. (Ed.), *Incontinence and its management* (2nd ed., pp.76–93). Dover, NH: Croom Helm.

Read, N. W. (1987). Faecal incontinence: The pathophysiology of anal leakage. In Gooszen H. G., Ten Cate Hoedemaker H. O., Weterman I. T., & Keighley M. R. B. (Eds.), *Disordered defaecation: Current opinion on diagnosis and treatment* (pp. 133–144). Boston: Martinus Nijhoff Publishers.

Rudy, E. B. (1984). *Advanced neurological and neurosurgical nursing*. St. Louis: C. V. Mosby Company.

Ruge, D. (1969). Neurological evaluation. In Ruge D. (Ed.), *Spinal cord injuries* (pp. 51–62). Springfield: Charles C Thomas.

Shepherd, A. M., & Blannin, J. P. (1986). The role of the nurse. In Mandelstam D. (Ed.), *Incontinence and its management* (2nd ed., pp. 160–183). Dover, NH: Croom Helm.

Smout, A. J. P. M. (1987). Physiology: Colonic motility. In Gooszen H. G., Ten Cate Hoedemaker H. O., Weterman I. T., & Keighley M. R. B. (Eds.), *Disordered defaecation: Current opinion on diagnosis and treatment* (pp. 51–60). Boston: Martinus Nijhoff Publishers.

Somjen, G. (1983). *Neurophysiology: The essentials*. Baltimore: Williams & Wilkins.

Swash, M. (1987). Faecal incontinence: Neurological causes. In Gooszen H. G., Ten Cate Hoedemaker H. O., Weterman I. T., & Keighley M. R. B. (Eds.), *Disordered defaecation: Current opinion on diagnosis and treatment* (pp. 111–115). Boston: Martinus Nijhoff Publishers.

18

Architectural Adaptations

During rehabilitation, a great deal of effort is expended in teaching and learning the physical skills required to function independently after discharge. Much of this effort is wasted, however, when people leave rehabilitation centers to reside in inaccessible environments. Such features as narrow doorways and appliances that are positioned out of reach can prevent people from functioning independently. An individual whose dwelling lacks an entrance route through which he can enter and leave without assistance may find himself imprisoned in his own home. Inaccessible architecture can handicap people as profoundly as can physical disability itself.

Because the physical environment of a person's home can have such a strong impact on his ability to function, this area should be addressed during rehabilitation. The team's involvement can include evaluation of the home, education on architectural barriers and adaptations, problem solving regarding home modification, and education about legal rights and advocacy.

This chapter will present typical design features that make a home wheelchair accessible and adapted to function with impaired grasp. However, there is no single design that will be perfectly suited to all disabled people. The ideal home design for a given individual will depend on his physical capacities. Such features as the optimal height of controls, appliances and plumbing fixtures, and the required width of doorways will depend on whether the person is ambulatory, uses a wheelchair for all activities, or uses a wheelchair for certain activities. If a wheelchair is used, the chair's overall length and width will dictate minimal doorway widths and turning spaces that must be present. The disabled individual's reaching capacity will depend on whether he walks or uses a wheelchair and will also be influenced by his body build, range of motion, and motor abilities. Motor function will also determine his capacity for grasping and manipulating controls and doorknobs.

Because disabled people vary in their body build, ambulatory status, equipment use, reach capacity, and ability to grasp and manipulate, an adapted home that is ideal for one disabled individual may be totally unsuitable for another. When a home is being designed or modified for a particular person, the environment should be tailored to suit his needs. Rather than providing "standard" accessible features, the home's design should reflect the individual's requirements.

Laws Regarding Architectural Accessibility

The Architectural Barriers Act (1968) mandates that virtually any[1] newly constructed, federally owned or federally funded public buildings, as well as federally funded alterations on existing buildings, must be accessible to people with physical disabilities. Of relevance to this chapter, at least 5% of all units, as well as all common areas, in residential facilities (hotels, motels, apartment buildings, etc.) must be accessible.

The Fair Housing Amendments Act of 1988 prohibits discrimination against people with disabilities in the area of rental or sale of housing. It also gives disabled tenants the right to modify rental property *at their own expense*. The tenant may be required to restore the property to its original condition (within reason) when the lease expires. As of March 1991, newly constructed multifamily dwellings with at least four units must be adaptable (Mental Health Law Project, 1989).

The Americans With Disabilities Act of 1990[2] mandates that all public facilities must be accessible to people with disabilities. This act differs from the Architectural Barriers Act in that it applies to privately owned facilities. Thus all newly constructed or renovated restaurants, stores, and other businesses open to the general public must be accessible (Galvin, 1989). Moreover, physical barriers in ex-

---

[1] Certain military facilities are exempted.

[2] In addition to architectural access to public accommodations, the act prohibits discrimination in employment, transportation, and telephone services (Galvin, 1989; Harker, 1990; U.S. Department of Justice, 1990).

isting structures must be removed if this removal can be achieved readily. These requirements are effective as of January 1993 for new construction and as of January 1992 for existing buildings (U.S. Department of Justice, 1990).

The laws mentioned above mandate accessibility. But what architectural features make a building accessible? Two widely used sets of standards are available that specify in detail the design features required to make a facility accessible to people with disabilities.

The standards for compliance with the Architectural Barriers Act are delineated in the Uniform Federal Accessibility Standards (UFAS, 1988). The standards cover accessible design in a variety of areas, including but not limited to apartment complexes, public restrooms, auditorium seating, public phones, street crossings, and swimming pools.

The second set of standards for design and construction is published by the American National Standards Institute (ANSI). The ANSI standards, used by the private sector, are similar to the UFAS standards. ANSI standards are commonly utilized in state laws on architectural accessibility.

Unfortunately laws regarding architectural accessibility are not always followed. People who feel that their rights have been violated can contact their local Protection and Advocacy System office for assistance. The Protection and Advocacy System, mandated by the Developmental Disabilities Act of 1977, provides advocacy services to people with disabilities.[3] Additional alternatives include filing a complaint with the Department of Housing and Urban Development (HUD),[4] contacting a fair housing agency, or filing a complaint in state or federal court (MHLP, 1989).

DESIGN FEATURES

For an apartment or house to be truly wheelchair accessible, it needs to have more than wide doorways and a ramp at the front door. An accessible environment allows a person to propel his wheelchair from the parking area or public transportation site to the home's entrance, to enter the door, and to move through the home. Within and around the home, the environment is structured so that the disabled person can perform everyday functions such

as getting the mail, cooking, operating lights, doing laundry, using the toilet, and bathing. Appliances, lighting and environmental controls, plumbing fixtures, work surfaces, and storage areas are designed and arranged for use from a wheelchair.

General Features

Certain features are common to all wheelchair-accessible environments: provision for negotiating any changes in floor or ground level, adequate width in doorways and halls to allow passage of a wheelchair, floors that do not provide excessive resistance to wheelchair propulsion, clear floor space and knee space to allow maneuvering the wheelchair and gaining access to various features of the home (appliances, storage areas, work surfaces, etc.), and design and location of these features allowing their access and use.

Paths and Ramps. Before taking advantage of the accessible features within a home, one must be able to get to it. An accessible home must have at least one accessible route leading to it. This route should connect the home with an accessible parking area, as well as with the sidewalk and public transportation stops when present. Paths should be at least 36 inches wide and smooth and level. (American National Standards Institute, 1986; Ford & Duckworth, 1987; UFAS, 1988).

Unless the home's entrance is level with the ground, provision must be made for the differences in level. Usually a ramp is the most practical solution for wheelchair users.

A ramp meeting ANSI (1986) and UFAS (1988) specifications for accessibility has a maximum slope of 1:12, or 1 foot of rise for 12 feet of horizontal distance. The minimum width of a ramp is 36 inches. If the ramp's slope is steeper than 1:15, horizontal landings must be provided at the top of the ramp, at the bottom, and at 30-foot intervals in the ramp. These landings must be at least as wide as the ramp and at least 60 inches long. When a ramp changes direction at a landing, the landing must be at least 60-inches square. Ramps greater than 6-feet long should have 2 handrails, between 30 and 34 inches high. If a cross slope (slope perpendicular to the direction of the ramp) is present, it must not exceed a 1:50 incline. Ramps and landings that are elevated above ground level must be constructed in a way that prevents people from falling off. Protection at the edges of such ramps and landings can be provided by curbs (at least 2 inches high), walls, or railings. All ramp surfaces must be slip resistant.

A ramp built according to the standards presented above will be negotiable by most people

---

[3] Protection and Advocacy offices are located throughout the nation. Anyone wishing to contact his local office can obtain the phone number from directory assistance.

[4] The phone number of the Fair Housing Complaint Hotline is (800) 424-8580.

using wheelchairs and will be *safe*. Such features as a slip-resistant surface, absence of excessive cross slope, landings when the ramp is long, and barriers to prevent falling from the ramp will enhance the safety of any ramp. However, private homes do not have to meet the exact specifications listed above. Considerations relevant to the individual concerned may make it most practical to deviate from these specifications. A ramp with a 1:12 slope could take up a great deal of space, and this gradual an incline may not be necessary for the person using it. On the other hand, a 1:12 slope is too steep for some people; a grade as gradual as 1:20 (Ford & Duckworth, 1987) is most appropriate for some. Before a ramp is built for a particular individual, it should be determined how gradual a slope he will require.

Three additional features can enhance the function and safety of a home ramp. Lighting the ramp will make it safer to negotiate at night. A roof over the ramp will protect both the ramp and the user from the weather. This may be particularly helpful in regions that have a good deal of ice and snow in the winter. Finally, when a ramp leads to a door, a platform at the top of the ramp will make it easier and safer to get in and out of the door (Ford & Duckworth, 1987; Hale, 1979; Somerville & Pendleton, 1985). Such a platform will make it possible to unlock the door and open or close it without having to stabilize the wheelchair on the ramp while doing so. The platform should be large enough to allow the person to maneuver his wheelchair and operate the door. The exact size and shape of platform needed will depend on the door (size and direction of opening) and the direction of approach.[5]

People needing ramps can purchase them prefabricated or can have them custom built out of concrete or wood. Prefabricated ramps should come with nonslip surfaces. To create a nonslip surface on a concrete ramp, the surface can be roughened slightly with a trowel or a broom before it dries (Somerville & Pendleton, 1985). A variety of options are available for creating a nonslip surface on a wooden ramp. These include firmly attaching indoor-outdoor carpeting, rough-surfaced roofing paper, or strips of other nonslip material; painting the ramp with epoxy paint mixed with crushed walnut shells or sand; or painting the ramp and sprinkling sand on it before the plaint has dried (Ford & Duckworth, 1987; Hale, 1979; Somerville & Pendleton, 1985).

Ramps are considered by some to be necessary evils for an adapted home because they can be un-attractive. However, when attention is paid to design and landscaping, a ramp need not detract from a home's beauty. A wooden ramp attached to a deck or porch can be designed and constructed to blend with the structure. An earth berm[6] with a concrete or asphalt ramp surface is an attractive alternative to a standard ramp. Whether a wooden ramp or earth berm is constructed, its beauty can be enhanced by shrubbery or a garden bordering or bordered by the ramp or by hanging plants or planters attached to the ramp (Bostrom, 1987).

Ramps can also be constructed to accommodate elevation changes within a home. Interior ramps are feasible only when the vertical distance between the levels is small—a few inches at most.

Escalators and Elevators. When the vertical distance between levels is too great, or space limitations make a ramp impractical, an escalator or elevator can be used.

Escalators, or inclined lifts, can be installed over existing stairs in straight or curved stairways. Some models have the advantage of leaving the stairs available for use when the escalator platform is positioned out of the way (Ford & Duckworth, 1987; Somerville & Pendleton, 1985).

Elevators and platform lifts raise a wheelchair vertically from one level to another. Unfortunately uniform safety standards have not yet been developed for platform lifts. People purchasing lifts should be aware of this and should select lifts that will be safe for both the people using the lifts and those nearby (UFAS, 1988). Safety features include mechanisms that prevent lifts from descending on people standing below and safety rails for those riding the lifts.

Doorways. Perhaps the most critical feature of an accessible doorway is its width. To be accessible, a doorway must have adequate clear space when the door is open to allow passage of a wheelchair. Clear space is the actual unobstructed space available for passage. Most doors are hinged so that even when open they partially block the doorway (Fig. 18–1). As a result, the clear space is narrower than the doorway itself.[7]

---

[5] ANSI (1986) provides detailed guidelines for maneuvering clearances at doors.

[6] An earth berm is a mound of dirt. It can be placed in an appropriate location and contoured to serve as a ramp. Bostrom (1987) provides guidelines for constructing earth berms.

[7] The space available for negotiating a doorway is the space between the door itself where it lies within the doorway when open and the inside of the jamb on the opposite side. With standard doors and hinges, this space is generally from 1.5 to 2 inches narrower than the full width of the doorway (Hale, 1979).

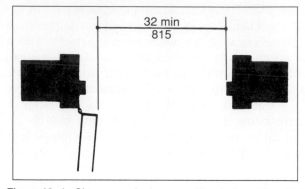

Figure 18–1. Clear space in doorway. *(Reproduced from Uniform Federal Accessibility Standards: U.S. Government Printing Office, 1988.)*

UFAS (1988) and ANSI (1986) standards specify that an accessible doorway must provide a clear space that is at least 32 inches wide. Private homes do not necessarily need doorways this wide. In general, a doorway that is 30 inches wide (clear space) will provide adequate clearance if the door can be approached directly. A door which must be approached at an angle may need to be wider (Ford & Duckworth, 1987). Most standard doorways provide adequate width for manual wheelchairs, with the exception that many bathroom doors are too narrow.

The exact doorway width needed by an individual is determined primarily by the overall width of his chair. Wheelchair widths are highly variable. As a rule, power wheelchairs are significantly wider than manual chairs. Additional factors determining a wheelchair's overall width include the seat width, wheelchair brand, type of tire, canting of the wheels, and handrim style. When making decisions about home modification, the wheelchair user and rehabilitation team should determine the minimal doorway width that the individual can negotiate in *his* wheelchair.

If one or more doorways in a home is too narrow, several options are available. If a doorway needs to be widened only slightly, replacing the hinges may suffice. Offset hinges allow the door to swing completely out of the doorway. This makes the entire width of the doorway available for passage, effectively increasing its width without major structural changes or expense (Hale, 1979). Alternatively, the door may be removed and replaced with a curtain. Removing the molding surrounding the doorway will further increase the clear space slightly (Somerville & Pendleton, 1985). When a door must be widened more than a couple of inches, the doorway itself must be rebuilt and a wider door installed.

The threshold is another feature of a doorway that influences its accessibility. Thresholds, or sills, lie at the base of doorways. A threshold that is too tall or shaped inappropriately (rising vertically from the floor with 90-degree angles between the top and side surfaces) can be an impassable barrier. An accessible door can have a threshold of up to one-fourth inch in height without beveling. Thresholds between one-fourth and one-half inch high must be beveled. A ramp is required when a threshold is greater than one-half inch tall[8] (ANSI, 1986; UFAS, 1988).

Thresholds of interior doorways may be removed to allow easier passage through doors. The thresholds of doors leading to the outside, however, should not be removed, as they generally are needed to seal doors against rain and drafts. If a threshold of a door leading to the outside is too tall or shaped inappropriately, it should be modified (shortened or beveled or both) or replaced with beveled thresholds. Weather stripping attached to the base of the door itself can help to seal out the weather (Somerville & Pendleton, 1985).

For a door to be accessible to someone with impaired grasp, adaptation of the knob may be required. Knobs can be adapted by affixing foam rubber to their surfaces, making them easier to grip. If this adaptation is not adequate, attachments can be placed on knobs that allow them to be operated as levers. Alternatively, door knobs can be replaced with lever-type door handles (Fig. 18–2). Finally, doorknobs can be eliminated altogether and replaced with catches that allow doors to be operated without manipulating any knobs or handles. This type of door catch, commonly used with kitchen cabinets, makes it possible to open and close the door by applying pressure against the door's surface (Hale, 1979; Somerville & Pendleton, 1985).

When a lock is present, it must be accessible. For someone who has good grasping and manipu-

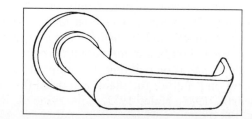

Figure 18–2. Lever-type door handle. *(Reproduced from Handbook for Design: Specially Adapted Housing [VA Pamphlet No. 26-13]. U.S. Government Printing Office, 1978.)*

---

[8] These specifications for changes in level apply to all accessible ground and floor surfaces.

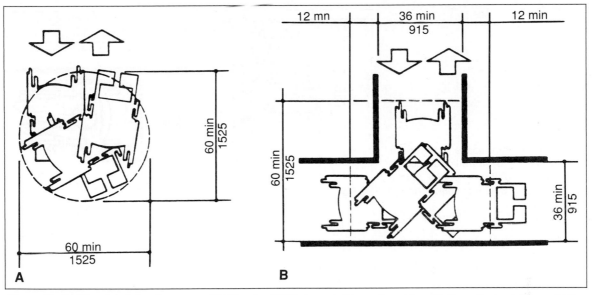

Figure 18–3. Wheelchair turning space. **(A)** Circular. **(B)** T-shaped. *(Reproduced from* Uniform Federal Accessibility Standards: *U.S. Government Printing Office, 1988).*

lating capabilities or who can function with an adapted key or key holder, the lock need only be placed within reach. Someone who cannot operate a standard lock may require a specialized lock. Options to consider include push-button combination locks, locks operated with access cards, and voice-activated locks (Somerville & Pendleton, 1985).

Finally, an accessible door is one that the individual can open and close independently. For most people the modifications described above are sufficient; given door handles and locks that they can operate, most are able to open and close standard doors. Mechanical devices for opening and closing doors are alternatives for those who are unable to do so (Somerville & Pendleton, 1985).

Hallways. Although a 32-inch–wide clear space will allow passage through a doorway, a hallway of this width is too narrow for wheelchair users. A hallway 36-inches wide will allow propulsion of a wheelchair (ANSI, 1986; UFAS, 1988). For access to rooms opening onto the hallway from the side, provision must be made for turning the chair. This can be accomplished with a wider hallway or wide doorways.

Clear Floor Space. To function in a room, one must be able to maneuver within it. For a room to be accessible to wheelchair users, it must have adequate clear floor space to allow this maneuvering. To allow turning 180 degrees in a wheelchair, the floor should be unobstructed in an area large enough to enclose either a circle of at least 60 inches in diameter (Fig. 18–3A) or a T-shaped area with di-

mensions as shown in Figure 18–3B (ANSI, 1986; UFAS, 1988). A 60-inch–diameter clear floor space is preferable, since it allows easier maneuvering than does a T-shaped area.

Clear floor space is also required in front of a home's appliances, light switches, electric outlets, environmental controls, plumbing fixtures, work spaces, and storage areas. This clear floor space allows access to these features from a wheelchair. An unobstructed rectangular floor space measuring 30 by 48 inches will accommodate a stationary wheelchair (ANSI, 1986; UFAS, 1988). The orientation of this space will determine whether the person must approach the object head on (front or forward approach) or from the side (parallel approach; Fig. 18–4).

As is true with other accessible features, a private home may not need to meet the exact specifications described above. Depending on his wheelchair's dimensions and his skill, a given person may be able to maneuver in a slightly smaller space. When adapting an existing home for a particular individual, that person's requirements for clear floor space should be taken into account.

Clear floor space does not imply that the area is unobstructed from floor to ceiling. Where there is adequate clearance under low cabinets and plumbing fixtures to allow free passage of the feet or feet and knees,[9] this floor space can be used for maneuvering.

---

[9] A space 9-inches high will allow the feet to pass. A 27-inch high space will permit passage of the knees (Veterans Administration, 1978).

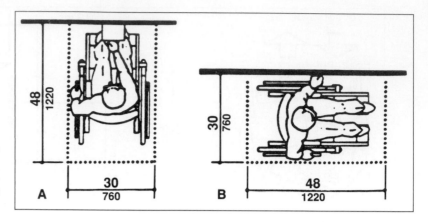

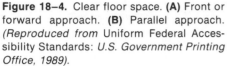

Figure 18–4. Clear floor space. **(A)** Front or forward approach. **(B)** Parallel approach. *(Reproduced from* Uniform Federal Accessibility Standards: *U.S. Government Printing Office, 1989).*

Clear Knee Space. Certain appliances and features such as sinks and kitchen work spaces are most readily used by people in wheelchairs if they can be approached closely front on. This close access requires the presence of clear knee space to allow the wheelchair user to place his knees under the object. A clear knee space is an unobstructed space that is at least 30-inches wide, 27-inches high, and 19-inches deep under the sink, appliance, or counter. The knee space must be part of or contiguous with a 30- by 48-inch clear floor space to accommodate the wheelchair (Bostrom, 1988; UFAS, 1988).

Reach Range. The height of an object that a person can reach from his wheelchair will depend upon whether he reaches forward or to the side. A forward reach is more limited; the person reaching forward cannot reach as high or as low. The arrangement of the clear floor space in front of an object will determine whether a side reach (parallel approach) or a forward reach (front approach) can be used. ANSI and UFAS standards specify that accessible objects such as thermostats, appliance controls, and electric outlets can be no higher than 48 inches and no lower than 15 inches above the floor when a forward approach must be used. When a parallel approach is possible, accessible objects must be no higher than 54 inches and no lower than 9 inches above the floor (ANSI, 1986; UFAS, 1988; Fig. 18–5).

Forward and side reach ranges are also influenced by body build, range of motion, and motor capabilities. When remodeling an existing home for a particular individual, his capacities in forward and side reach should be considered.

Controls and Outlets. Electric outlets and all controls, including thermostats, light switches, appliance controls, and door latches must be placed

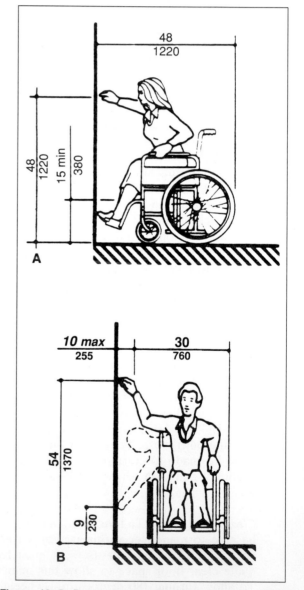

Figure 18–5. Reach ranges. **(A)** Forward reach. **(B)** Side reach. *(Reproduced from* Uniform Federal Accessibility Standards: *U.S. Government Printing Office, 1988).*

within either the forward- or side-reach range, depending on which approach the clear floor space allows. Controls should be designed so that they can be used with one hand and should not require wrist motion or a strong grasp or pinch. The force required for operation must not exceed 5 pounds (ANSI, 1986; UFAS, 1988).

Floors. Floors in accessible homes should be smooth and level, with surfaces that do not offer excessive resistance to wheelchair propulsion. Wood, linoleum, or unglazed tile floors provide the easiest surfaces for wheelchair propulsion and are easy to care for. If carpeting is used, it should be firm, affixed to the floor, and have a very short pile. Removal of foam padding under carpeting will make propulsion over the carpet easier (Ford & Duckworth, 1987; Hale, 1979; Somerville & Pendleton, 1985). If a cushion or pad is used under carpeting, it should be firm. The combined thickness of the carpet and cushion should not exceed one-half inch (UFAS, 1988).

Windows. To be accessible to people with impaired grasp, windows must be operable with 5 pounds or less of force. All hardware (locks, levers, cranks) must meet the specifications for controls given above (ANSI, 1986). A variety of options are available for window operation. Sliding, awning, and casement windows are relatively easily opened and closed (Johnson, 1988). If a new accessible home is being built or if a new addition is being added, perhaps the most practical way to select the window style best suited to an individual is for him to try the different types and see which is easiest to manage.

Storage Space. An accessible home has storage areas that can be reached from a wheelchair. Storage areas include kitchen and bathroom cabinets, linen closets, and bedroom and hall closets. An accessible storage area has adequate clear floor space to allow access and is within the appropriate reach range (ANSI, 1986; UFAS, 1988; Fig. 18–6).

Much of the storage space in a standard home does not fall within the reach range of a person sitting in a wheelchair. For this reason, providing for adequate storage space can be a challenge. A variety of minor alterations can be used to maximize accessible storage space in an existing home. New shelving can be constructed, and those shelves that are within reach can be enlarged. The interiors of cabinet and closet doors can be fitted with small shelves. Some closets can be made accessible simply by lowering closet bars. Commercially available

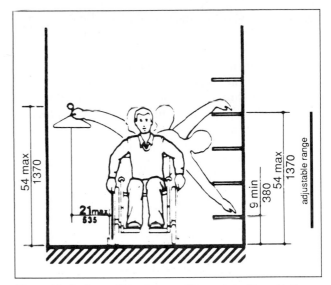

Figure 18–6. Accessible storage. *(Reproduced from* Uniform Federal Accessibility Standards: *U.S. Government Printing Office, 1988).*

closet organizers can maximize the functional use of available space. Hardware on doors and drawers can be adapted or replaced to accommodate users with impaired grasp or to accommodate space limitations (Ford & Duckworth, 1987; Hale, 1979; Johnson, 1988).

Durability, Protection of the Environment. The walls and doors of a wheelchair user's home are likely to be subject to more than their share of abuse as the chair periodically scrapes or bumps their surfaces. To minimize wear and tear on the home, surfaces that are likely to come in contact with the wheelchair can be protected with durable material. This will preserve the home's beauty and minimize upkeep.

Walls are most likely to get damaged in areas where there is tight maneuvering space. Corners and hall walls are likely spots for this damage. These areas can be protected by plastic guards (Somerville & Pendleton, 1985).

People who open and close doors with their wheelchairs may wish to install kickplates on their doors. A kickplate covering the bottom 16 inches of a door should provide adequate protection (ANSI, 1986; UFAS, 1988).

Aesthetics

A wheelchair-accessible home need not (and should not) look like an institution. With attention to color, furniture arrangement, lighting, accessories, wall decorations, and window treatments, the accessible environment can be homey and reflect the tastes of the people who live there (Johnson, 1988; Fig. 18–7).

Application in Specific Rooms

The accessible features described above should be present throughout the home of someone who uses a wheelchair. In a fully accessible home, all rooms have accessible doorways, adequate clear floor space, and floors that can be traversed in a wheelchair. Controls, storage areas, and electric outlets are within reach. When needed, all controls are adapted for use by someone with impaired grasp.

Kitchens, bathrooms, and laundry facilities require special attention because of the nature of their use. Suggestions for accessible design in these areas are presented below. Unless otherwise noted, the specifications for accessible design presented above (dimensions for clear floor and knee space, reach ranges, design of controls, etc.) apply.

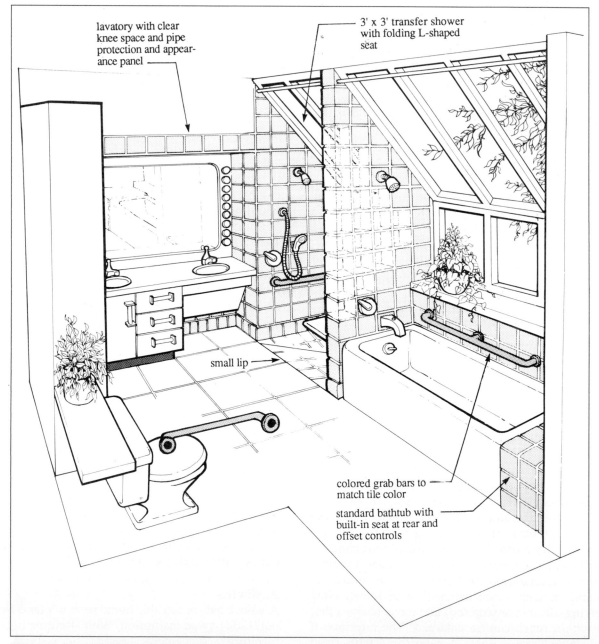

lavatory with clear knee space and pipe protection and appearance panel

3' x 3' transfer shower with folding L-shaped seat

small lip

colored grab bars to match tile color

standard bathtub with built-in seat at rear and offset controls

Figure 18–7. Accessible bathroom without institutional look. *(Reproduced from Bostrom, Mace, & Long:* Adaptable Housing: A Technical Manual For Implementing Adaptable Dwelling Unit Specifications: *Department of Housing and Urban Development, 1987.)*

Kitchen. An accessible kitchen is designed for cooking and cleaning from a wheelchair. Its features include adaptations in its work surfaces, cooking areas, sink, dishwasher (if present), storage areas, and refrigerator. Adequate clear floor space is available for maneuvering a wheelchair. Ideally the various appliances and work surfaces are arranged for the most efficient use of the kitchen. Figure 18–8 illustrates many of the accessible features described below.

An accessible kitchen must have at least one work surface on which to perform such tasks as cutting and mixing. A standard countertop is too high to be used from a wheelchair. In addition, the cabinets and drawers present beneath the counters in most kitchens make it impossible to approach the counters face-on in a wheelchair (Brostom, Mace & Long, 1987).

Perhaps the ideal work surface for a wheelchair user is a lowered countertop with adequate clear knee space underneath and clear floor space allowing a front approach. This design makes counter space available for working and makes it possible to reach items stored in overhead cabinets and on the back of the counter. To accommodate a wheelchair, lowered countertops must be at least 30 inches wide; greater widths are preferable (Bostrom, 1988; Ford & Duckworth, 1987).

Pullout shelving is a second design feature that can be used to provide accessible work surfaces. These shelves can be used as an alternative or adjunct to lowered countertops. As a third option, a table can serve as a work surface when financial constraints preclude remodeling (Hale, 1979).

Whether lowered counters, pullout shelves, or tables are used, the height of most lowered work surfaces should be between 30 and 32 inches high. Some find that certain activities such as beating and mixing can be performed most easily on a work surface that is even lower. A pullout shelf is often the best means of addressing this need. Cutouts in the shelves can be useful for stabilizing mixing bowls (Bostrom, 1988; Bostrom, Mace & Long, 1987; Ford & Duckworth, 1987; Hale, 1979).

Accessible kitchens must also have cooking facilities that can be used from a wheelchair. As a minimum, an accessible kitchen will have adequate clear floor space in front of the cooking appliances, the appliances and their controls will be within the appropriate reach range, and all controls will be located so that they can be manipulated without reaching across burners. A cook with impaired grasp will also require suitable controls on the appliances. Where knee spaces are available beneath cooking appliances, there must be adequate insulation present to prevent burns (ANSI, 1986; UFAS, 1988).

Among conventional ovens, side-opening wall ovens[10] are most convenient for people using wheelchairs, as this type of oven allows the cook to get close to the oven. The door should be hinged so that it opens toward a countertop. Installing the oven slightly lower than is standard will place its lowest shelf at a more convenient height. A pullout board or trolley in front of the oven and an adjacent countertop at the level of the lowest oven shelf will make it easier to place and remove dishes from the oven. When an existing oven is inaccessible and funding for remodeling is limited, a toaster oven can be used in place of a wall oven. It can be placed on a low countertop, table, trolley, or sturdy pullout board (Ford & Duckworth, 1987; Hale, 1979).

A drop-in stove built into a low counter with clear knee space underneath provides a convenient accessible cooktop (Fig. 18–9). European burners (burners incorporated into a large, flat surface) are easily cleaned and allow pots to be slid on and off readily. To reduce the danger of reaching over hot burners to reach pots in the rear, burners may be arranged either in a line parallel to the counter edge or in a staggered pattern. Portable burners on a low countertop, table, trolley, or sturdy pullout board can be used in place of a built-in stove. These options require more lifting (Ford & Duckworth, 1987; Hale, 1979).

Microwave ovens are a great convenience in any kitchen. They are particularly useful for people with impaired sensation in their hands, since the oven and dishes do not heat up during cooking (Ford & Duckworth, 1987; Hale, 1979).

Meal preparation as well as clean-up requires the use of a sink. An accessible sink is low, shallow (6 ½-inches deep or less), and has adequate clear knee and floor space to allow a forward approach to the sink (Fig. 18–10). The sink, drain, and hot water pipes must be insulated to prevent burns, and the area under the sink must be free of sharp or abrasive surfaces. The faucet controls should be within easy reach. If the sink is to be used by someone with impaired grasp, the controls must be designed appropriately (ANSI, 1986; Bostrom, 1988; Ford & Duckworth, 1987; UFAS, 1988). A retractable spray hose is an additional convenient feature. It makes rinsing food and dishes easier and can be used to fill pots on an adjacent counter so that the pots do not have to be lifted from the sink after being filled (Ford & Duckworth, 1987; Hale, 1979).

An accessible dishwasher will, of course, re-

---

[10] Self-cleaning ovens are of course easiest to maintain.

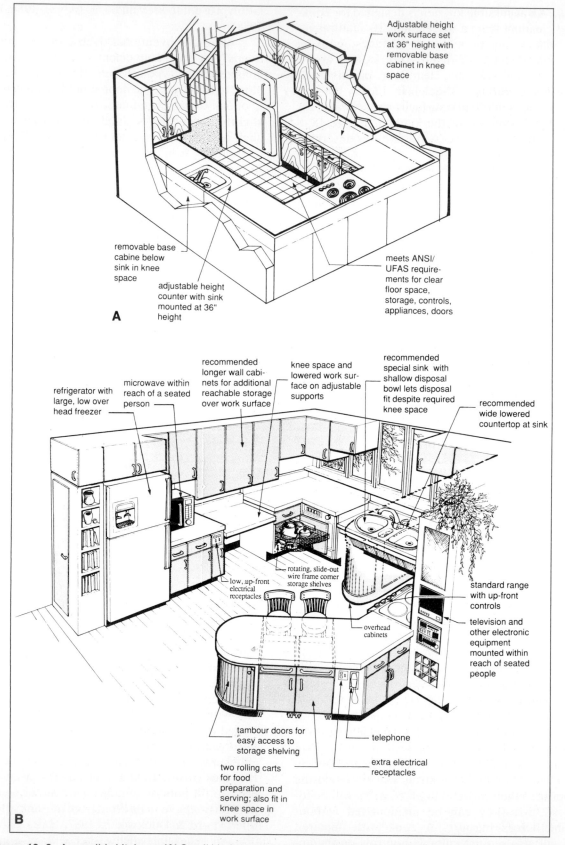

Figure 18–8. Accessible kitchens. **(A)** Small kitchen with minimal modifications. **(B)** Elaborate kitchen. *(Reproduced from Bostrom, Mace, & Long:* Adaptable Housing: A Technical Manual For Implementing Adaptable Dwelling Unit Specifications: *Department of Housing and Urban Development, 1987.)*

duce the work load of the disabled cook. To be accessible, a dishwasher must have adequate clear floor space in front and controls within reach. Front-loading models with self-clearing drains and shelves that pull out individually are most convenient. Especially if the cook has difficulty lifting and requires a continuous countertop for sliding objects, the dishwasher should be low enough that it does not protrude above the level of the counter (UFAS, 1988; Ford & Duckworth, 1987; Hale, 1979).

Adequate storage can be problematic in any kitchen—is there ever enough space to store the staples, pots and pans, cooking implements, dishes, cleaning supplies and assorted whatnot that are used in meal preparation, serving and cleaning up? Providing enough storage space can be particularly challenging in an accessible kitchen, since so much of the space that is used for storage in standard kitchens is either out of reach from a wheelchair or has to be eliminated to provide clear knee space.

Some storage space can be gained by constructing shelves at the back of low counters that have clear knee space underneath. Shelves in cabinets can be used if there is adequate clear floor and knee space to allow access and if the shelves are between 15 and 48 inches above the floor. Handles on the cabinet doors should be within reach. Storage space on shelves and in the refrigerator can be maximized with lazy susans and revolving shelf units. Drawers, slideout bins, and sliding racks can increase the area available for storage in base cabinets. When a kitchen is being adapted for use by someone with impaired upper-extremity strength, cabinet door catches should be operable with minimal force and manipulation (ANSI, 1986; Bostrom, 1988; Ford & Duckworth, 1987; Johnson, 1988; Hale, 1979; UFAS, 1988).

An accessible kitchen must have a refrigerator and freezer that can be used from a wheelchair. This need can be met with either a side-by-side refrigerator/freezer or an over/under unit that has all of the refrigerator and at least half of the freezer within reach. The temperature controls must also be within reach. Both the controls and the door catch should be designed so that they can be worked with minimal force and manipulation. Refrigerator/freezer shelves that slide out make foods stored at the back easier to reach. With over/under models that have sliding shelves, a pullout shelf installed adjacent to the refrigerator will make it possible to slide items from the refrigerator instead of lifting them[11] (ANSI, 1986; Ford & Duckworth, 1987; UFAS, 1988).

---

[11] The refrigerator door must be hinged so that the door opens toward the slideout shelf.

Because of differences in body build and motor ability, people differ in the exact features of a kitchen that are most suitable to them. For example, the optimal counter height varies between people. Some require different levels of work surface for different activities. Others who have difficulty lifting may function best in kitchens where the counters are all at the same height so that they can slide objects from place to place (Bostrom, 1988; Ford & Duckworth, 1987). People also vary in their requirements in other kitchen features, such as appliance and sink controls, sink height and depth, and reach range for storage. When building or remodeling a kitchen for a particular person, care should be taken to design the kitchen in such a way that it is most suitable for that individual. When a kitchen is being designed to be used by a variety of people (as would be the case in a rental unit), adjustable features will make it possible to adapt the kitchen as needed.

Bathroom. The bathroom is often the least accessible room in the house. Typically the door is too narrow to allow a wheelchair user to enter the room. In addition, the layout and the limited space within most bathrooms is such that a wheelchair cannot be maneuvered within the room and cannot be positioned close enough to the plumbing fixtures for their use. An accessible bathroom must have an accessible door and adequate clear floor space, as well as plumbing fixtures that can be accessed from a wheelchair (Figs. 18–7 & 18–12**B**).

The door of an adapted bathroom should have the features of any accessible door: adequate width, small or no threshold, and hardware that can be worked with minimal force and manipulation. Additional privacy and safety considerations are unique to bathroom doors. The wheelchair user should be able to close the door once inside the bathroom. If the door opens into the bathroom, closure from within requires additional clear floor space. Folding doors do not require as much added clear floor space but have the disadvantage of significantly reducing the functional width of the doorway (Hale, 1979). Sliding doors and standard doors that swing outward do not require any added clear floor space to be closed from within the bathroom. These doors also have a safety advantage: they are not blocked when someone falls against them in the bathroom (Ford & Duckworth, 1987). As a final alternative, a bathroom's door can be removed altogether and replaced with a curtain. This solves the problems of closure and blocking from within but does not provide the level of privacy afforded by a door.

An accessible bathroom must have a toilet onto

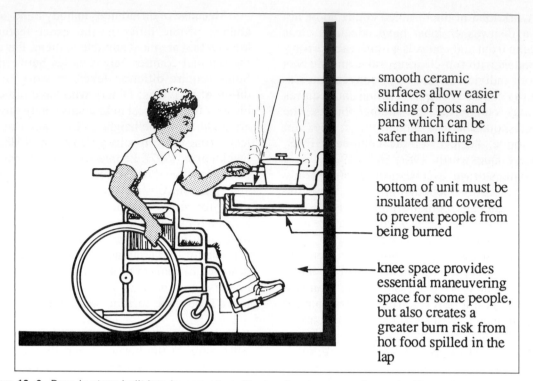

Figure 18–9. Drop-in stove built into low counter with clear knee space underneath. *(Reproduced from Bostrom, Mace, & Long:* Adaptable Housing: A Technical Manual For Implementing Adaptable Dwelling Unit Specifications: *Department of Housing and Urban Development, 1987.)*

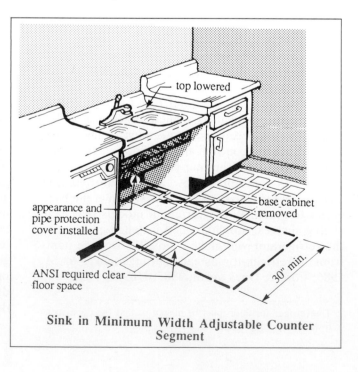

Figure 18–10. Accessible sink. *(Reproduced from Bostrom, Mace, & Long:* Adaptable Housing: A Technical Manual For Implementing Adaptable Dwelling Unit Specifications: *Department of Housing and Urban Development, 1987.)*

which a person can transfer from a wheelchair. Access to the toilet requires adequate clear floor space on one side to accommodate a stationary wheelchair. The toilet seat must be at a height that allows safe transfers to and from the wheelchair. UFAS (1988) and ANSI (1986) standards specify that the top of a toilet seat should fall between 15 and 19 inches above the floor. Transfers will be easiest if the toilet and wheelchair seats are the same height. Appropriate height of the toilet seat can be accomplished by placing the existing toilet on a wooden platform (Hale, 1979). Often a removable raised seat is the most practical solution; these seats are relatively inexpensive, do not require renovation, and can be removed for traveling. Additional features that make a toilet accessible include grab bars when needed and a toilet paper dispenser within reach. A cabinet beside the toilet can be convenient both for aiding balance and holding bowel and bladder management equipment (Ford & Duckworth, 1987).

An accessible bathing facility is another requirement of an adapted bathroom. This requirement can be met with either a tub or a shower. For a bathtub to be accessible, there must be adequate clear floor space by it to allow transfers. Faucet controls must be within reach when sitting in the tub, and if they are to be used by someone with impaired grasp, they should be designed accordingly. Depending on their motor function and skill level, many individuals require grab bars may also require either a tub bench or a built-in tub seat. A hand-held shower-spray unit is convenient in any accessible tub and is required if a tub bench or built-in seat is used.

In general, a shower is more convenient than a tub. There are two types of accessible showers: roll-in showers and those with built-in seats. Either type must be bordered by adequate clear floor space to allow access. The shower enclosure must not obstruct entrance into the shower, and the controls must be within reach (ANSI, 1986; UFAS, 1988).

A roll-in shower is designed to be used while sitting in a wheelchair.[12] UFAS (1988) and ANSI (1986) standards specify that this type of shower must measure at least 30 by 60 inches,[13] and there must be no curb at its border. The absence of a curb allows the bather to propel his wheelchair in and out of the shower and makes the floor of the shower available as clear floor space for maneuvering within the bathroom.

The standards for showers with seats specify

that the stall measures 36-inches square, and the controls must be positioned opposite the shower seat. The seat must be positioned between 17 and 19 inches above the floor and extend the full depth of the stall (ANSI, 1986; UFAS, 1988). The seat can be built to fold out of the way (Veterans Administration, 1978).

Wherever grab bars are installed, their placement should be designed to meet the needs of the individual using them. The bars must be affixed to either the floor, wall studs, or wood that has been attached to the studs; standard wall board is not strong enough to anchor grab bars. Likewise, towel racks and soap dishes cannot be used to substitute for grab bars.

An accessible bathroom lavatory has the same basic requirements as a kitchen sink: insulated hot water and drain pipes, an underside free of sharp or abrasive surfaces, and faucet and drain controls that are easily operated and within reach. The accessible basin must also be relatively low; the upper surface must be no higher than 34 inches. Adequate clear floor space must be present to allow forward approach in a wheelchair, and a clear knee space that is at least 8 inches deep is needed (ANSI, 1986; UFAS, 1988).

Additional features of accessible bathrooms include storage areas and electric outlets within reach and mirrors mounted low. A mirror that is mounted with its lowest edge no higher than 40 inches above the floor will be usable from a wheelchair (ANSI, 1986; UFAS, 1988). Alternatively, a mirror can be tilted to make it accessible (Johnson, 1988; VA, 1978).

Because bathrooms are often small and because of the relative difficulty of moving plumbing fixtures, it is often more practical to build a new bathroom than to remodel an existing one (Ford & Duckworth, 1987). Whichever option is chosen, the design should reflect the individual's requirements. For example, the ideal toilet seat height for a given person will depend on the level of his wheelchair's seat. His transfer techniques will dictate the clear floor space requirements by the toilet. An individual skillful in transfers may be able to transfer with his wheelchair positioned diagonally in front of the toilet and thus will not require the clear floor space to be directly to the side of the toilet. In like manner people vary in their requirements for other bathroom features, such as the type of tub or shower and the position of clear floor space needed for its access.

Laundry. Laundry facilities must be located along an accessible route, with adequate clear floor space to allow access to the machines. Washers and dryers

---

[12] The bather uses a "shower chair," not his standard wheelchair.

[13] This size shower will fit in the space required for a standard bathtub (UFAS, 1988).

should be front loading and have their controls easily operated and positioned within reach (ANSI, 1986; UFAS, 1988). Side-hinged doors allow access to the interior of the machines for loading and unloading laundry (Hale, 1979).

Adaptable Design
Adaptable housing is an option that may appeal to owners of rental units who wish to minimize their vacancy rates by renting their accessible units to able-bodied people. It is also of interest to homeowners who wish to make their homes accessible but who are concerned about the resale value of their homes.

An adaptable home has permanent accessible features such as wide doors and hallways, a ground-level entrance, and controls mounted low enough to be reached from a wheelchair. In addition, it has

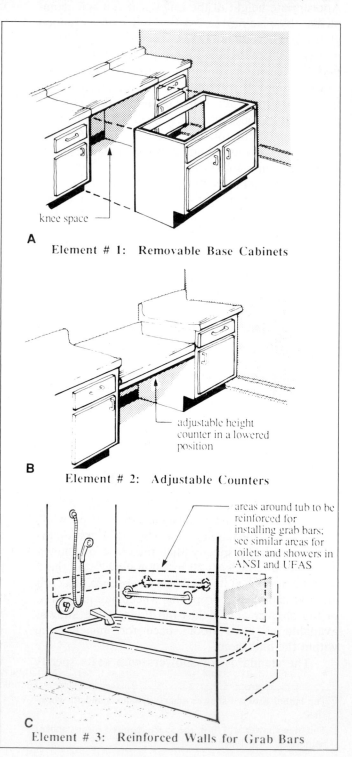

Figure 18–11. Adaptable features. **(A)** Removable base cabinets. **(B)** Adjustable-height counters. (Sinks also adjustable.) **(C)** Reinforced walls for grab bars. *(Reproduced from Bostrom, Mace, & Long:* Adaptable Housing: A Technical Manual For Implementing Adaptable Dwelling Unit Specifications: *Department of Housing and Urban Development, 1987.)*

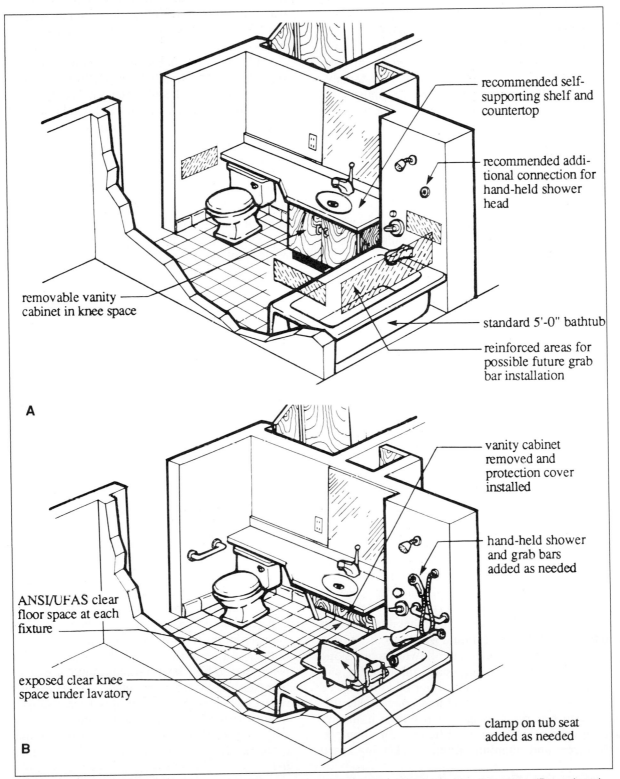

recommended self-supporting shelf and countertop

recommended additional connection for hand-held shower head

removable vanity cabinet in knee space

standard 5'-0" bathtub

reinforced areas for possible future grab bar installation

A

vanity cabinet removed and protection cover installed

hand-held shower and grab bars added as needed

ANSI/UFAS clear floor space at each fixture

exposed clear knee space under lavatory

clamp on tub seat added as needed

B

Figure 18–12. Small adaptable bathroom. **(A)** Conventional configuration. **(B)** Adjusted configuration. *(Reproduced from Bostrom, Mace, & Long:* Adaptable Housing: A Technical Manual For Implementing Adaptable Dwelling Unit Specifications: *Department of Housing and Urban Development, 1987.)*

features such as removable base cabinets and adjustable-height counters and sinks that can be altered with minimal time and expense to suit either able-bodied or disabled residents. Bathroom walls are reinforced in appropriate places to accommodate grab bars (Fig. 18–11). The bars themselves can be removed or installed as needed. An adaptable home looks like any other home when adjusted for an able-bodied resident but can be made fully accessible without major structural changes[14] (Bostrom, Mace, & Long, 1987; Fig. 18–12).

STRATEGIES

No standard set of specifications can be used to create an accessible environment that would be perfect for all disabled people. An ideal home is one designed to match the unique needs and preferences of the person living there. This outcome is possible only with careful analysis and planning, with the disabled person and the rehabilitation team working closely together.

The first issue to be addressed is where the person will live after discharge. Will he or his family own or rent the property? Will he live alone or with friends or relatives? How permanent will his living arrangement be? Modification of a rented home will require the approval of the owner. A child or adolescent returning to his parent's home may not need the kitchen and laundry facilities to be accessible, particularly if he was not responsible for kitchen or laundry chores prior to his injury. And if a person's immediate postdischarge living arrangement will be temporary, the modifications to that environment should be kept to a minimum.

Once it has been determined where an individual will live following discharge, modifications should be made only after careful planning. The first step in planning involves determination of the person's unique requirements. The rehabilitation team and the disabled person should work together to discover his requirements in the following areas: slope of ramp that he can negotiate, door width and threshold requirements, clear-floor and knee-space dimensions needed, maximal and comfortable forward- and side-reach ranges, capabilities in manipulating controls, and optimal heights for counters, appliances, and plumbing fixtures. Planning based

on this information will make it possible to minimize home modifications, thus minimizing expense. It may be found that many of the home's features, though not accessible by UFAS and ANSI standards, are accessible to the individual concerned.

Planning for home modification requires assessment of the home's features. Before alterations are planned, the disabled person and the rehabilitation team should determine which features of the home need modification. Perhaps the best way to make this determination is for the individual to spend some time at home. Then it will become apparent, for example, which doorways need to be widened and what appliances are out of reach. It should be kept in mind, however, that the person's exact accessible requirements are likely to change as rehabilitation progresses. His needs will change as he grows stronger and more skillful and when his permanent wheelchair arrives. Thus it is important to avoid making major modifications to the home prematurely.

To supplement the information gathered in the informal home assessment described above, a health professional or family member should perform a detailed evaluation of the home. Ideally the disabled person will be present during the evaluation. The evaluation should involve assessment of all relevant features of the home: layout of the entrance paths and immediate area surrounding the home; height of entrances above the ground; dimensions of structures and available space surrounding entrances; changes in floor and ground level within and around the home; thresholds and clear space within all doorways; force and manipulation required to work all controls and hardware (cabinet handles, door knobs, and locks); height of these controls and hardware; clear floor space available for maneuvering in hallways and rooms and for access to plumbing fixtures, appliances, storage areas, windows, and thermostat controls; height of and clear knee space under counters, appliances, and plumbing fixtures; and height of all electrical outlets and light switches. Whether the evaluation is performed by a health professional or by a family member, the evaluator should first receive guidance regarding what to measure, how to measure it, and how to record the evaluation findings. The evaluation results will be most useful if the findings are recorded in a detailed sketch as well as in a checklist.

Based on a careful assessment of the individual and his home, the disabled person and the rehabilitation team can work together to plan home modifications. Unfortunately funding is another factor that must be taken into account. Certainly all pos-

---

[14] *Adaptable Housing: A Technical Manual For Implementing Adaptable Dwelling Unit Specifications* (Bostrom, Mace, & Long, 1987) provides detailed instructions for designing adaptable housing features and obtaining products for adaptable homes.

sible funding sources should be investigated. When funds are limited, expense must be a major consideration when choosing between options. Home modifications may have to be prioritized, with remodeling being done in stages as finances allow.

The rehabilitation team's role takes on another dimension with individuals who plan to live in rental units following discharge. These people should be educated regarding their housing rights and should know how to ensure that these rights are not violated. Specifically, they should learn about federal and local housing laws relevant to accessibility and should be informed about the advocacy services available to them.

SUMMARY

The accessibility of a home environment has a great impact on a disabled person's ability to function. Certain design features are required for a home to be accessible. This chapter describes the characteristics of accessible homes and provides strategies for planning home modifications.

REFERENCES

American National Standards Institute. (1986). *American national standard for buildings and facilities—Providing accessibility and usability for physically handicapped people.* New York: American National Standards Institute. (Available from American National Standards Institute, 1430 Broadway, New York, NY, 10018.)

Architectural Barriers Act of 1968, 42 U.S.C. (As Amended through 1984) 4151–4157. (1984).

Bostrom, J. (1987). Attractive ramps. *Mainstream: Magazine of the Able-Disabled, 12*(4), 18–20.

Bostrom, J. (1988). Creating a workable kitchen. *Mainstream: Magazine of the Able-Disabled, 12*(7), 25.

Bostrom, J.; Mace, R., & Long, M. (1987). *Adaptable housing: A technical manual for implementing adaptable dwelling unit specifications.* Washington, DC: Department of Housing and Urban Development.

Corbet, B. (Ed.). (1985). *National resource directory: An information guide for persons with spinal cord injury and other physical disabilities* (2nd ed.). Woburn, MA: National Spinal Cord Injury Association.

Ford, J., & Duckworth, B. (1987). *Physical management for the quadriplegic patient* (2nd ed.). Philadelphia, F. A. Davis Company.

Galvin, J. (1989). Capital update. *RESNA News.* Washington, DC.

Hale, G. (Ed.). (1979). *The source book for the disabled: An illustrated guide to easier more independent living for physically disabled people, their families and friends.* New York: Paddington Press.

Harker, C. (1990). ADA passes house with bi-partisan accord. *APTA Progress Report, 19*(7), p. 10.

Johnson, P. (1988). *Creation of the barrier-free interior.* Millville, NJ: A Positive Approach, Inc.

Mental Health Law Project. (1989). *Rights of tenants with disabilities under the fair housing amendments act of 1988: A guide for advocates, consumers and landlords.* Washington, DC: Mental Health Law Project. (Available from Community Watch at MHLP, 2021 L Street NW, Suite 800, Washington, DC 20036.)

Somerville, N., & Pendleton, H. (1985). Evaluating and solving home access problems. In Adkins H. (Ed.), *Spinal cord injury* (pp. 243–270). New York: Churchill Livingstone.

U.S. Department of Justice. (1990). Americans with disabilities act requirements fact sheet. (Available from the U.S. Department of Justice, Civil Rights Division, Coordination and Review Section, P.O. Box 66118, Washington, DC 20035-6118.)

Uniform Federal Accessibility Standards. (1988). Washington, DC: US Government Printing Office. (Available from the Special Advisor for Handicapped Programs, Department of Housing and Urban Development, 451 7th Street, SW, Room 10140, Washington, DC 20410.)

Veterans Administration. (1978). *Handbook for design: Specially adapted housing* (VA Pamphlet No. 26-13). Washington, DC: US Government Printing Office.

19

Equipment

Equipment can make the life of a disabled person easier, enable him to do things that he otherwise could not do, and conserve the time and energy used for mundane tasks to free him to do other things. But equipment is a double-edged sword: it can also create dependence on itself, reducing the user's ability to function without it. A person who is dependent upon a piece of equipment has to put up with its drawbacks (bulk, cosmesis, maintenance, etc.). He will also be unable to function in the event that the equipment is lost, broken, misplaced, or left behind.

In recent years there has been a virtual explosion in the adaptive equipment market. There is much variability in the quality and usefulness of available products; some are excellent, others have little value. Additionally, a given piece of equipment may be beneficial for some and useless or even detrimental to others. To maximize functional status, health, satisfaction, and gain most for their equipment dollar, health professionals and disabled people should select equipment carefully.

DECISION MAKING

The first step in ordering equipment is establishing a need. A person's need for equipment may be functional or medical.

Functional Need. A functional need exists if an individual requires equipment to perform functional activities. Equipment such as door knob adaptors, leg orthoses, and vehicular modifications can meet functional needs.

If someone cannot perform an activity satisfactorily without equipment, he *may* benefit from equipment designed to aid in the task. Judgment regarding the functional need for equipment should take the individual's future potential into consideration. In cases where it is possible that a person could learn to function without a particular piece of equipment, the equipment should be purchased only after a thorough rehabilitative effort has failed to enable him to function independently without it. Therapists should be wary of equipment that at first appears to improve function but that the patient could learn to do without. Often equipment can make a task easier while someone is first learning a skill, like training wheels on a bike. The problem is that therapists often leave these "training wheels" on, thinking that the need remains. The result is that the need does remain and the person is left using unnecessary equipment.

Once it has been determined that someone cannot function well without a given piece of equipment, he and the therapist should ascertain whether he *can* function better *with* it. Through the years much money has been wasted on equipment that turned out to be of limited or no benefit to the intended users. Prior functional training with and "test drives" of equipment prior to purchase could help to eliminate this problem.

Medical Need. A medical need exists if a piece of equipment is required for an individual to maintain or return to a healthy state. Wheelchairs, wheelchair cushions, and vertebral orthoses are examples of equipment that meet medical needs.

Some medical needs are temporary. For example, during the acute phase of rehabilitation, a cord-injured person may experience orthostatic hypotension as his body readjusts to upright sitting. While this occurs he may require a wheelchair with a reclining back and elevating legrests. Within a brief period of time, however, he will most likely adjust to upright sitting and will not need these features in a wheelchair. With a temporary medical problem such as this, the needed equipment should be rented or borrowed rather than purchased.[1]

Choosing Equipment

Once a functional or medical need has been established, the health professional and patient must de-

---

[1] This is not possible with all types of equipment. Vertebral orthoses, for example, must be purchased.

termine which piece of equipment best meets this need. For most types of equipment, there is a large selection from which to choose. The various brands generally offer different options and vary in quality, price, durability, maintenance required, availability of replacement parts and qualified maintenance facilities, warranty specifications, and other characteristics. With the market constantly expanding, clinicians who are involved in prescribing and advising on equipment must keep current.[2]

When deciding on a piece of equipment, it is best to keep in mind the fact that *any* equipment has both advantages and disadvantages. For example, pneumatic wheelchair tires are better than hard rubber tires in the following respects: smoother ride and easier propulsion over uneven surfaces, easier negotiation of curbs, and greater traction. However, pneumatic tires also have their drawbacks. They go flat if punctured, increase the overall width of the wheelchair, cost more than hard rubber tires, track more dirt into buildings, and must be filled with air periodically. Like the pneumatic tire, any equipment or component will have positive and negative qualities. Clinicians involved in prescribing or advising on equipment should investigate the benefits and drawbacks of the available equipment options.

When possible, equipment (or an identical model) should be used for a trial period before it is purchased. Ideally several different models will be made available for trials.[3] This practice increases the likelihood that the equipment chosen is really the best fit for the individual concerned.

The decision about any piece of equipment should be based on its advantages and disadvantages, considering the needs and priorities of the prospective user. Ultimately the final choice between equipment options is based on values. When weighing the positives and negatives of different options, should ease of use take priority, or should greatest consideration be given to convenience, durability, maintenance requirements, price, or aesthetics? Because equipment choice is a value-laden decision with no universal right and wrong answers, the person for whom the equipment is being ordered must be involved in the decision. Otherwise the piece of equipment chosen by the clinician may not be the one most suitable to the values and priorities

of the user. Involving the prospective user in equipment selection also promotes independence and encourages personal responsibility and consumerism.[4]

EQUIPMENT OPTIONS

There is a tremendous variety of equipment that is designed to enable disabled people to function more independently and comfortably. (There seems to be a gadget or doodad for every conceivable functional task.) Adaptive equipment ranges in complexity from simple reachers or light-switch adaptors to voice-activated environmental control units that perform multiple functions. Whatever the equipment being considered, the principles of selection described above apply: the equipment should satisfy a true need, the options currently available should be investigated, the potential benefits and drawbacks of each option should be considered, the equipment should be tried when possible, and the clinician and prospective equipment user should decide together which equipment will be most suitable.

This chapter will address the durable equipment used most commonly by cord-injured people: wheelchairs, cushions, orthoses, and adapted driving equipment.

WHEELCHAIRS

Wheelchair selection involves deciding between dozens of options in size, style, and components. The wheelchair's size and features must be chosen carefully; an improperly prescribed wheelchair can result in decubiti, deformity, and impaired functional status. A properly prescribed and adjusted wheelchair will maximize its owner's function and health.

When prescribing a wheelchair, the clinician(s) and prospective user determine the size, style, and components most suitable to the individual. Another choice that the clinician and prospective owner must make is the manufacturer of the wheelchair. The manufacturer of choice will in part be

---

[2] Information on product evaluation and comparison of assistive devices and rehabilitation equipment can be obtained from REquest, Rehabilitation Engineering Center, National Rehabilitation Hospital, 102 Irving Street NW, Washington, DC, 20010-2949.

[3] Vendors are often accommodating when asked to provide equipment for trial.

[4] Involving patients in ordering equipment does not mean ordering them everything that they want. An individual may want something that is not truly needed or that will be detrimental to his physical or functional status. In an instance such as this, the health professional would be doing the patient a disservice by ordering the requested equipment. The clinician also has a responsibility to third party payers to recommend equipment only when it can be justified as meeting a true need.

determined by the wheelchair's specifications. Generally a limited number of manufacturers will produce a chair with the desired characteristics. Other factors to consider when selecting brands include cost, availability of replacement parts and service facilities, warranty specifications, and reputation of the manufacturer.

When the prospective user has a recent spinal cord injury, wheelchair prescription should be delayed until functional training is well under way. During the weeks and months after injury, a cord-injured person's physical status and functional abilities are likely to change dramatically. As a result his equipment needs will change significantly: a wheelchair that is appropriate for someone just beginning his rehabilitation may be completely unsuitable two months later. If a wheelchair is prescribed prematurely, it is not likely to be optimally matched to the individual's ultimate needs.

Options. Power and manual chairs are the two major classes of wheelchair. Power, or electric, wheelchairs can provide a means of independent mobility for people who are unable to propel manual chairs. Power-recline models are available for people who cannot perform independent pressure reliefs. Different control options are available for power chairs, allowing the user to control the chair using his breath or motions of his upper extremities, chin, or mouth. Because of the different control options, power chairs can make independent mobility possible for virtually anyone, no matter how severe the physical disability.

Power wheelchairs are necessary equipment for people who cannot propel manual wheelchairs. However, these wheelchairs have drawbacks that make their use unwise for people who are capable of functioning without them. Power chairs are bulky, requiring more space to maneuver than manual wheelchairs. They are also extremely heavy. Because of their size and weight, power chairs are restricted to wheelchair-accessible environments. (A manual wheelchair can often be propelled through narrow doorways and taken up and down stairs or curbs independently or with assistance.) The bulk and weight of an electric wheelchair also precludes the use of a car.[5] Perhaps the major disadvantage of a power chair is that its user does not receive the physical benefits that are gained from propulsion of a manual wheelchair.

Manual wheelchairs are lighter and smaller than power chairs, so they can be transported in cars and can be taken into environments that are not accessible to wheelchairs. More importantly, manual wheelchairs can have beneficial physical effects on those who propel them. Manual wheelchair propulsion can result in cardiovascular conditioning (Tahamont, Knowlton, Sawka, & Miles, 1986) as well as strengthening of the musculature used in propulsion. These effects can in turn lead to improved performance in functional tasks.

Manual wheelchairs are available in standard weight, lightweight, and ultralight models. Standard weight chairs are heavy, and they have relatively limited options in size and components. Lightweight chairs are somewhat lighter but are still relatively heavy and have limited options. Ultralight wheelchairs are made of durable lightweight materials and are generally available with more options in size, adjustability, and components. Ultralight chairs allow more efficient propulsion, reducing the energy demands on the user (Hilbers & White, 1987).

The components of a manual wheelchair are illustrated in Figure 19–1. Virtually all of these components have several options from which to choose when selecting a wheelchair. The commonly prescribed options for these components are summarized in Chart 19–1.

In choosing between the available options, the clinician and prospective owner should weigh the positives and negatives of each option. Trial runs in wheelchairs that have the features under consideration are critical to this choice. Each manufacturer has its own designs for such features as the wheel locks and the armrests. What seems to be a good option when looking at the manufacturer's literature may turn out to be unsuitable when the chair arrives. Until an individual (particularly one with impaired hand function) tries out a given design, it is often impossible to determine with certainty that he will be capable of using it. Someone who tries a "similar" wheelchair but does not actually sit in, propel, and transfer in and out of the exact model being considered for purchase may find that he cannot function optimally when his own chair arrives.

Although aesthetics were not formerly considered to be an important consideration in wheelchair design or selection, the significance of this area is now recognized (Taylor, 1987). Modern wheelchairs come in a variety of colors and styles. The ultralight models, in addition to their numerous other advantages, tend to look better than other chairs. Their sporty colors and designs can make the user look less impaired. This in turn can make him more socially acceptable, facilitating his reintegration into the community.

---

[5] For this reason the owner of a power chair should have a manual wheelchair as a back-up for times when travel in a car is necessary.

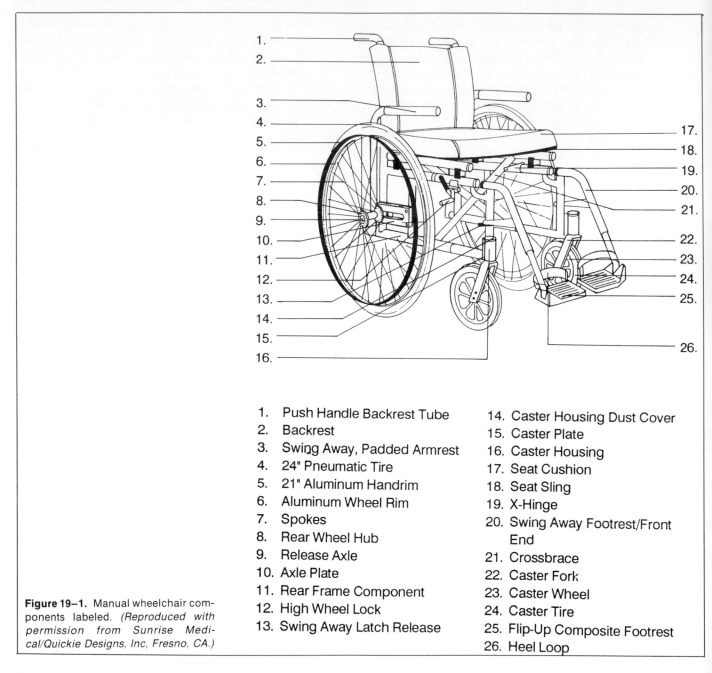

1. Push Handle Backrest Tube
2. Backrest
3. Swing Away, Padded Armrest
4. 24" Pneumatic Tire
5. 21" Aluminum Handrim
6. Aluminum Wheel Rim
7. Spokes
8. Rear Wheel Hub
9. Release Axle
10. Axle Plate
11. Rear Frame Component
12. High Wheel Lock
13. Swing Away Latch Release
14. Caster Housing Dust Cover
15. Caster Plate
16. Caster Housing
17. Seat Cushion
18. Seat Sling
19. X-Hinge
20. Swing Away Footrest/Front End
21. Crossbrace
22. Caster Fork
23. Caster Wheel
24. Caster Tire
25. Flip-Up Composite Footrest
26. Heel Loop

Figure 19–1. Manual wheelchair components labeled. *(Reproduced with permission from Sunrise Medical/Quickie Designs, Inc, Fresno, CA.)*

Wheelchairs have become less institutional-looking. The new chairs are sporty-looking, lighter, faster, and take up less space, making me look less conspicuous. The first chair I had made me look like a tank.

Dean Ragone (1987).

Size Selection. The fit of a wheelchair is important to both function and health. A seat that is too wide can promote the development of scoliosis, create problems in pressure distribution under the buttocks, and can make propulsion of the chair more difficult. A seat that is too narrow can create ex-

cessive pressure over the greater trochanters. Excessive depth of the seat (seat too long from front to back) can promote lumbar kyphosis and restrict circulation below the knees. A seat that is too shallow (seat too short from front to back) will result in excessive pressure on the weight-bearing surfaces due to the limited area over which pressure can be distributed. A seat that is not high enough off the floor will make appropriate leg positioning impossible, creating excessive pressure over the ischial tuberosities (Wilson, 1986). A backrest that is too short will not provide adequate support to the back, making upright sitting and wheelchair propulsion more difficult. One that is too high will limit shoul-

Chart 19—1 Options Available in Manual Wheelchair Components

Components	Options	Characteristics
Backrest	Fixed height	Back height cannot be adjusted
	Adjustable height	Allows custom adjustment to maximize function and comfort; can change back height as needs change
Seat	Hammock (sling)	Allows folding; causes hip adduction, reducing postural stability
	Solid	Firm support for better posture; some models allow folding
Wheels	Standard attachment	Require tools for removal and replacement
	Quick release	Wheels easily removed and replaced for car transfers or adjusting axle position
	Vertical (standard)	Overall chair width narrower
	Cambered wheels	Allows pushing movement to occur in one plane; may be more efficient
Axle	Fixed position	Axle position cannot be altered
	Adjustable position	Allows custom adjustment for optimal function and posture
Frame	Folding	Requires less space when folded; does not require good hand function to load into car; provides shock absorption; allows all wheels to contact the ground on uneven terrain
	Rigid	Frame stiffness makes propulsion more efficient; wheels must be removed to load into car
Armrests	Desk length	Allows closer approach to tables and desks
	Full length	Provides support to entire length of forearm
	Fixed	Only stand-pivot transfers are possible
	Removable, swing away	Can be removed or repositioned for transfers; some styles add to chair's overall width; different styles have varying difficulty of management
	Adjustable height	Can be adjusted to suit the individual; can be raised to make standing from wheelchair easier; may be noisy, less durable
Front rigging	Legrests (elevating)	Allow propulsion with legs elevated; heavy; add length to chair; awkward to reposition; must be removed for transfers
	Footrests	Easily repositioned; do not have to be removed for transfers
	Heel loops	Keep feet from sliding off footplates; make removal of feet from footplates more difficult
Tires	Pneumatic	Best shock absorption; require more maintenance (puncture, require periodic inflation); do not "bog down" in sand or soft soil; make chair's overall width greater; treaded pneumatic provide good traction
	Solid	Most durable; do not go flat; add less width to chair; less cushioned ride; make obstacle negotiation more difficult; "bog down" in sand or soft soil
Wheel and caster design	Wire spokes	Light; require periodic alignment
	Mag	More durable; do not lose true; more easily cleaned; entire wheel/caster must be replaced if damaged
		Metal: more expensive; heavy
		Plastic: light

(continued)

Chart 19—1 Options Available in Manual Wheelchair Components (*continued*)

Components	Options	Characteristics
	Adjustable position	Allows accommodation for axle adjustment (rear wheel)
Caster tires	Pneumatic	Best shock absorption; require more maintenance (puncture, require periodic inflation); do not "bog down" in sand or soft soil
	Semipneumatic	Intermediate shock absorption; do not puncture or require inflation; do not "bog down" in sand or soft soil; heavy
	Solid	Most durable; do not puncture or require inflation; lightest; provide least resistance to turning on even surfaces; less cushioned ride; "bog down" in sand or soft soil
Caster size	8-inch diameter	Heavier, easier to propel over uneven terrain
	5-inch diameter	Lighter, easier to maneuver on even surfaces
Handrims	Standard	Durable surface
	Vinyl coated	Increase friction, making propulsion easier when hand function is impaired; surface not durable, gets nicks with sharp edges
	Pegged	Handrim projections make propulsion easier when arms are very weak; pegs can interfere with pushing rhythm; increase overall wheelchair width

Chart 19—1 references: Hilbers & White (1987); Nixon (1985); Wilson (1986).

der mobility, making propulsion uncomfortable and more difficult.

Historically, appropriate wheelchair dimensions for an individual have been determined using a tape measure. This method is inefficient and is subject to error. A more efficient and accurate method involves having the individual try out wheelchairs of different dimensions. When sitting in a wheelchair, the seat width should be such that the hips do not contact the wheels or skirt guards, but there is not excessive space beside the hips. The seat depth should be such that there is a space of approximately 1 to 2 inches between the calves and the edge of the seat. The seat should be high enough above the floor to allow proper adjustment of the footplates with at least 2 inches of clearance between the floor and the footplates. The appropriate back height will depend on the wheelchair user's ability to stabilize his trunk in the chair. An optimal fit can be found by experimenting with different back heights.

The height of cushion on which a person sits will affect his requirements for backrest and seat height. For this reason the cushion should be selected before the wheelchair is ordered.

Evaluation. Once a wheelchair arrives, the clinician should evaluate it, addressing the following questions. Are the wheelchair's dimensions appropriate, and are its features suitable? Does the chair match the prescription? If not, are the substitutions acceptable to both the clinician and the person for whom the chair was ordered?

Adjustment. Virtually all wheelchairs have at least one adjustable feature: footrest height. This adjustment is critical to both posture and pressure distribution. The footrests should be adjusted with the person sitting in the wheelchair on his cushion. If he ever changes cushions, the footrest height should be checked and readjusted if needed. The footplates should be positioned at a height that places the knees at or slightly below the level of the hips. This position will help to optimize posture and pressure distribution. Footplates that are positioned too high lift the thighs off the seat, resulting in excessive pressure over the ischial tuberosities. Footplates positioned too low cause excessive pressure on the distal thighs and reduce postural support.

If the wheelchair has an adjustable backrest, the optimal backrest height should be determined. To find the best backrest height, the wheelchair user can sit in and propel the chair with the backrest adjusted to various heights. The clinician and wheelchair user should determine which height results in the best posture, comfort, and function.

If the wheelchair has an axle with adjustable position, the clinician and wheelchair user should work together to find the optimal axle position. Anteroposterior adjustments can have a profound effect on function, especially in cases where the wheelchair user is only marginal in his propulsion ability (Tomlinson, 1990). A relatively anterior wheel position makes propulsion easier by reducing the chair's rolling resistance and tendency to turn downhill[6] and by increasing its propulsion efficiency. Posterior placement of the axle has the opposite effect. Anteroposterior adjustments of the wheel's position also affect the chair's "tippiness." Anterior placement of the axle makes the chair less stable: the chair is more likely to tip over backwards, and it is easier to lift the casters for obstacle negotiation (Brubaker, 1990). Optimal adjustment for an individual may involve finding a balance between propulsion efficiency and stability (Tomlinson, 1990).

Vertical axle adjustments affect the tilt of the seat and backrest: a more superior axle position effectively tilts the seat and backrest backward. A slight backward tilt can be helpful to the wheelchair user who has difficulty maintaining trunk stability.

Unfortunately axle position adjustments that benefit propulsion and posture can interfere with transfers to and from the wheelchair. Moving the wheels to an anterior or superior position reduces the distance that the seat extends anterior to the wheels. This reduces the space available for lateral transfers to and from the wheelchair (Tomlinson, 1990). For the individual who is marginal in both transfer and propulsion skills, optimal wheelchair adjustment will involve finding a balance between transfer and propulsion abilities.

Alterations in axle position change the position of the wheel locks relative to the wheels, interfering with the locks' function. Thus the locks must be adjusted after the axles have been positioned. Axle position also affects the orientation of the casters, which in turn impacts on wheelchair propulsion. When adjustments are made in a wheelchair's axle position, the caster angle should be adjusted to achieve a vertical orientation of the caster stems (Tomlinson, 1990).

When a power wheelchair is used, adjustment also includes the chair's controls. The controls' spatial orientation, physical configuration, and control parameters should be adjusted to suit the needs of the individual involved (O'Neil & Seelye, 1990).

CUSHIONS

Most nonambulatory spinal cord-injured people require wheelchair cushions to aid in the prevention of decubiti. These cushions are specifically designed for pressure distribution, minimizing the pressure on the skin of the buttocks by spreading the supporting forces over a greater area. Cushions that minimize shear forces on the skin also help to maintain skin integrity.

Cushions vary in their effectiveness in reducing pressure and shear forces, as well as in the degree to which they cause buildup of heat and moisture on the skin.[7] They also differ in weight, maintenance required, cost, and the amount of difficulty that they cause during transfers. Cushion selection is critical because of the cushion's enormous impact on both the user's skin integrity and on his ability to function.

A cord-injured person's wheelchair cushion should reduce the pressure on his buttocks enough to enable him to function in a normal day (sitting and performing his accustomed activities all day, *with pressure reliefs*) without skin breakdown. The most critical factor in cushion selection is the cushion's effect on skin integrity. A cushion that is not adequate in this respect is inappropriate for the individual in question.

People with spinal cord injuries are highly variable in the degree to which their skin can tolerate pressure without breaking down. Factors that can impact on skin tolerance include age, body build, blood pressure, edema, anemia, and nutritional status (Garber, 1985; Nixon, 1985). The only way to determine a given cushion's appropriateness for an individual is to have him use the cushion (or an identical model) for a period of time. If at all possible, he should use a cushion for several days before one is ordered. During the trial period, his skin should be checked frequently to determine whether the cushion provides adequate pressure distribution. The cushion's influence on the patient's functional status should also be noted.

Unfortunately, the cushions that distribute pressure most effectively tend to be heavier and interfere more with transfers. These factors must also be considered when selecting a cushion. A heavy cushion adds to the overall weight that the individual must push when propelling his chair and may be difficult or impossible for him to take in and out of his chair independently. A cushion that interferes

---

[6] Sidewalks usually to have a cross slope, with the sidewalk surface tilting slightly toward the street. A wheelchair being propelled over this slope tends to turn in the downhill direction, making propulsion more difficult.

[7] Pressure, shear forces, moisture, and elevated temperatures contribute to the development of decubiti (Nixon, 1985).

with transfers may create dependence when the person could otherwise function without assistance. Thus a cushion can have tremendous impact on functional status. Cushion selection involves finding the cushion that provides adequate pressure distribution for the individual in question while creating the least interference with his functioning.

The maintenance required by a cushion should also be considered. Cushions that require frequent maintenance to retain their effectiveness are appropriate only for people who will take the responsibility to provide or to obtain this maintenance (Ferguson-Pell, 1990).

Expense may also be considered when selecting a cushion. This factor should be of the lowest priority, however, since cushions have such a significant impact on health and function. The cost of even the most expensive cushion is negligible when compared to the potential cost of a single decubitus.

Options. The three classes of commonly used wheelchair cushions are polymer foam, air-filled, and flotation cushions.[8] Different brands are available in each class of cushion.

Polymer foam cushions are made of a dense foam.[9] They come in different densities, thicknesses, and seat dimensions. Density and thickness are chosen according to the user's weight and skin tolerance. Foam cushions are light, do not greatly inhibit function, are relatively inexpensive, and can absorb moisture. Options include contoured cushions and cushions composed of two or more layers of different densities. Foam cushions are the least effective in distributing pressure but are adequate for many cord-injured people. The disadvantages of this class of cushion include the following: they cannot be washed, they tend to cause elevated skin temperatures, and they may need to be replaced as often as every 6 months (Ferguson-Pell, 1990; Garber, 1985; Nixon, 1985; Wilson, 1986).

Gel cushions provide better pressure distribution than do foam cushions. Additionally, gel cushions can reduce heat buildup (Ferguson-Pell, 1990) and may be the most effective type of cushion in minimizing shear forces on the skin. This characteristic is particularly advantageous to the active person, who is more likely to have skin problems due to shearing. Unfortunately gel cushions are heavy and can cause moisture buildup on the skin, elevation of local skin temperature after prolonged sitting, reduced sitting stability, and a fair amount of difficulty during transfers (Ferguson-Pell, 1990; Garber, 1985; Nawoczenski, 1987; Nixon, 1985).

Air-filled cushions provide excellent weight distribution if they are inflated properly. Their disadvantages include the following: they are relatively heavy, are easily punctured, can reduce sitting stability, and they make transfers *much* more difficult. Some designs can cause buildup of moisture on the skin (Garber, 1985; Krouskop, Williams, Noble, & Brown, 1986; Nixon, 1985). Perhaps the greatest disadvantage of air-filled cushions is that they are ineffective in pressure reduction if they are over-inflated or underinflated. To optimize pressure reduction, the inflation pressure should be checked daily (Krouskop, Williams, Noble, & Brown, 1986).

Cushion covers should also be selected carefully, as the cover can influence a cushion's effectiveness in pressure distribution. Covers can also increase or decrease moisture and heat buildup on the skin (Ferguson-Pell, 1990; Wilson, 1986).

Cut-out boards under cushions can be used to improve postural support and to decrease pressure (slightly) under the ischial tuberosities. A cut-out board can be made by cutting a piece of plywood to fit the seat and by cutting a U-shaped piece from under the ischial tuberosities. Proper dimensions of the board and the cut are imperative (Nawoczenski, 1987).

Education. People who require wheelchair cushions for pressure distribution should be thoroughly instructed in their use. The instruction should cover care and maintenance requirements and schedule of use. (Use whenever sitting!) Most importantly, people should be instructed about their cushions' limitations. *No cushion can guarantee the prevention of decubiti* because none lowers pressure on the skin enough to keep it below capillary pressure. No matter what type of cushion a person uses, periodic pressure reliefs are required to allow circulation in the areas that are subjected to pressure in sitting (Nawoczenski, 1987; Nixon, 1985).

ORTHOSES

A variety of orthoses are commonly used following spinal cord injury. Spinal orthoses are often used to maintain vertebral alignment. Orthoses can also be used to position the extremities as part of therapeutic programs aimed at preventing or correcting

---

[8] Dynamic systems, which provide alternating pressure, are less commonly used because they are cumbersome and require a power source (Garber, 1985).

[9] They are *not* to be confused with standard foam rubber, which provides virtually no pressure distribution. The foam rubber cushions that often come with wheelchairs do not provide adequate pressure distribution for cord-injured people.

deformity. Finally, a wide range of orthoses are used to maximize functional capabilities.

Clinicians should be aware of the potential harm that orthoses can inflict. Because an orthosis works through application of forces to the body, it can restrict circulation and cause pressure sores, nerve damage, skin rashes, pain, and deformity. Orthoses should be evaluated carefully when first received and should be checked periodically in follow-up visits to minimize the risk of complications.

Orthotic training should always accompany an orthosis. The nature of this training will depend on the orthosis. It may include education about the wearing schedule and practice donning and doffing. Instruction in the benefits of orthotic use is likely to enhance compliance. Functional training will be needed to gain maximal benefit from orthoses designed to enhance functional status. Finally, orthotic users should be warned of the potential hazards of their orthoses. They should be taught how to avoid complications and should be told what to do if complications occur.

Vertebral Orthoses

Vertebral orthoses are often used to stabilize the spine for a variable period of time following spinal injury. This orthotic stabilization promotes fusion, prevents deformity, and protects the cord from further neurological damage. Vertebral orthoses may be used prior to, following, or in lieu of surgical stabilization. The various designs differ in the degree to which they immobilize the different levels of the spinal column and the direction of motion that they can control. Vertebral orthoses must be selected carefully, with consideration given to the location and degree of immobilization required.

As is true with any orthosis, the wearer of a vertebral orthosis should be educated about (and *convinced* of) the importance of wearing the device. Otherwise the orthosis may not be worn. Even a halo, which is attached directly to the skull, can be removed by its wearer (Glaser, Whitehill, Stamp, & Jane, 1986).

Cervical Orthoses

An assortment of cervical orthoses are available. The halo, Minerva, SOMI, and Philadelphia collar are commonly used for stabilization of the cervical spine.

Halo. A halo orthosis consists of a metal ring that encircles the skull and is affixed to the skull by pins and is attached caudally via metal uprights to a prefabricated adjustable plastic vest lined with sheepskin (Fig. 19–2). With the possible exception of the

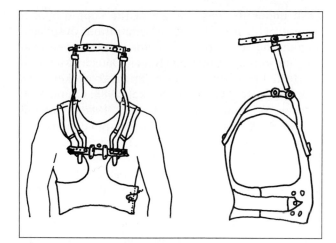

Figure 19–2. Halo orthosis. *(Reproduced with permission from* Spinal Orthotics: *New York University Post-Graduate Medical School, 1983.)*

Minerva, the halo is the orthotic device most effective in preventing cervical motion. It is particularly effective in limiting rotation and lateral flexion of the entire cervical spine and flexion and extension in the higher cervical levels. It can also be used to apply longitudinal distraction (Johnson, Hart, Simmons, Ramsby & Southwick, 1977; Wang, Moskal, Albert, Pritts, Schuch, & Stamp, 1988). The halo provides maximal stabilization, but not complete immobilization, of the cervical spine. It allows some gross motion as well as "snaking," flexion or extension at one cervical level with compensatory opposite motion in adjacent segments (Benzel, Hadden, & Saulsbery, 1989).

Halo devices may be used following or in lieu of surgical stabilization of the spine, depending on the nature of the vertebral and ligamentous injury. The high degree of stabilization afforded by a halo apparatus makes it possible for the wearer to get out of bed and initiate functional training earlier than would otherwise be possible. This may result in earlier home visits and discharge (Garfin, Botte, Waters & Nickel, 1986; Glaser, Whitehill, Stamp, & Jane, 1986; Parry, Delargy, & Burt, 1988). Unfortunately, although halo orthoses make earlier mobilization possible, they make functional training more difficult because they limit shoulder motions and raise the wearer's center of gravity (Millington, Ellingsen, Hauswirth, & Fabian, 1987; Nawoczenski, Rinehart, Duncanson & Brown, 1987).

Complications experienced by people wearing halo devices include loss of reduction, pin loosening, infection at the pin sites (in turn occasionally resulting in septicemia, osteomyelitis, and subdural abscess), decubiti in skin underlying the vest, skin rash under the vest, injury of the supraorbital or supratrochlear nerve, dural penetration, dysphagia, disfiguring scars, pin discomfort, and temperomandibular joint dysfunction (Bucci, Dauser, Maynard, & Hoff, 1988; Garfin, Botte, Triggs & Nickel, 1988; Garfin, Botte, Waters, & Nickel, 1986; Crum, 1990; Glaser, Whitehill, Stamp, & Jane, 1986; Whitehill, Richman, & Glaser, 1986). Proper application, care, and monitoring can minimize the occurrence and severity of these complications.

The majority of complications associated with halo orthoses originate at the pins. Pin loosening is of concern for two reasons: it can result in loss of stability, and it often precedes infection at the pin site. Application of pins with higher torque results in reduced frequency of loosening and infection (Botte, Byrne, & Garfin, 1987). Pins that loosen should be tightened or replaced with a pin in a different site. Proper hygiene at the pin sites will minimize the occurrence of infection. When an infection occurs, it should be treated early (Botte, Garfin, Byrne, Woo, & Nickel, 1989; Garfin, Botte, Triggs & Nickel, 1988; Garfin, Botte, Waters, & Nickel, 1986).

Complications involving the skin underlying the vest can also be minimized with proper care and monitoring. The skin over the scapulae, ribs, acromion processes, and spinous processes are at greatest risk. These areas should be checked frequently when possible. The liner between the skin and vest should be kept dry and changed monthly (Nawoczenski, Rinehart, Duncanson, & Brown, 1987).

A halo should be comfortable. If pain occurs, the health care team should investigate the cause. Pain at the pin sites is likely to be caused by loosening or infection. Pain in the trunk is likely to be due to excessive pressure from the vest.

Despite the complications that halos can cause and the functional limitations that they impose, most people tolerate these orthoses well. Halos remain a popular orthotic option for people who require maximal stability of their cervical spines.

Minerva. The thermoplastic Minerva body jacket (TMBJ, or Minerva) is a custom-molded orthosis that encases the chin and the posterior aspect of the skull and extends caudally either to the inferior costal margin or to enclose the pelvis, depending on the stability required. A headband encircles the skull to hold the head in place (Fig. 19–3).

Like the halo, the Minerva restricts cervical motion in all planes and can provide distraction forces (New York University, 1983). Neither the halo nor the Minerva provides perfect immobilization of the cervical vertebrae; both allow some gross

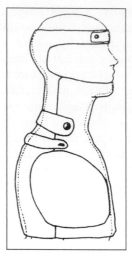

Figure 19–3. Minerva orthosis. *(Reproduced with permission from Fishman, S., Berger, N., Edelstein, J., & Springer, W. [1985]. Spinal Orthoses. In: American Academy of Orthopedic Surgeons: Atlas of Orthotics: Biomechanical Principles and Application [2nd ed.]. Princeton, NJ: C. V. Mosby Company.)*

motion and "snaking." The Minerva orthosis has been reported to provide better stabilization of the cervical spine than does the halo, except between C-1 and C-2 (Benzel, Hadden, & Saulsbery, 1989).[10]

As is true with halo orthoses, the excellent stability afforded by Minerva orthoses allows early initiation of functional training. Since the Minerva allows good range of motion in the shoulders, it does not interfere as much with functional progress. Minervas are also reported to be more comfortable and cosmetically acceptable than halos (Benzel, Hadden, & Saulsbery, 1989; Millington, Ellingsen, Hauswirth, & Fabian, 1987).

Fewer complications are associated with Minerva orthoses than with halos. Since a Minerva is not screwed into the wearer's skull, it does not cause any pin-related problems. The Minerva's design may also reduce skin complications. Custom molding can result in better pressure distribution than is achieved with the prefabricated halo vest. Additionally, half of a Minerva can be removed at a time (with the wearer positioned in prone or supine) for skin inspection, bathing, and cleaning of the orthosis. If an area of excessive pressure is noted, the orthosis can be modified (Millington, Ellingsen, Hauswirth, & Fabian, 1987).

---

[10] In the study cited, the measurement of cervical motion allowed by the Minerva was done 3 weeks after measurement with the halo (Benzel, Hadden, & Saulsbery, 1989).

SOMI. A SOMI, or sterno-occipital-mandibular-immobilizer, consists of a padded metal sternal plate to which are attached three adjustable uprights that support occipital and mandibular supports (Fig. 19–4).

The SOMI allows significantly more vertebral motion in all planes than is allowed by the halo and Minerva. SOMIs are more effective than Philadelphia collars (described below) in restricting cervical flexion, but they do not restrict extension as well (Fisher, Bowar, Awad, & Gullickson, 1977; Johnson, Hart, Simmons, Ramsby, & Southwick, 1977).

When someone wearing a SOMI moves between supine and upright postures, the position of the mandibular support should be adjusted. Proper adjustment is required for both comfort and optimal restriction of motion (Nawoczenski, Rinehart, Duncanson & Brown, 1987).

Philadelphia Collar. Philadelphia collars are two-piece collars made of polyethylene foam reinforced by rigid plastic struts and joined by velcro. The anterior piece cups the mandible and extends caudally to the upper chest. The posterior piece cups the occiput and extends caudally to the upper back (Fig. 19–5).

Philadelphia collars limit cervical motion to

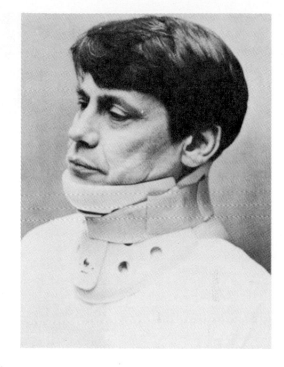

Figure 19–5. Philadelphia collar. *(Reproduced with permission from Marsolias, E. [1985]. Spinal Pain. In: American Academy of Orthopedic Surgeons, Atlas of Orthotics: Biomechanical Principles and Application [2nd ed.]. St. Louis: C. V. Mosby Company.)*

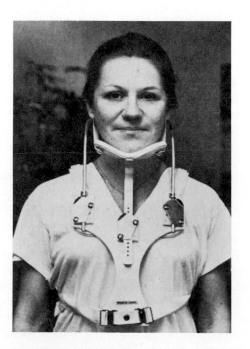

Figure 19–4. SOMI orthosis. *(Reproduced with permission from Shurr, D., & Cook, T. [1990]. Prosthetics & Orthotics. Norwalk, CT: Appleton & Lange.)*

some degree but do not effectively immobilize the spine. Thus they should not be used in the presence of vertebral instability (Fisher, Bowar, Awad, & Gullickson, 1977; Johnson, Hart, Simmons, Ramsby, & Southwick, 1977).

Thoracolumbosacral Orthoses

Like cervical orthoses, thoracolumbosacral orthoses vary in their effectiveness in restricting motion. Molded plastic body jackets, Jewett orthoses, and Knight-Taylor orthoses are described below.

Molded Plastic Body Jacket. A molded plastic body jacket encases virtually the entire trunk (Fig. 19–6). It is made of two pieces of plastic, molded to fit the individual and attached to each other with velcro straps. The abdominal area may be covered or exposed. (A window in the abdominal region makes assisted coughing possible.)

This type of orthosis provides maximal stability to the trunk, limiting motion in all planes in the thoracic, lumbar, and lumbosacral vertebrae. If the orthosis encases the abdominal region, it decreases the vertical load on the spinal column by increasing

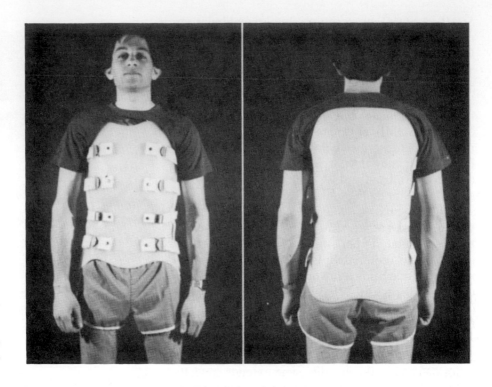

Figure 19–6. Molded plastic body jacket. *(Reproduced with permission from Fishman, S., Berger, N., Edelstein, J., & Springer, W. [1985]. Spinal Orthoses. In: American Academy of Orthopedic Surgeons: Atlas of Orthotics: Biomechanical Principles and Application [2nd ed.]. St. Louis: C. V. Mosby Company.)*

intercavity pressure (Fishman, Berger, Edelstein, & Springer, 1985; New York University, 1983).

The location of the inferior and superior borders of the anterior portion of the jacket determines the degree to which the orthosis restricts hip and shoulder motion. If the jacket is shaped appropriately in these regions, hip flexion should be possible to at least 90 degrees, and shoulder motions should be unrestricted. As rehabilitation progresses, hypertrophy of the shoulder musculature may necessitate trimming of the jacket's superior border (Nawoczenski, Rinehart, Duncanson, & Brown, 1987).

A cotton T-shirt worn under the orthosis will absorb perspiration to increase comfort and prevent skin maceration. When the wearer is prone or supine, half of the orthosis can be removed to allow inspection and washing of the skin and cleaning of the orthosis (Nawoczenski, Rinehart, Duncanson, & Brown, 1987).

Jewett. A Jewett orthosis is a prefabricated orthosis made of a metal frame to which pads are attached (Fig. 19–7). The suprapubic, sternal, and thoracolumbar pads exert forces on the trunk that restrict flexion and encourage hyperextension. The hyperextension of the spine places the vertebrae in a close packed position. With the vertebrae "locked" in this manner, lateral flexion and rotation

are restricted (Fishman, Berger, Edelstein, & Springer, 1985; New York University, 1983).

Well-adjusted Jewett orthoses effectively prevent flexion in the thoracic and lumbar regions and restrict lumbosacral flexion to a limited degree. Extension is free at all levels. Rotation and lateral flexion are controlled to an intermediate degree at best, depending on the amount of hyperextension that the orthosis maintains (Fishman, Berger, Edelstein, & Springer, 1985; New York University, 1983).

Improper adjustment of the orthosis can result in loss of vertebral stabilization and pressure on the throat or genitals when sitting.

Knight-Taylor. The framework of a Knight-Taylor orthosis consists of pelvic and thoracic bands worn posteriorly, connected to two pairs of vertical uprights. Axillary straps encircle the shoulders from behind. An abdominal support is attached to the lateral uprights (Fig. 19–8).

In the thoracic region, Knight-Taylor orthoses allow unrestricted rotation and provide an intermediate level of restriction of flexion, extension, and lateral rotation. Lumbar rotation is restricted to an intermediate degree. Motions in other planes are effectively restricted in the lumbar spine. In the lumbosacral region, flexion and extension are essentially unrestricted, rotation is limited to an in-

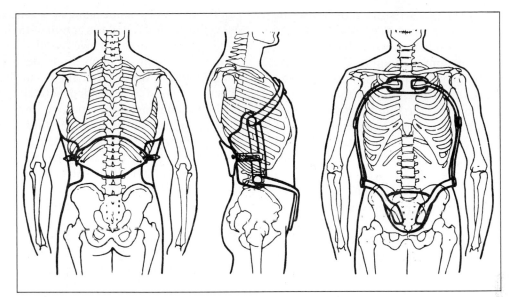

Figure 19–7. Jewett orthosis. *(Reproduced with permission from* Spinal Orthotics: *New York University Post-Graduate Medical School, 1983.)*

termediate degree, and lateral flexion is effectively restricted (Fishman, Berger, Edelstein, & Springer, 1985; New York University, 1983).

Upper Extremity Orthoses

Upper extremity orthoses may be used following spinal cord injury to prevent overstretching and contractures, correct contractures when they develop, and enhance functional abilities. Upper-extremity orthoses, also called splints, may be static or dynamic. Static splints have no moving parts. They work through immobilization of the joints that they encompass. Dynamic splints, in contrast, cause motion in at least some of the joints that they encompass (Fess, Gettle, & Strickland, 1981).

During the acute phase of rehabilitation, static splints may be used to protect joints and muscles from overstretching and prevent the development

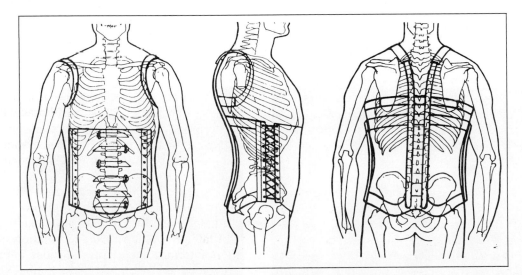

Figure 19–8. Knight-Taylor orthosis. *(Reproduced with permission from Fishman, S., Berger, N., Edelstein, J., & Springer, W. [1985]. Spinal Orthoses. In: American Academy of Orthopedic Surgeons: Atlas of Orthotics: Biomechanical Principles and Application [2nd ed.]. St. Louis: C. V. Mosby Company.)*

of deformity. For example, wrist-hand orthoses can prevent deformity and protect the wrist and finger extensors from overstretching when the wrist extensors are weak or nonfunctioning. These splints should be made to position the wrists in slight extension, the metacarpophalangeal joints of the fingers in slight flexion, and the thumbs in opposition. This will preserve the natural tenodesis action of the hand and wrist. The hand's potential for useful functioning will be maximized if the splint is fabricated to preserve the thumb's web space and the hand's transverse palmar arch (Baumgarten, 1985; Nawoczenski, Rinehart, Duncanson, & Brown, 1987).

Static splints are also used to increase range of motion when tightness develops. For example, when limitation in elbow extension has developed, a splint can be fabricated that exerts mild stretching forces around the elbow.

Many static splints used for prevention and correction of deformity interfere with use of the extremity while being worn. This creates a problem for people who are out of bed and active. In these cases independence and progress in rehabilitation may be enhanced if splints that interfere with function are worn only at night.

Not all static splints are used to prevent or to correct deformity. Some are used to enhance functional abilities. For example, a simple cuff (universal cuff) that attaches to the hand can be used to hold small objects such as eating utensils.

The tenodesis splint is a dynamic orthosis that can be used to achieve a palmar pinch between the thumb and the first two fingers. This orthosis is appropriate for people who lack innervation of the finger flexors and cannot achieve a functional grasp using the natural tenodesis action of their wrists and hands. A wrist-driven hinge splint (Fig. 19–9) positions the thumb in opposition and the interphalangeal joints of the first two fingers in slight flexion. When the wrist is extended actively, metacarpophalangeal flexion of the first two fingers brings the distal pads of the fingers and thumb in contact. When the wrist extensors relax, gravity assists the wrist into flexion, and the fingers open. This orthosis is most likely to be used after discharge if the wearer is able to don and doff it independently and quickly (Freehafer, 1985). A variation of this orthosis, the ratchet wrist-hand orthosis, creates a pinch grasp in the same manner except that the wrist is positioned passively. This orthosis can be used when wrist extensor strength is less than 3+/5 (Baumgarten, 1985).

Upper extremity orthoses should be used to augment, not substitute for, a therapeutic exercise program. They must be fabricated well and monitored carefully to minimize the risk of decubiti. Anesthetic areas of the skin are particularly at risk and should be given special attention. Clinicians should be extremely cautious about splinting an upper extremity in which an intravenous (IV) needle is in place distally. Swelling can develop rapidly in these cases, and a previously well-fitting splint will no longer fit appropriately.

Lower Extremity Orthoses

After spinal cord injury, lower extremity orthoses are commonly used for ambulation. Ambulation following complete cord injury remains controversial,

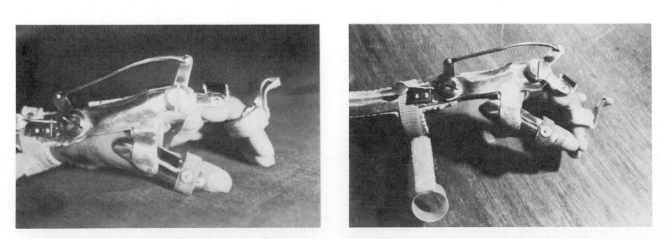

Figure 19–9. Wrist-driven hinge splint. *(Reproduced with permission from Ford, J., & Duckworth, B. [1987]. Physical Management for the Quadriplegic Patient: Philadelphia: F. A. Davis Company.)*

since many who train with orthoses do not use them after discharge.[11]

Materials. Lower extremity orthoses can be made of metal, plastic, or a combination of the two.

Metal orthoses are made of lightweight aluminum and leather. These orthoses are heavier than their plastic counterparts, but they allow easier and greater adjustability. The shoe is built into a metal orthosis, and the shoe itself must be sturdy. Thus someone who wears metal orthoses has little choice in shoe design and cannot change shoes readily (Nixon, 1985; New York University, 1986).

Plastic orthoses are lighter than metal orthoses. The control that a plastic orthosis provides is determined by the rigidity of the plastic used and the configuration of the orthosis. A variety of shoes may be worn, since the shoe is not a part of the orthosis and does not have to provide all of the stabilizing forces. As a rule, plastic orthoses are not readily adjusted, so the proper alignment must be determined prior to fabrication. Since plastic orthoses contact a large area of the skin, they must be fabricated to provide a precise fit with appropriate distribution of pressure. Fluctuating edema precludes the use of these orthoses, as changes in limb volume may result in excessive pressure on the skin. Since plastic is nonabsorbent, excessive perspiration can result in skin maceration (Nawoczenski, Rinehart, Duncanson, & Brown, 1987; Nixon, 1985; New York University, 1986; Peterson, 1985).

Metal-plastic designs are often made of metal components proximally, with plastic components used distally. For example, the metal uprights of an orthosis may attach to a plastic shoe insert instead of attaching to the shoe itself. With this design, ankle adjustments are readily made and the orthotic user can wear a variety of shoes (New York University, 1986).

Ankle-Foot Orthosis. Ankle-foot orthosis (AFOs) are primarily used for people who have the ability to stabilize their knees in stance using their quadriceps but need stabilization at their ankles. The orthotic control needed at the ankle will depend on the motor function present.

When the dorsiflexors are weak, the dorsiflexion assist at the ankle will prevent foot drop during swing. A dorsiflexion assist will also allow plantar flexion at heel strike for a more normal gait pattern. In the presence of gastrocsoleus spasticity, a plantar flexion stop should be used instead of a dorsiflexion assist.

Weakness in the plantar flexors may necessitate a dorsiflexion stop to stabilize the tibia on the foot during stance, preventing excessive dorsiflexion as the center of gravity passes anterior to the ankle. A stop limiting dorsiflexion to 10 degrees will provide adequate stability and allow a relatively normal gait pattern (Peterson, 1985).

An AFO that restricts both dorsiflexion and plantar flexion can also be used to provide control at the knee. When the quadriceps are weak, an ankle joint positioned in slight plantar flexion can help to stabilize the knee. An ankle held in a neutral or slightly dorsiflexed position can prevent genu recurvatum (O'Daniel & Krapfl, 1989).

Knee-Ankle-Foot Orthoses. Knee-ankle-foot orthoses (KAFOs) are used when orthotic stabilization is required at the knees and the ankles. KAFOs are often used by people who lack muscular stabilization not only of the knees and ankles but of the hips and trunk as well.

A conventional metal KAFO has double uprights that are connected posteriorly by two thigh bands and a calf band. Anterior thigh and leg cuffs and a knee cap stabilize the leg in the orthosis. Typically, drop-ring locks are used at the knees. The ankles generally stop plantar flexion, and dorsiflexion may be stopped or left unrestricted.

A Scott-Craig KAFO (also called a Craig-Scott KAFO) is designed to provide maximal stability at the ankle and foot (Fig. 19–10). A T-shaped foot plate is embedded in the sole of the shoe, extending from the heel to the area of the metatarsal heads. This plate provides excellent anteroposterior and mediolateral stability, making the shoe a stable base for the rest of the orthosis. An adjustable double-stop ankle holds the ankle immobile in approximately 10 degrees of dorsiflexion. This fixed dorsiflexion at the ankles places the hips in a stable position during stance.[12] The optimal angle for a given individual's ankle is determined during initial gait training. In addition to the stable shoe and ankle, a Scott-Craig KAFO has two metal uprights, a single posterior thigh band, pawl locks with bail control, a hinged pretibial band, and a cushioned heel. The sole of the shoe is shaped to allow both stability and a smooth roll-over in stance. After the orthotic user has developed his ambulatory skills and the optimal ankle position has been determined,

---

[11] This controversy is presented in Chapter 14.

[12] In the absence of hip extensors, the hips are stable when the center of gravity falls posterior to the hips. This is achieved by standing with the hips anterior and the lumbar spine in lordosis. Techniques for standing and walking with KAFOs are presented in Chapter 14.

a sturdy plastic AFO can be substituted for the components below the knee (Lehmann, 1986; O'Daniel & Krapfl, 1989; New York University, 1986).

Whether a Scott-Craig orthosis or a conventional KAFO is used, an orthosis with a long sole plate and an ankle that is positioned rigidly in dorsiflexion makes walking easier. With these features, balanced standing does not require upper extremity effort. Additionally, the magnitude of the center of gravity's vertical oscillations during gait are less than occur with KAFOs which allow free dorsiflexion. The end result is that less energy is consumed during ambulation (Lehmann, 1986; O'Daniel & Krapfl, 1989).

Thoracolumbosacral-Hip-Knee-Ankle-Foot Orthoses. A reciprocating gait orthosis immobilizes the knees, ankles and feet and causes reciprocal motions of the hips during ambulation. The orthosis consists of plastic KAFOs with locking knees and reinforced ankles, attached proximally to a molded pelvic band with thoracic extensions (Fig. 19–11). Hip motions are controlled by cables that connect the hip joints. These cables are designed to transfer forces between the hips. Motion at one hip causes motion in the opposite direction to occur in the contralateral hip: to take a step forward, the wearer shifts his weight off the leg and extends the contralateral hip (Lehmann, 1986; New York University, 1986).

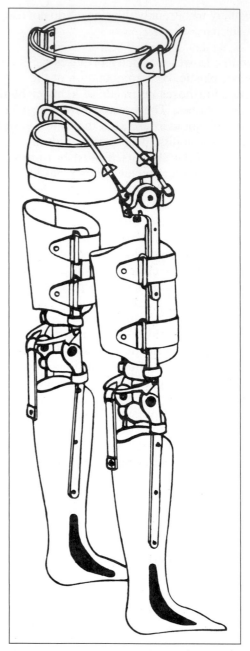

Figure 19–11. Reciprocating gait orthoses. *(Reproduced with permission from Nick Rightor, CO and the LSU Medical Center. [1983]. In LSU Reciprocating Gait Orthosis: A Pictorial Description and Application Manual. Chattanooga, TN: Durr-Fillauer, Medical.)*

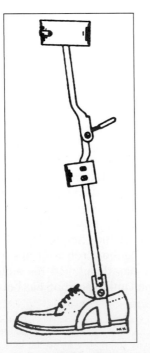

Figure 19–10. Scott-Craig KAFO. *(Reproduced with permission from Lower-Limb Orthotics: New York University Post-Graduate Medical School, 1986.)*

VEHICULAR MODIFICATIONS

When spinal cord injury results in significant motor impairment in the lower or upper extremities or both, adapted driving equipment is required for independent driving. While driving may at first seem to be a low priority ability, it is an important area of concern that deserves the attention of the rehabilitation team. Private transportation is considered by many to be a necessity of life in the United States. In many areas public transportation is either not available or not accessible. Even where public transportation is available and accessible, a private vehicle allows greater freedom in terms of destinations and timing. Personal transportation can be a necessity for work, recreation, social activities, and tasks such as grocery shopping or transporting children to and from day care. Thus independent driving may be required for reintegration into family and community life after spinal cord injury.

Equipment Options

Cars, Vans, and Minivans. Cars, vans, and minivans can be adapted for disabled drivers. Each type of vehicle has advantages and disadvantages for the driver.

Cars are usually less expensive than vans to buy and modify. They are also less expensive to operate, since they get better gas mileage. Cars have better resale value than converted vans and do not require as much space for parking. To use a car independently, the driver must be able to transfer in and out and store his wheelchair unassisted. The chair may be stored behind the driver's seat, on the passenger side of the front seat, or on top of the car. To make transfers and wheelchair placement easier, a buyer purchasing a car should consider the following features: two-door model, tilting steering wheel, bench-style front seat, and a reclinable driver's seat (Kent, 1986; REquest, 1990).

Vans make independent driving possible for people who cannot transfer in and out of a car without assistance. Vans can also be fitted with a greater variety of adapted driving equipment. An adapted van must have a ramp or lift to allow exit and entry.[13] It must also have restraints that stabilize the wheelchair(s) in the van and the driver in the wheelchair. Additional modifications that may be required include lowered floors and raised roofs and doors. Unfortunately vans are more expensive than cars. They cost more than cars initially, can be extremely expensive to modify, and are more costly to operate. They also require larger parking spaces. These disadvantages make vans less practical than cars for people who are capable of functioning independently with cars (Bowker, Edwards, & Smeltzer, 1985; Gacioch, 1989; Kent, 1986; REquest, 1990).

---

[13] An exception to this rule is a van driven by a person who has intact upper extremities and is able to transfer in and out of the van independently.

Minivans provide an alternative to vans for people who cannot transfer in and out of cars. The modifications required for their conversion are similar to those required for vans (Gacioch, 1989). Like vans, minivans are expensive to convert. However, the purchase price for minivans tends to be slightly less. They also have better gas mileage than vans, with some models being comparable to large cars in their gas mileage. These vehicles also fit into smaller parking spaces.

Adapted Controls. Automatic transmission and power brakes are required for a vehicle to be adapted with hand controls. Power steering is a necessity for drivers with impaired upper extremity strength. It is also helpful for people with intact upper extremities, since these drivers steer one handed while using the other hand to control braking and acceleration. Additional features that can be helpful to cord-injured drivers include cruise control; air conditioning; rear window defoggers; remote-controlled outside mirrors; and power-controlled driver's seat adjustments, windows, door locks, and trunk or hatch release. All of the vehicle's essential controls must be within the driver's reach when his lap and shoulder belts are on (Kent, 1986; Nixon, 1989; REquest, 1990). Additional vehicular modifications for disabled drivers include adapted steering, braking, accelerator, and accessory function (lights, horn, etc.) controls.

The steering modifications required by drivers with paraplegia or low quadriplegia are minimal. Simple handles attached to standard steering wheels make one-handed steering possible with or without intact hand function. Modified steering wheels are available for drivers who lack the strength or range of motion needed to manage a standard steering wheel. Options include steering wheels that are smaller than standard or are mounted horizontally or a combination of both and systems requiring reduced forces to operate. "Zero-effort" systems make it possible to steer with as little as one ounce of force (Gacioch, 1989; Kent, 1986).

Accelerator and brake controls are usually combined. Most are operated by pushing and pulling, but some are worked by pushing and twisting. Whatever motions are used, the brake and accelerator are operated by moving the control lever in different directions. Hand controls are safest if the brakes are activated by a forward push. (During an emergency situation, rapid deceleration will cause the driver to be thrown forward.) Ultrasensitive accelerator and braking systems are available for drivers who cannot manage standard hand controls

(Bowker, Edwards, & Smeltzer, 1985; Kent, 1986; REquest, 1990).

For drivers with severe upper-extremity impairment, ultrasensitive systems are available that combine steering and braking/accelertion in one control. Several designs are available in these combined control systems, with the various models utilizing different control motions (Bowker, Edwards, & Smeltzer, 1985; Gacioch, 1989).

Driving involves more than acceleration, braking, and steering. Safe driving also requires the ability to use the vehicle's lights, horn, turn signal, parking brake, doors, windshield wipers, defroster, and washer. The driver should also be able to control the vehicle's locks, windows, radio, and heater/air conditioner. The controls for all of these accessory functions must be within the driver's reach and appropriate for his manipulation abilities. Adapted switches are available that make these controls usable by people with impaired hand function. For drivers unable to manipulate standard or adapted keys, magnetic and digital code entry and ignition systems are also available (Bowker, Edwards, & Smeltzer, 1985; Gacioch, 1989).

Lifts. A large selection of lifts are available for vans and minivans. The different models vary in their placement (rear or side), door-width requirements, load capacities, parking-space requirements, safety features, price, and degree to which they interfere with front passenger seat adjustments and entry and exit by nondisabled people. Some lifts are fully automatic. Others require operation by an attendant (Gacioch, 1989; Kent, 1986).

Selection

A disabled driver's requirements for vehicular modification will be determined by his range of motion, strength, and transfer abilities. The diverse options available on the market make it possible to drive despite profound musculoskeletal limitations, but safe driving requires a good match between the driver's abilities and the equipment. To ensure that the prospective driver obtains the equipment best suited to his needs, the rehabilitation team must be involved in the selection. As is true with any equipment selection, the prospective driver and the rehabilitation team should work together to find the optimal driving system.

SUMMARY

Following spinal cord injury, equipment can have a significant impact on function and health. Thus equipment procurement is an important component of a rehabilitation program. The clinician and patient should work together to identify functional and medical needs, investigate and evaluate the available options, and reach an agreement regarding choice of equipment.

The adaptive equipment market is constantly changing. The clinician who keeps up with these changes will be best prepared to assist disabled people in finding the equipment most suited to their needs.

REFERENCES

Baumgarten, J. (1985). Upper extremity adaptations for the person with quadriplegia. In H. Adkins (Ed.), *Spinal cord injury* (pp. 219–242). New York: Churchill Livingstone.

Benzel, E.; Hadden, T., & Saulsbery, C. (1989). A comparison of the Minerva and halo jackets for stabilization of the cervical spine. *Journal of Neurosurgery, 70*, 411–414.

Botte, M.; Byrne, T., & Garfin, S. (1987). Application of the halo device for immobilization of the cervical spine utilizing an increased torque pressure. *Journal of Bone and Joint Surgery, 69-A*(5), 750–752.

Botte, M.; Garfin, S.; Byrne, T.; Woo, S., & Nickel, V. (1989). The halo skeletal fixator: Principles of application and maintenance. *Clinical Orthopedics and Related Research, 239*, 12–18.

Bowker, J.; Edwards, C., & Smeltzer, J. (1985). Orthotic and adaptive devices for recreation and driving. In Bunch W., Keagy R., Kritter A., Kruger L., Letts M., Lonstein J., Marsolias E., Matthews J., & Pedeganna L. (Eds.), *Atlas of orthotics: Biomechanical principles and application* (2nd ed., pp. 487–512). Princeton, NJ: C. V. Mosby.

Brubaker, C. (1990). Ergonometric considerations. *Journal of Rehabilitation Research and Development, Clinical Supplement #2*, 37–48.

Bucci, M.; Dauser, R.; Maynard, F., & Hoff, J. (1988). Management of post-traumatic cervical spine instability: Operative fusion versus halo vest immobilization: An analysis of 49 cases. *Journal of Trauma, 28*(7), 1001–1006.

Buchanan, L., & Ditunno, J. (1987). Acute care: Medical/Surgical management. In Buchanan L., & Nawoczenski D. (Eds.), *Spinal cord injury: Concepts and management approaches* (pp. 35–60). Baltimore: Williams & Wilkins.

Crum, N. (1990). Signs of temporomandibular joint dysfunction in spinal cord injured patients wearing halo braces: A clinical report. *Physical Therapy, 70*(2), 132–137.

Cybulski, G., & Jaeger, R. (1986). Standing performance of persons with paraplegia. *Archives of Physical Medicine and Rehabilitation, 67*, 103–108.

Fess, E.; Gettle, K., & Strickland, J. (1981). *Hand splinting: Principles and methods*. St. Louis: C. V. Mosby.

Fisher, S.; Bowar, J.; Awad, E., & Gullickson, G. (1977). Cervical orthoses effect on cervical spine motion: Roentgenographic and goniometric method of study. *Archives of Physical Medicine and Rehabilitation, 58,* 109–115.

Fishman, S.; Berger, N.; Edelstein, J., & Springer, W. (1985). Spinal orthoses. In Bunch W., Keagy R., Kritter A., Kruger L., Letts M., Lonstein J., Marsolias E., Matthews J., & Pedeganna L., (Eds.), *Atlas of orthotics: Biomechanical principles and application* (2nd ed., pp. 238–256). Princeton, NJ: C. V. Mosby.

Ferguson-Pell, M. (1990). Seat cushion selection. *Journal of Rehabilitation Research and Development, Clinical Supplement #2,* 47–73.

Freehafer, A. (1985). Orthotics in spinal cord injuries. In Bunch W., Keagy R., Kritter A., Kruger L., Letts M., Lonstein J., Marsolias E., Matthews J., & Pedeganna L., (Eds.), *Atlas of orthotics: Biomechanical principles and application* (2nd ed., pp.287–296). Princeton, NJ: C. V. Mosby.

Gacioch, M. (1989). Vans, vans, and more vans. *Mainstream, Magazine of the Able-Disabled 14*(3), 7–17.

Garber, S. (1985). Wheelchair cushions: A historical review. *American Journal of Occupational Therapy, 39*(7), 453–459.

Garfin, S.; Botte, M.; Triggs, K., & Nickel, V. (1988). Subdural abscess associated with halo-pin traction. *The Journal of Bone and Joint Surgery, 70-A*(9), 1338–1340.

Garfin, S.; Botte, M.; Waters, R., & Nickel, V. (1986). Complications in the use of the halo fixation device. *Journal of Bone and Joint Surgery, 68-A*(3), 320–325.

Glaser, J.; Whitehill, R.; Stamp, W., & Janc, J. (1986). Complications associated with the halo-vest: A review of 245 cases. *Journal of Neurosurgery, 65,* 762–769.

Harris, J. (1986). Cervical orthoses. In Redford J. (Ed.), *Orthotics etcetera* (3rd ed., pp. 101–121). Baltimore: Williams & Wilkins.

Hilbers, P., & White, T. (1987). Effects of wheelchair design on metabolic and heart rate responses during propulsion by persons with paraplegia. *Physical Therapy, 67*(9), 1355–1358.

Johnson, R.; Hart, D.; Simmons, E.; Ramsby, G., & Southwick, W. (1977). Cervical orthoses. A study comparing their effectiveness in restricting cervical motion in normal subjects. *Journal of Bone and Joint Surgery, 59-A*(3), 332–339.

Kent, H. (1986). Automobile modifications for the disabled. In Redford J. (Ed.), *Orthotics etcetera* (3rd ed., pp. 595–622). Baltimore: Williams & Wilkins.

Krouskop, T.; Williams, R.; Noble, P., & Brown, J. (1986). Inflation pressure effect on performance of air-filled wheelchair cushions. *Archives of Physical Medicine and Rehabilitation, 67,* 126–128.

Lehmann, J. (1986). Lower limb orthotics. In J. Redford (Ed.), *Orthotics etcetera* (3rd ed., pp. 278–351). Baltimore: Williams & Wilkins.

Millington, P.; Ellingsen, J.; Hauswirth, B., & Fabian, P. (1987). Thermoplastic minerva body jacket—A practical alternative to current methods of cervical spine stabilization. *Physical Therapy, 67*(2), 223–225.

Nawoczenski, D. (1987). Pressure sores: Prevention and management. In Buchanan L., & Nawoczenski D. (Eds.), *Spinal cord injury: Concepts and management approaches* (pp. 99–121). Baltimore: Williams & Wilkins.

Nawoczenski, D.; Rinehart, M.; Duncanson, P., & Brown, B. (1987). Physical management. In Buchanan L., & Nawoczenski D. (Eds.), *Spinal cord injury: Concepts and management approaches* (pp. 123–184). Baltimore: Williams & Wilkins.

New York University. (1986). *Lower-limb orthotics*. New York: New York University Post-Graduate Medical School.

New York University. (1983). *Spinal orthotics*. New York: New York University Post-Graduate Medical School.

Nixon, V. (1985). *Spinal cord injury: A guide to functional outcomes in physical therapy management*. Rockville, MD: Aspen.

Nixon, V. (1989). Environmental modifications. In Scully R., & Barnes M. (Ed.), *Physical therapy* (pp. 1073–1103). Philadelphia: J. B. Lippincott.

O'Neil, L., & Seelye, R. (1990). Power wheelchair training for patients with marginal upper extremity function. *Neurology Report, 14*(3), 19–20.

O'Daniel, B., & Krapfl, B. (1989). Spinal cord injury. In O. Payton (Ed.), *Manual of physical therapy* (pp. 69–172). New York: Churchill Livingstone.

Parry, H.; Delargy, M., & Burt, A. (1988). Early mobilization of patients with cervical cord injury using the halo device. *Paraplegia, 26,* 226–232.

Peterson, M. (1985). Ambulation and orthotic management. In H. Adkins (Ed.), *Spinal cord injury* (pp. 199–217). New York: Churchill Livingstone.

Ragone, D. (1987). It is worth it?: A personal perspective. In Buchanan L., & Nawoczenski D. (Eds.), *Spinal cord injury: Concepts and management approaches* (pp. 249–265). Baltimore: Williams & Wilkins.

Request. (1990). Driving with a disability. Washington, DC: National Rehabilitation Hospital Rehabilitation Engineering Center. (Available from Request, Rehabilitation Engineering Center, National Rehabilitation Hospital, 102 Irving Street NW, Washington, DC, 20010-2949.)

Summers, B.; McClelland, M., & El Masri, W. (1988). A clinical review of the adult hip guidance orthosis (ParaWalker) in traumatic paraplegics. *Paraplegia, 26,* 19–26.

Tahamont, M.; Knowlton, R.; Sawka, M., & Miles, D. (1986). Metabolic responses of women to exercise attributable to long term use of a manual wheelchair. *Paraplegia, 24,* 311–317.

Taylor, S. (1987). Evaluating the client with physical disabilities for wheelchair seating. *American Journal of Occupational Therapy, 41*(11), 711–716.

Tomlinson, J. (1990). Maximizing manual wheelchair propulsion for the marginal user. *Neurology Report, 14*(3), 14–18.

Wang, G.; Moskal, J.; Albert, T.; Pritts, C.; Schuch, C., & Stamp, W. (1988). The effect of halo-vest length on stability of the cervical spine. *Journal of Bone and Joint Surgery, 70-A*(3), 357–360.

Whitehill, R.; Richman, J., & Glaser, J. (1986). Failure of immobilization of the cervical spine by the halo vest. A report of five cases. *Journal of Bone and Joint Surgery, 68-A*(3), 326–332.

Wilson, A. (1986). *Wheelchairs: A prescription guide.* Charlottesville, VA: Rehabilitation Press.

Index

Page numbers followed by c or f indicate
charts or figures, respectively.

B

Page numbers followed by *c* or *f* indicate charts or figures, respectively.

Page numbers followed by c or f indicate charts or figures, respectively.

Page numbers followed by c or f indicate
charts or figures, respectively.

Page numbers followed by *c* or *f* indicate charts or figures, respectively.